Praise for
Debbie Merrill

"Debbie Merrill is a great teacher and dancer. I would have been lost without her."

—Steve Martin
Actor, Comedian

"Debbie Merrill has taken the fruits of her life in order to transform other people's lives! Her book is off the charts and touches people's hearts. I highly recommend it to everyone!"

—David Wolfe
Author of *Eating for Beauty* (North Atlantic Books), *Naked Chocolate* (Sunfood Nutrition), *The Sunfood Diet Success System* (Maul Bros. Pub.) and *Amazing Grace* (North Atlantic Books). www.sunfood.com

"Debbie Merrill is an outstanding and beautiful example of the power of live foods. She demonstrates how to elevate health to its highest level, to create the energy of youthing and to activate regeneration on every level. Debbie is a wonderful example of living the culture of life. In her book, The Raw Truth to the Fountain of Youth, *she reveals some of her secrets as to how this rejuvenation process works."*

—Gabriel Cousens M.D., M.D. (H),
Diplomat American Board of Holistic Medicine, Diplomat Ayurveda and Author of *Rainbow Green Live Food Cuisine*, *Conscious Eating, Spiritual Nutrition* and *There is a Cure for Diabetes* (North Atlantic Books), www.treeoflife.nu

"Debbie's boundless energy on skates and on the page can't cover up her brilliance, wisdom and insight when it comes to health and wellness in the vegetarian/vegan/raw lifestyle. Her new book, The Raw Truth to the Fountain of Youth, offers the readers all of that and some! A very fulfilling read!"

—Patricia Bragg, N.D., PhD,
Health Crusader, Daughter of the Originator of Health Food Stores. Author of *The Bragg Apple Cider Vinegar Miracle Health System* (Health Science), www.bragg.com

"I have known Debbie for more than 40 years. We went to the same high school in Yonkers, New York and trained early mornings before school at the same rink for years. Her message is not just about diet and health, it is about participating in and living life, and creating the life you want. If you want to enjoy physical pursuits, such as skating, tennis, skiing, biking, volleyball, swimming and maintain your full-mental faculties into your later years you can't rely on luck, you have to earn it. Debbie's a real fitness and health guru and her book reveals the secrets to her success."

—Joel Fuhrman, M.D.,
Author of *Eat To Live and Eat For Health*
(Little, Brown and Company) www.DrFuhrman.com

"Debbie's method really worked for me and my family. The Learn to Skate video was a great way of keeping up with the lessons."

—Peter Chelsom, Film Director

"Debbie is a fantastic teacher, we had an absolute ball with her!"

—Melanie Griffith, Actress

"Debbie's technique made my skating fun, easy and effective for NYPD Blue."

—Kim Delaney, Actress

"*Debbie Merrill's instruction was a life changing experience for me. She is my lifestyle guru for exercise and diet.*"
—Jane Velez-Mitchell, TV Correspondent and Author

"*We love Debbie's energy and her new book,* The Raw Truth to the Fountain of Youth, *is definitely going to help heal the planet.*"
—Juliano and Ariel of Juliano's Raw Restaurant, author of *RAW*, (William Morrow), www.planetraw.com

"*The fountain of youth bubbles in the bloodstream of our anatomy. Each cell is formed and developed by nourishing them with charged nutrients. Over the decades, I have observed hundreds of thousands of people when consuming raw and living food recapture their vitality and youth. The spark of life that is contained in these powerful morsels offers us the original fare that our bodies and minds were meant to flourish on. Debbie Merrill is a pioneer leading the way for the rest of humanity to reinvigorate themselves and conquer premature aging. In the near future, you will find science validating the words inked on the pages of this important guide. Come back to yourself, by honoring the very premise of food as thy medicine.*"
—Dr. Brian Clement, N.M.D., Ph.,D., L.N., Hippocrates Health Institute, author of *The Hippocrates Health Program for Healing and Longevity, Lifeforce, Living Foods for Optimum Health*

"*We all need inspiring, motivating, informative people in our lives. Debbie Merrill is definitely one of those people. From her skating excellence to her dedication to fitness and health, her new book belongs on every ones shelf. We are grateful for her being a lover of real food daily restaurant and teaching our children to skate great! I support her legend to roll and rawk on, for the well being of our planet.*"
—Ann Gentry, author of *The Real Food Daily Cookbook: Really Fresh, Really Good, Really Vegetarian* (Ten Speed Press) www.realfood.com

"Debbie Merrill brings great insight, inspiration and intelligence to the subject of health with her new book *The Raw Truth to the Fountain of Youth*. She is a living example of vitality and expresses herself beautifully with wit and wisdom. We can all learn so much from this amazing lady!"

—Brigitte Mars
Author of *Rawsome!*, (Basic Health Pub.), *Beauty By Nature*, (Book Pub Co.) and *The Desktop Guide to Herbal Medicine*, (Basic Book Pub.), www.BRIGITTEMARS.com

"Debbie taught me to skate with style and grace."

—Mayor Richard Riordan

"Debbie Merrill's zest for life, quick witted humor and profound quips are unforgettable! She is a great source of inspiration and motivation for anyone wanting to live life to the fullest and her new book, The Raw Truth to the Fountain of Youth, reflects that."

—Cherie Soria
Director of Living Light Culinary Arts Institute, www.rawfoodchef.com, Author of *Raw Food Diet Revolution and Angel Foods*, (Book Pub Co.)

"Debbie Merrill brightens up our Whole Foods market & brings amazing energy to introduce delicious raw food products, while educating customers on the benefits of raw food. We absolutely love having Debbie come to host classes & demonstrations, as she has an incredible engaging energy that draws customers in to learn about products & raw foods. Debbie is a wealth of information on raw food, the picture of health, and a delight to have around!"

—Kelly Layne
Marketing Supervisor
Whole Foods Market, Santa Monica

THE RAW TRUTH TO THE FOUNTAIN OF YOUTH

THE RAW TRUTH TO THE FOUNTAIN OF YOUTH

Step-by-step transitioning to a fabulous vegetarian/vegan/raw vegan diet, for living a life of vibrance, fitness and beauty at any age!

Foreword by Gabriel Cousens, M.D.

DEBBIE MERRILL

America's Raw Veggie Vegan Diva

This book is available at special quantity discounts for bulk purchase for sales promotions, premiums, fund-raising, and educational needs.

For more information, please contact us at debbiemerrillshow.com or skategreatusa@gmail.com and friend me on facebook: DebbieMerrill.

Disclaimer

This book is not intended to replace the services of a licensed health care provider in the diagnosis or treatment of illness or disease. This book is not intended as medical advice because both the author and publisher of this book are not medical practitioners. The author, publisher and distributor of this book are not responsible for any advice, effects or consequences from the use of any suggestions, foods, substances, products, procedures or lifestyle prescribed thereafter. Any application of the material set forth in the following pages is at the reader's discretion and sole responsibility.

ISBN-13: 978-1477548394
ISBN-10: 1477548394

Cover and interior design: Ghislain Viau

To the Readers

Dear Readers and Seekers,

I want you to know that I am not a doctor, nutritionist, or medical expert. I am someone who offers inspiration, motivation and knowledge; I'm also a professional athlete, health educator, dancer and certified skating instructor. For 28 years I've been eating and living a vegan lifestyle, and 18 of those years have been as a 100% pure, raw vegan. What I am offering you is my experience, strength, strategies and wisdom for attaining great health, fitness, creativity, and spirituality. The tools I am sharing have worked for me and I have enjoyed tremendous success in living an enlightened, creative, healthy, fit and spiritual life. My wish for you is the same – that you too will attain all the power and health you want in every area of your life. Good luck and good health!

Love – Raways and Forever,

Debbie Merrill
America's Raw Veggie Vegan Diva

Table of Contents

Section 3 Entrée: Creating

Section 4 Dessert: *Living and Giving*

Foreword

T he *Raw Truth to The Fountain of Youth* is an inspirational masterpiece written on a humorous level that speaks to everyone. It appeals to me as a holistic physician, psychiatrist, livefoodist for 26 years, yogi, rabbi, Native American sundancer and spirit dancer, as well as an inductee in the National Football Hall of Fame. Perhaps most of all, it appeals to me as a spiritual athlete because this perhaps best captures Debbie Merrill's life story which she so elegantly shares as a narrative for her teachings throughout this excellent book.

In her life journey she takes you through all the steps and lessons she personally learned as a professional athlete and as a person who transitioned to life foods and the fountain of youth one inch at a time. In this process, she addresses all the basic issues, one bite at a time, one faces in the transition to a full and inspiring life fueled by live foods. Her "Merrillisms" add a great deal of heartfelt depth and understanding to the process. They reveal much philosophical depth, love, spiced with a subtle humor…all of which add to the inspirational and grounded practical offering this book is. Her raw bites advice at the end of each section brings a nutritional and psychological common sense to her story that makes it compelling reading.

Debbie's recipes are excellent and her *Raw on the Roll Success System* food plan and super food list empower the reader with the materials and skills to be successful on the physical plane of actually walking their talk. In this book one is encouraged, but not forced to live a full, joyful, loving, healthy life with every bite of food, with every breath, from the making of love to every drop of exercise sweat.

The power of this book is the delightful and insightful way Debbie has shared her years of experience, her life's wisdom and strategies, for building a nutritionally healthy body, mind, and spirit. The world is truly a better place because she has walked into it and has written this outstanding book. She empowers us to create a healthy functioning five-sense bio-computer body and mind so that our spirits can soar in creativity and spiritual pleasure beyond the mind. We will be recommending *The Raw Truth to the Fountain of Youth* to all our clients at the Tree of Life Rejuvenation Center. It is a winner.

Gabriel Cousens, M.D., M.D. (H)
Holistic physician, Diplomat American Board of Holistic
Medicine, Diplomat in Ayurveda. D.D., Rabbi, director of
the Tree of Life Rejuvenation Center, and author of Spiritual
Nutrition, Conscious Eating, Rainbow Green Live Food
Cuisine, and Creating Peace By Being Peace.

Preface

This book is my gift to you...

I know none of us are getting out of here alive; I know, I lost both of my parents due to eating-related diseases. That's one of the reasons why I chose to lead such a healthy life and to educate others in the pursuit of vibrant health, fitness and beauty.

Living the raw lifestyle with my *Raw Truth to the Fountain of Youth*™ *Food-For-Life Plan* helped me to become a self-healer and overcome the illnesses I struggled with in my life: hepatitis A, osteopenia, stress fractures in my legs, irritable bowel, chronic constipation, bloating and gas, hormonal imbalances, low blood sugar, acne, candida, anemia, bad eating habits and emotional pain. Plus, I lost my constant cravings for sugar, carbs, preservatives, bad fats, caffeine, alcohol and cigarettes...all without drugs, diets and surgery—AND I LOST 20 POUNDS!"

In the process, I got my body, full creative expression, health and my spiritual connection back.

My wish is that you let this *Raw on The Roll Success System* seep into your consciousness, spirit and body for a fleeting moment and that you achieve great success. When YOU work it, it WORKS!

Good luck and good health!

Acknowledgments

I'd like to give special thanks to all those who have gone before me, continue to go with me and support me in making my dream to educate the world back to health and fitness a reality:

- First, I'd like to thank my Higher Spirit for giving me the divine right order of my life and the right to choose this rawsome lifetyle, with all the miracles I've been given.

- My parents, Angelo and Elvira DiGiacomo, who brought me into this world, loved me, and dedicated their lives to me.

- Mother Nature for giving me everything freely, absolutely and perfectly.

- Tary Duarte, who believed in and encouraged me.

- All my friends in the 12-Step Programs.

- Joan Gutierrez and Winton Churchill, who gave me the tough love I needed to write this book.

- Dan Carlson, for his abundant love and support.

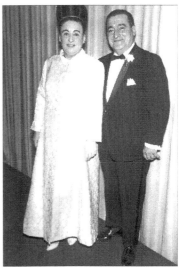

I dedicate this book to my loving and beautiful parents who taught me about health and fitness and who supported me creatively, physically and lovingly their entire lives, and then lost their lives to eating-related diseases.

- Doris Goldman, for her daily support and love on the phone.
- Don Kidson (The Godfather of Raw Foods) for introducing me to the raw vegan lifestyle and encouraging me to produce *The Debbie Merrill Show: Raw Foods on the Roll, Getting America Healthy*
- Paul Nison, David Wolfe, Dr. Gabriel Cousins and Juliano (Juliano's Raw Restaurant) who all went before me and inspired me to go 100% raw vegan.
- Kristen Heimo, for her joy, health, spirit and workability.
- Erewhon Natural Foods Markets who have sponsored, supported and believed in me.
- Time Warner Cable throughout Southern California for the production and airing of *The Debbie Merrill Show* and all the channels nationwide that aired *The Debbie Merrill Show* and helped spread the message, not the mess.
- Marlena Zaro and Rejuvenative Foods for giving me the opportunity to educate and enjoy such a great line of raw food products including cultured veggies and nut butters.
- Zack at Navitas Naturals for sponsoring my TV show and lectures by providing some of the best super foods on the planet.
- Many thanks to Robert at Ultimate Super Foods for his ultimate raw pristine quality products and support.
- Alan Heinze for being my Webmaster genius and getting me global while I act local.

- John and Bill at Blue Ink for their amazing minds, hands and patience with me. Guru.com for getting me started in the writing process.
- Barry Rick at Brick Entertainment Talent Agency for getting me some fun, great creative jobs.
- St. Ann's Church in Santa Monica, CA for giving me a place to commune with my source and soul.
- Deborah Reno, Jeff Lewis and Charles Copeland for keeping me smart and business savvy.
- To all of my raw veggie vegan friends, thank you for being you and for accepting me.
- George George for supporting me in being a risk taker.
- Marsha Epstein for her unconditional love and support.
- The entire Tocco Family for being my only true family and always being there for me.
- Essential Living Foods for supplying me with my needs and super foods so I can supply the world with theirs.
- My cousins and godchildren for loving me no matter what I eat.
- Richard and Melody Chakar – owners of Perry's Cafe in Santa Monica, CA (the Mecca of skating) for welcoming my skating school, Skate Great USA, and putting me on the map for over 20 years.
- Rollerblade, Inc. for putting wings on my feet for over 20 years.
- Cynthia Hamilton for casting me on the first raw TV show and encouraging me to do my own.
- Bobby Denard for transforming me from a tomboy to a "Miss Bling" with rhinestones, glitter and sequins.

- All of my clients and students who I attribute to transforming me into the best possible teacher and health educator I can be.
- Franna Diamond for my sanctuary to write, heal and rest.
- Rawsheed, Rod Rontondi of Leaf Cuisine, Matt Amsden of Rawvolution, Nwenna, Juliano of Juliano's Raw, and Chef Melissa Mango for their delicious raw food, feeding Californians, and leading by example with their rawvolution of raw delicacies.
- Dr. Michael Klaper, M.D. for convincing me to eat a plant based diet after his appearance on my TV show.
- Yogi Susi and James Tejada of Ancient Sun for keeping me green and in high vibe with Blue Manna, Crystal Manna and Ancient Sun Bars.
- Lydia's Organics and her delicious raw goodies, especially my favorite Tropical Mango Bars.
- Finally, I'd like to thank all those geniuses who I have followed and who have given me a new view of life, for my spirit and my environment; they have enlightened my possibilities of life including: Marianne Williamson for lecturing and teaching me about *A Course in Miracles*; Shatki Gawain, Louise Hay for *You Can Heal Your Life*; Wayne Dyer for all of his books, seminars and tapes; The Landmark Forum Education; *The Bible, The Twelve Steps, The Secret* and many more I will encounter in my lifetime journey towards great health, wealth, knowledge and peace.

Thank you all.

Introduction

"Nobody can go back and start a new beginning,
but anyone can start today and make a new ending."
—Maria Robinson

You could say that I got into ice-skating just so I could wear the beautiful costumes. Since I was five years old, I've loved the feel of chiffon—the way those beautiful pinks, blues, yellows and reds draped across my body—sequins, rhinestones, chiffon and glitter sparkling as I flew across the ice. Forget about pirouettes, double axels and the Olympics, I wanted to be Cleopatra, Barbie, or at the very least, Peggy Fleming.

I only owned two kinds of clothes—fancy or sporty—there was nothing in between. I either felt beautiful and special or like a jockaholic—skating all the time. I guess that's what happens when you're a figure skater growing up in Yonkers. Of course, I dressed like an ordinary girl when I had to—to school and back—but as soon as I got home, I rushed upstairs to put on those bold, colorful costumes that made me feel as if the world were watching me as I jumped on my bed and danced in front of the mirror. I imagined scores of admirers lined up along the sidewalk, pushing and shoving to get a glimpse of me as I paraded down Lockwood Avenue, each of them secretly wishing they could live my life and be me. It was a fanciful childhood dream, but somewhere inside me, I knew it was more than that. I wanted to stand out, perform, be different, unique and special, and walk the runway. I wanted to make my mark in the world. I can

1

still see my father's face, as I'd walk through the door in my latest chiffon or hip and trendy outfit, adorned with glitter, feathers, fringes, sequins or rhinestones. He'd shake his head, his eyes would peer over the reading glasses that dropped down his nose, then shout the same thing he always did, "Would you look at that Sarah Bernhardt getup she has on now?" And, as if he knew how much I liked to hear it, he'd always say it one more time. "Would you just look at that getup?" Then, like clockwork, he'd say, "Are you going out like that?" That was high praise coming from my dad, a gesture of love to me. I felt loved, admired, cherished and adored, which is how I wanted to be treated by my imaginary audience. It was never a dress or a costume, but always a "getup." I loved the words. They made me feel bigger than life. I felt the same way when my father proudly described to his friends how I walked into a room. "My little monkey—she's like a boom walking into a room making her grand entrance," he would say. And then one more time for effect, "A boom walking into a room, making her grand entrance."

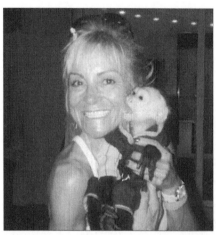

My favorite animal is the monkey because they are so cute and remind me of myself since that was my Dad's nickname for me growing up. I ask that we please stop using horrific experiments to test needlessly on monkeys. We must work on ending animal suffering!

For me, it was the ultimate compliment. Those words summed up my life. It was everything I hoped to achieve. To walk into a room and know that the world was a better place because I had walked into it. Like everyone else who shares this planet, I wanted to be special. I didn't know at the time, however, that it would take me half a lifetime to get there. I didn't know that the road from our dreams to reality isn't always a straight line. It can be crooked, or even circular, often leading us—like a fad diet—right back to where we started. I should know. For over 28 years, I walked in circles and banged into walls. I lived through isolation, loneliness, disorders, self-hatred and feeling defective. At various times, I was overweight, underweight, compulsive and apathetic. I was like a racehorse with blinders on. I spent, what seemed like an eternity, trying to be perfect in every way. I spent my life over giving, over-compensating, over achieving, overworking, over exercising—then promising never to do it again. I was a skater, a dancer and a model; I told myself I had no choice. It was my job to look good and be perfect. I had to be the first, the best and the only—no matter what the cost. In the end, it cost me a pile of mental baggage that created unbearable pressure and almost took my life.

Starting when I was 18, and for nearly a decade, I was training as a competitive ice skater, then I turned professional, and toured the world with professional ice shows. Then I returned to New York City to pursue an acting career and appeared in my first Broadway play, "The Marriage of Figaro" starring Christopher Reeve and Mary Elizabeth Mastrantonio. At the end of the run, my self-esteem plummeted, along with my energy, creative expression, joy and health. I wasn't in a hospital bed with tubes down my throat, but I was miserable, unhappy, depressed and moody, proving first hand that you don't need terminal cancer to be dying. I was a <u>MESS</u>: <u>M</u>ystified <u>E</u>mpty <u>S</u>elf-centered <u>S</u>piritually Sick. I told myself I was FINE, but I was: <u>F</u>ed Up <u>I</u>nsecure <u>N</u>eurotic and <u>E</u>motional. I was eating unhealthy, processed junk food, thinking negatively and it affected my well-being, creativity, self-esteem and performance.

Every step of the way, my descent into illness and depression was fueled by the twin poisons of our society: the crap I fed my brain and the crap I fed my body. I told myself I was fat,

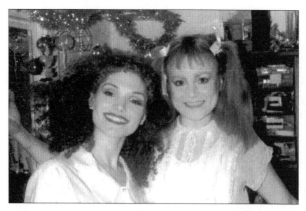

My lucky break starring in the "Marriage of Figaro" on Broadway with great artists Mary Elizabeth Mastrantonio and the late Christopher Reeve. Flying off a 9 foot high swing on roller skates and into a curtain in a black out was a challenge for me. With their help and encouragement I made it every performance.

ugly, unworthy, and a failure. While I was filling my mind with negativity, I was just as quickly filling my body with fried cheese, cheeseburgers, pizza, champagne, aspirin, processed foods, preservatives, and washing it all down with a case of diet soda. My most satisfying and intimate relationships were with Baskin Robbins and Entenmann's Cakes. I was killing myself with my thoughts and my fork. Being a professional figure skater, I slowly saw my creativity start to decline. Suddenly, I wasn't in the mood to skate or create. I was in the mood to eat sugar. That was it. Lots and lots of sugar and fat, that's where I was at. And the more sugar and fat I ate, the less I skated and the less I created. I hated myself so I ate, and I ate because I hated myself. My skating took a detour to fear and destruction, becoming a symbolic figure eight that had me going in circles on and off ice.

I know my story is not unique and I don't pretend it to be. Just turn on the television and you'll find unlimited stories of addiction,

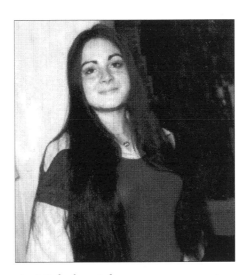

At 18 before I became a vegetarian. I was carrying around 20 extra pounds, felt miserable, depressed and had no self-esteem or fulfillment except food. I was living dead, eating dead, and it all turned to dread.

self-destruction and bad health. We've become so desensitized to poor health and lack of vitality in our country that we've begun to con ourselves into believing it's normal to look and feel the way we do. How else do you explain why we now have over 60 million overweight Americans, and that there is now a 15% annual rise in children's obesity?

The real tragedy is that what we're doing to our bodies, we're doing to our spirits and our minds at the same time. With failing health, the quality of our lives has drastically suffered. And while we hear story after story of self-destructive behavior, we don't hear enough stories of lasting redemption, hope and long-term solutions. It's all about drive-through rehab, fad diets, nips and tucks and the 10 secrets to success. While such popular remedies may work for a while, unless they're built on a foundation of inner personal character building, awareness, strength, transformation, and sound nutritional principles, most will eventually fail; causing those trusting individuals to spiral back into the same destructive behavior as before, leaving them not only discouraged, but right back to the same con as before—that how we look and feel is normal. We tell ourselves, "I'll fix it tomorrow, or later." We go into denial, procrastination, and defiance to get ourselves off the hook of truly taking care of ourselves. Well, I'm here to tell you that disease, atrophy, lethargy, depression, heartache and self-loathing are not our natural birthright. They are a disease, a dysfunction, a disorder in the body. There is nothing normal about waking up and feeling less than you know you are capable of feeling. You know in your heart that you came here to be extraordinary and if you're not doing that, then know that you can be. Health, in all its manifestations—a fit body, a healthy mind and a happy spirit—is your birthright. In spite of what you see around you, or what others may tell you, you deserve to be healthy, happy and full of joy. You not only deserve it, you can have it. It's closer than you think. We get our power, beauty and intelligence back, by getting our health back, not the other way around. If we want our country and world to be a better place, we all must be in better health and spirit.

As the old cliché goes, "If I can do it, you can do it." The only difference between you and me is that over the last 28 years, I have developed a system that helped me take back my health. I call it *The Raw on the Roll Success System*, and it's built around the simple idea that we should eat only a plant-based diet and raw (uncooked) food in its pure organic state, the way Mother Nature offers it up to us. You are what you eat. Now, before you start running for the hills, or the nearest barbecue joint, there's no reason to be afraid of the word *raw*. Nobody's asking you to grab a handful of goji berries and head for the high desert for a colonic and a 40-day fast, enjoyable as that may sound to some of us. All I'm asking is for you to keep an open mind to what raw is and what it's not. *The Raw on the Roll Success System* is about more than eating raw, it's about *living raw*—in the pure, organic, raw state of health and love from which we came into this world. It's about a return to the organic lifestyle, where less is more and abundance is for everyone. Gluttony, greed and fear are not a part of our true nature. RAW spelled backwards is WAR, and backwards thinking is what causes war within our bodies and minds, as well as eating cooked, preservative-filled foods. Think RAW, not WAR. We need to think life backwards and live life forwards.

The Raw on the Roll Success System is not just about what you eat, but how you think, the way you move your body, your creative expression and your spiritual connection—these are the keys, tools, and principles that will lead you right to the Raw Truth to the Fountain of Youth! It's about waking up to your spiritual self and reclaiming the health that will allow you to enjoy life. Would I love for you to be a 100% raw vegan by the end of the book? Absolutely. In fact, some of you may already be considering it or at least heading down the path. Does it matter? Absolutely not. What matters is that you discover and accept where you are right now, then use the principles in this book to begin to transform your unhealthy behaviors towards a healthier lifestyle. What matters is that you move toward a lifestyle that embraces healthy choices and a *less is more*, raw state of mind. Eat less, live more. Absorb the message, not the mess. The less you carry around, the longer you are around.

I've lived through every type of diet there is. I've gone from red meat to chicken to fish, from vegetarian to macrobiotic to lacto-ovo to vegan to raw vegan, and it is certainly not for me to say where you should end up. As I say to my students, if your life is working for you and you feel healthy, happy, energetic, and have a positive self-image, then by all means keep doing what you're doing. I wish you a wonderful life. On the other hand, if there is the slightest twinge in your soul that you are not where you want to be—that there is more to life than what you are presently experiencing—that you feel you are not the best you know you can be, then I invite you to take this wonderful journey with me back to a raw state of mind, body, spirit and creative expression.

Be clear of one thing: It is not my intention to tell you what to do, I'm just sharing with you what I've done. And if the suggestions I offer within these pages resonate within your heart, go for it. As I mentioned at the very beginning of this book, I'm not a doctor or a nutritionist, nor do I pretend to be. I am a professional athlete, teacher, 100% raw vegan, performer and health educator. I am happy to say I have not had a cold in over 28 years and have had great success with my health and fitness. I figure skate (ice/inline/roller), practice yoga, cycle, weight train, hike, sing, act, dance, write, educate and teach. I have more energy, peace of mind and joy in my life than I had when I was 20 years old. And my body is as fit and shapely as it was back then as well. As a matter of fact, I have my 18-year-old "figure-eight" back. And that's not to brag, but to serve as a testament to what a raw lifestyle of diet, fitness, creative and spiritual expression can offer. It's *The Raw Truth To The Fountain of Youth* for me.

Ultimately, this book is about helping you discover for yourself what works for your health and what doesn't. And the only way you'll fully grasp this is to put into action the principles you'll learn in this book. All you need is an open mind and willingness, which you can begin to stretch by embracing the first of many Merrillisms, notes, quotes, skills, drills, tips and tricks which I will be sharing throughout this book:

Merrillism #1: "Don't Deny It 'Til You Try It and Apply It."

While formal education is valuable and, in our society, mandatory, experience is very often our best teacher. We can read, learn and study all we want, but at the end of the day, we alone know what's best for our health. The purpose of this book isn't about going fast or being first. It's about slow and measured progress. There is more to life than making it go faster. I encourage you to take one step at a time.

The chapters in this book are small, but the lessons are large. Understand each chapter, incorporate it, own it and then, and only then, move on. The more you allow yourself to feel success and experience growth, the more likely you will be fueled with the motivation, inspiration and energy you need to embrace the next step on your journey. Prove to yourself that you are moving in the right direction. Let your body, your spirit, and your intuition be your guide. It doesn't matter if you take a week, a month, a year or ten years to finish this book. After all, it took me 28 years to live it and write it. I'm not where I want to be, but I am a heck of lot closer than I was. What matters is that you keep moving forward toward the life you were meant to lead, and toward the life you imagine. It's the domino effect. The more you do the more you are able to do. Remember that miracles are out there, you just have to recognize them; they are all around you, expect them every day. You don't have to earn them or deserve them, they just happen because you are a child of the Universe.

> *"The greatest good you can do for another is not just to share*
> *your riches, but to reveal to him his own."*
> —Benjamin Disraeli

John Lennon once said, "The love you take is equal to the love you make." This has become my motto, my way of life, my teaching, and the rallying cry for the second half of my life. It's the reason I wrote this book. I'm selfish. I want to get to heaven, but I have to take someone with me, and, like John Lennon, I believe we only get when we give; I live to give now. The healthier I have become in my life, the more I have realized how important it is to help others. Be selfless and be about "we," not just "me."

As an only child, I stood on stage alone, but as an adult, I have come to realize that sharing the stage with others is a lot more fun. Life is richer and more rewarding when I share it with those around me. It's not my stage; it's our stage. It's not my adventure; it's our adventure. It's not about me, but about community and unity. The world is not an island. The more I help you, the more you will help me, and together, the more we will help the world. As I give to the world, so the world gives to me. Today, I act locally and think globally. My thoughts and actions affect others and the world. If you don't get it, I don't get it, and we all need to get it.

Society tells us that once we get to a certain age, we should put away our childhood fantasies. We should grow up and get real. Well, I'm here to tell you that nothing could be further from the truth. The greatest gift we can give ourselves is our willingness to redis-cover the childhood dreamer and dreams we once had. It's time to bring color, glitter and rhinestones back to our life and uncover the artistic genius within. It's time to unlearn all the nonsense society has fed us, and to once again find the magic, adventure, playfulness and joy in our lives. My friends, it's time to take the stage. It's time for each and every one of us to get up and get rolling, wearing our own personal "getups." It's time to step into who you know yourself to be; it's time to be a leader, a force to be reckoned with and take a stand for life itself. It's time to reclaim yourself; it's time to be about something in your life. Like my father always said, it's time to be that "boom that walks in the room" and bring joy to the world and put a mile of a smile on everyone's face in the place.

The Raw Truth To The Fountain Of Youth is your invitation to an extraordinary life of health, joy, peace, freedom, fulfillment, miracles, prosperity, fun and full creative expression. Enjoy it, you deserve it. It's your birthright and my wish for you all.

Section 1

Appetizer: Awakening

Chapter 1

Create Your Own Treasure Map

*"What you visualize, vocalize and physicalize,
you can manifest in your life. I know it because I've done it.
Inch by inch it's a cinch, yard by yard it's very hard."*
—Debbie Merrill

From the moment we wake up in the morning, until we go to bed at night, most of us are in a state of perpetual motion. We are always moving to get things done—get dressed, make breakfast, pack lunches, get children off to school. There are carpools to drive, freeways to maneuver and meetings to attend, along with conference calls, business lunches, soccer practice, gym workouts, board meetings, homework, emails and phone calls to return. In between, we find time to go to the market, the bank and the hair dresser, tune cars, do laundry, pick up dry cleaning, workout and manicure our nails. Yes, we are part of a society that proudly knows how to pack it all in a day and get things done. We're moving all over the place, all of the time. When you add up all those days, stringing them into months, years and decades, we have to ask the inevitable questions: Are we moving in the right direction? Are we going where we truly want to go, dressed for success and in constant motion? Are we human doings instead of human beings? Are we taking on life, or is life taking us? Are we doing what we want to do, or is it what we *should* do, or just what someone else thinks we should do?

There are no accidents. You picked up this book for a reason. And the process is already working, because you are reading it. Some part of your inner being doesn't like where you are in your life and wants to get to another place. It's that simple. You want movement in your life—a different type of movement. Well, let me begin by saying, you should pat yourself on the back. Growth is the first step toward a healthy and conscious life. Successful people take action and then things line up for them. Unsuccessful people wait for things to line up before they take action.

Now comes the fun (and challenging) part: It's time to hone in on exactly where you want to go. So, where do you want to go? What do you envision for your future—what do you want your tomorrow to look like? How about next week, next year or ten years from now? If you have no idea of what you want, and where you want to go yet, then be open to the possibility of it being revealed to you, through people, places, things and your Higher Spirit. Not knowing what you want, or where you want to go, often keeps you safe, stuck, paralyzed, vague and blind to it. If you don't know where you are going, then you can't get there, and then you don't have to do the work that it takes to get there.

Not knowing where you want to go leads to unconscious living; a haphazard acceptance of life which can lead to all kinds of destructive behaviors such as unconscious eating, reckless spending, over-working, self abuse, drug abuse, abusive relationships, anger and frustration. It leads to the unconscious creation of your life. It's like getting into a taxi and telling the driver to take you anywhere. You'll get somewhere, all right; it just won't be a place that your inner being really wants to go. It won't be a place that's best for you, one driven by your passions and the higher part of your soul. It definitely won't be a place that is as beautiful and magical as it could be. Instead, it will be some place the taxi driver wants to take you, a place where you will live out someone else's dreams. Most tragically, it will often be a place that is a symbolic manifestation of your own fears and self-imposed limitations. And then what happens? You get what you never wanted. Because you did not declare clearly and specifically your wants and desires to the Universe, or anyone, not even yourself; you did not believe it was possible, you were blind to your own wants and desires.

Over many years—and with the power of selective memory—you might even talk yourself into believing that you were the one who told the taxi driver where you wanted to go. Sadly, many of us will go to our graves not even knowing that our life was a choice we didn't even know we had made. When you are living a life someone else designed for you, you are not really awake, alive, alert, aware and inspired. You become the living dead. That's how some people are, that's how I saw my life. I was the living dead, walking dead, skating dead. I was blind to who I was and what I wanted, and I kept it from myself and others. I blamed everyone else and I did not take responsibility for my own ability. I was very unhappy and didn't know why.

Of course, if we're lucky, somewhere along the line, we'll realize we're lost, wondering where we are and how we got there. It's like awakening in a fog, and suddenly becoming aware of who and where we are. That awareness often leads to despair, hopelessness, separation, depression, and even self-pity and addiction. The good news is: if we're strong enough to endure it, this same pain will often lead us to the realization that we need to stop and tell the taxi driver to pull over to the side of the road, that we need to shift our lives. We need to change direction. We need to tell the taxi driver where to go. To one degree or another, that's where many of you may be right now; on the side of the road, figuring out where you want to go and how to get there. Congratulations! It's a great place to be in, the tunnel with no ray of light. That's where you have to trust, it's where miracles and new possibilities begin.

All great journeys—inner and outer—begin with a dissatisfaction of where we are and a clear desire of what we want out of life, along with the willingness to transition our behaviors towards a healthier lifestyle. I believe the Universe provides us with exactly what we need. More than that, it gives us what we ask for. Look at the Universe like one infinitely wise and omnipotent Master who's handing you a treasure map of endless possibilities. Whatever you want, the Universe can send to you. And—guess what—that Master is on call 24/7. You can always ask for, and receive, exactly what you want. The trick is that you have to ask. Ask and you shall receive; act and you shall receive, as well.

Whether we know it or not, we are continuously requesting from the Universe. We are putting our requests in with what we think, feel and believe. And while we'll talk about this later in the book, for right now, I just want you to stop moving. Pull over to the side of the road, and start thinking about what you truly want from the Universe. Why did you buy this book? What do you want to experience? How do you want to look? Feel? Act? What do you want your life to stand for? Where do you want to go? How do you want to be of service? Who are the people you want in your life? What do you want to do with your life? What do you love to do? How do you like to express yourself? If you could have anything you want, what would it be? Take some time right now to make some notes while you think about these questions and your answers.

Just like that taxi, if we don't know what we want, the All-Knowing Master will steer you to what you **think you want** or what others think you want or should have. Or, if you allow it, the Master will give you what the guy next to you is having, who undoubtedly ordered the same thing as the person next to him. That's how we end up looking, feeling and acting like each other. Be clear, be communicative, be at cause in your life and be honest with yourself and others. Be a leader, not a follower. You know what happens when you follow the herd? You step in poop. To paraphrase the well known quote, "Leaders do what followers won't."

Sometimes when attempting to identify goals and dreams, it helps to think back to an earlier time in your life when you felt the world was open to infinite possibilities. What were your dreams then? What kind of goals did you have when you were not so afraid of failing? What kinds of plans did you have before someone else told you that you could not have them? Recently, I was looking through my high school yearbook, when I noticed even back in high school, I had an inkling of what I wanted.

"Let your dreams become your realities."
—My High School Yearbook quote

So, before we take this first big and wonderful step together, let's all be certain of what we want out of life. It's time to look at our own individual desires and create exactly what our future will be. Think of the life you want as buried treasure—and all you have to do is find it. But how?

Let's begin with creating a Treasure Map—one you will create yourself, on paper. This will help to fully embody the elements of the new life you wish to live, and how you want that life to look. You may have many areas to create, and several different maps. For instance, you may create a love map, a relationship map, the perfect body map, a vacation map, creative expression or spirituality map, whatever you want to have in your life. Now I want you to really dig deep into your heart's desires, and tell the Universe what you truly want. Be clear, and be specific in your details. Use a large piece of sturdy paper or board, as you will need plenty of room. Fill that sheet with your wants and desires. First use words. Use a pen, pencil, crayon or computer; write it, rhyme it, list it or draw it; but just do it. Then find images to include with your words. Create the images yourself or cut photos or illustrations from magazines or books and attach them. Do whatever works best for you—see it in your mind and feel it in your heart. At this stage, don't even worry about believing it. Use affirmations if you want. Describe and illustrate the details of your dreams. Include sizes, shapes, times and places. Think big and work big. Make it clear and make it colorful. Don't worry about making it perfect, just make it about you. Take that leap of faith and place your order for the life you want to lead, the love you want to have and give, and the future you imagine.

Below is a list of some of the affirmations I included in creating my own Treasure Map. I'm listing them here to help you get started. Get excited and creative about what *you* want.

My Affirmations

- I now have quality in my life, not quantity.
  Less is more.

- I now love myself.

- I am enough, I have enough, I do enough, there is enough.

- I am now doing my right work.

- I now live and express myself fully,
  freely and come from my heart and truth.

- I now live in abundance, prosperity, creativity and spirituality.

- I am now surrounded by people who nourish,
  support and love me.

- I now have conscious, committed,
accountable, awake relationships.

- I now live in nature and revel in raw.

- I now exercise my body, mind and spirit daily.

- I now live a life of service, contribution,
entitlement and worthiness.

- I now have a spiritual purpose and am full of creative expression.

- I now give back, and I now recover what was lost,
forgotten or injured to the world.

- I now enjoy peace, love, laughter and playfulness in my life.

- I now have more fun.

- I am a human being, not a human doing.

- And yes, I will dance and skate until I'm 98,
have sex until I'm 99, live to 100+ and die in my sleep.

Next, you will create a Treasure Box. This box will hold a written list of your wants and desires. You can create and decorate the box yourself, or find a box you like. Refer to your Treasure Map for items to include in your written list. Place the list in the box, and then turn the box over. What you are doing is turning it over to the Universal Masters and spirits to arrange and design for you.

Once you've finished your life's Treasure Map and Treasure Box, put them in a sacred place in your home—spiritual zone, altar, arena, stage—any meaningful and significant corner of your world. Post the Treasure Map where you will see it everyday, and affirm it. Share it with someone else if you want, or keep it to yourself, but make sure you will see it every day so you start conceiving it and creating it in your life. Remember, if you name it, then you can claim it and finally attain it. You can declare, "This is my Treasure Map to my heart's treasures, and my 'request' to the Universe for my treasures of pleasures." You are on a treasure hunt and you have designed your own Treasure Map. You will follow that map and do what works for you—and only you. You will find the treasure you were always looking for, and that treasure is YOU. You, in your divine right state, weight, and with your favorite food on your plate. Don't hesitate and don't wait because it's never too late. Please don't think of the "how" first, just think of "what" you want and the Universe will reveal to you the "how." You just have to trust that *it will*. And, most importantly, be kind and generous with yourself. If it doesn't scare you, it's not big enough. You'd be surprised at how generous the Universe can be when you decide to work with its infinite wisdom, power and love.

This exercise is just the beginning of an exciting and rawsome journey to *You*. Stick with me here and we will get through this together. Stay with *The Raw on the Roll Success System* and I promise you—your plate will be filled with everything you desire and require and more. The whole planet is going through a powerful transformation in collective consciousness. Join in and go with this effervescent time of now.

Merrillism #2: "You Can't Get What You Don't Know You Want."

To get you started right now, I am going to introduce you to what I call **RAW BITES.** They are tips, suggestions, inspirational thoughts, words of wisdom, encouragement, and helpful reminders to help guide, support and enlighten you along the way on your journey. They will give you concrete steps or actions you can take right now, today, to begin to move in the direction you want to go. I challenge you to jump in and make one small adjustment, or even two or three. Use my suggestions or create your own. Of course, I hope you will eventually incorporate these suggestions into the fabric of your life so that they become your habit but as I have said, begin where you are—one eyelash at a time. It doesn't have to be forever, or even for a month or a week, just try it for today. Dig in and chow down!

Raw Bites

- *Between bites, put your fork down and breathe.*
- *Chew your liquids; drink your solids.*
- *Cherish, relish and bless your food.*
- *Practice positive thinking: Don't allow negative thoughts while eating.*
- *Go to bed one hour earlier or sleep in one hour later. Your body will thank you and you'll feel better. I promise.*
- *Don't spend as much as you want, eat as much as you want or sleep as much as you want, and don't listen to anyone who doesn't have what you want.*

Chapter 2

Your Magical Recipes

"Life isn't about finding yourself.
Life is about creating yourself."
—George Bernard Shaw

Growing up, Sundays were always a busy time for my family. The phone rang a lot. And everybody wanted to stop by—aunts, uncles, friends, teachers, neighbors, long lost cousins, priests, pets and police officers. Even skating coaches would knock on our door! People weren't lining up to watch the football game with my dad, listen to our Sunday arguments or watch me prance around in a sparkly getup. Nope, we were popular for one reason and we all knew it. It was my mother's homemade spaghetti and lasagna dinners, and her Italian cheesecake. Mama Mia Sundays were legendary in my neighborhood and everybody wanted to be a part of our weekly ritual. The sauce was that good. If I close my eyes, I can still smell the tomatoes, peppers and onions, oregano, basil and garlic mingling and drifting down the block of my old neighborhood, and I can still see the smiles on the faces of those lucky enough to eat it—their eyes closing as they rolled another forkful of spaghetti and meatballs in the spoon. My mom made the spaghetti, meatballs and lasagna by hand.

Of course, everyone wanted to know how she made it, convinced that it originated in a tiny, long forgotten village in Naples and was passed down from generation to generation. They would beg her for the recipe, offering clothes, trips, money, husbands and first-born children as payment. If she liked you, and you were lucky, she might tell you how she made the best meatball sauce you'd ever tasted. First, she'd look around for eavesdroppers, then quickly usher you into the living room, where she'd turn on the TV so no one could overhear. There— under the Motorola cone of silence—she'd slowly cup her hand around your ear, then after a long and dramatic pause, she'd finally whisper the ancient secret: "Love. The recipe is love. And home grown. No cans, boxes, jars or bags. It's all Mother Nature."

This was always met with loud groans. The build-up and let down was unbearable. They were certain she was holding back or having a laugh at their expense. To prove herself, my mother would offer up the ingredients. "Try it yourself," she'd say. "But don't forget the love—and the homegrown flavor of Mother Nature's garden." Actually it was the DiGiacomo Garden of Vegan.

Over the years, there were many who took the ingredients home, but few ever came close to matching her results. There was speculation that she was leaving out one or two critical ingredients —that special pinch of something that turned tomatoes into gold. But that was my dad. He had a green thumb, and planted and cared for everything. He even planted and picked the tomatoes, herbs, veggies and flowers all by himself, awaiting Mom's spectacular creations. She'd sometimes invite those same doubting individuals to come to the house and watch her cook, but at the end of the day, no one believed her.

Today, I will set the record straight, putting an end to the myth behind her legendary sauce. The recipe was indeed love, and respect for Mother Nature. My mother never saw love as an abstract, lip service sort of sentiment. It was real, concrete and tangible. Love was in the care, attention, love and joy she put into every tiny aspect of her sauce. Love was in the details, starting with the ingredients she used, all of which came straight from the garden—parsley, oregano, thyme, garlic, basil, tomatoes and olives. She would have made her own salt if the ocean were closer. But since she couldn't, she left it out. She didn't use sugar either. My dad didn't just grow the ingredients; he grew them with meticulous care—the proper fertilizing and grooming, the right light and the precise amount of water. And my mom and dad picked everything at the perfect moment, waiting for the stars to align at precisely the right savory instant. There was no detail too small for her attention, right down to the old stainless steel bowl she used for her cooking and the huge Italian ceramic floral-patterned bowl for serving.

The next step was to "simmer with love." Mom's philosophy was that you could not rush something to completion. She was convinced that the deathblow for American cuisine was directly related to our need to have things instantly prepared in microwave timing. "The food will be ready when the food is ready," she always said "and not a moment before." She would let her sauce simmer all day, allowing the richness and uniqueness of each ingredient to blend into a beautiful melding of taste. What people really savored on Mama Mia Sundays wasn't the sauce; it was the love, art and dedication to the food, the compassion, creativity and the table setting—down to the fan-folded silk napkins, Italian china and real gold silverware from her wedding day. And she did this every Sunday, whether there were guests or not, rain or shine, snow or sleet. She would cook for eight hours before we ate, and afterwards there was always an empty plate.

Merrillism #3: "As You Give To The World, So The World Gives Back To You."

In Kevin Costner's movie, *Field of Dreams*, there is the famous line, "If you build it, they will come." It's a good line and it worked well for the movie, but anybody can build something, like anybody can make a spaghetti sauce. It doesn't mean they'll be clamoring at your door. There has to be more to what you're offering. There has to be intent, love and passion behind what you build. There has to be love, purpose and dedication. There has to be care, attention and joy. If my mother were still alive, she'd re-write that line in a heartbeat. "Debbie," she'd say, "If you build it with love, passion and joy, they will come." That's how I've tried to live my life. More importantly, that's how I've created my life.

Each one of us is a product of our own gifts and ingredients—the food, thoughts and beliefs we have taken in over the course of our lifetime. Each of us is gifted with unique gifts to regift back to the world. Ultimately, we decide what those ingredients will be, how to mix them and what seasonings to add. More importantly, we alone will decide what we will infuse into those same ingredients—the intent, love and compassion we decide to put into creating our life. It's our own personal recipe for the life we want to live.

Merrillism #4: "Reinvent Yourself, Recreate Yourself and Regenerate Yourself."

Now that you have finished your treasure map—somewhat knowing where you want to go and who you want to become—it's time to put together the ingredients that will help you realize your dreams. Regardless of what your treasure map may look and feel like, there are universal ingredients we all need in creating the lives we imagine. Feel free to add your own ingredients. The treasure you find will be the new you, the "you" you always knew you were.

The Recipe is Love: Ingredients For A New You

One Treasure Map. Imagine your future. We all need a picture of the divine design of how we envision our life. Keep a journal, and cut out pictures of your new life and put them on a board called your treasure map, give yourself something to aspire to. More will be revealed, one day at a time.

A Pinch of Patience. Let your life simmer. Be aware that all the changes you want in your life don't have to happen at once. Take baby steps towards your goals. Life is progress, not perfection; it's a process, not an event.

A Pound of Acceptance. Allow yourself the freedom to be all right with where you are at this moment, embrace it. You are right on course and exactly where you need to be in order to get where you want to go.

A Cup of Forgiveness for all your past failures, hurts and losses along with the realization that there are no failures, only slow successes, the past does not exist in the now.

An Adventurous Spirit and Courage to look at yourself in the mirror every day and say, "I love myself, I love my life and I love the world. I am the creation of peace, happiness, fun, love and abundance. I am the gift of life."

More than an Ounce of Strength and Willingness to act on what you know you need to do to become who you want to be. You have the courage and willingness to be fearless and unstoppable. Just put wings on your feet and soar.

A Generous Sprinkling of a Sense of Humor to understand that joy is the spice with which we season our life. Don't take yourself so seriously. Lighten up. Life can be more fun. It has to be. The more you play, the more life works. Always reward yourself with fun. Fun is the excuse for the run of the race.

An Open Mind to accept unexpected miracles and magic that are out there if you look for them. I am a miracle and so are you. And if you don't believe in miracles, come and be one. Be open to miracles everyday. Did you know you don't have to be worthy or deserving of miracles? They happen naturally, just because of your very existence. You only have to be willing to receive them. (According to the Merriam-Webster Dictionary, the definition of the word "miracle" is "An extraordinary event manifesting intervention in human affairs.")

An Abundance Of Love. Love yourself back to health, fitness, joy, creativity and spirituality. Let others love you until you can learn to love yourself. Then the way you love yourself is the way you love others and always.

These are the ingredients we'll start with for our journey. Don't worry on how to mix them, or where to start; just look them over, read them and re-read them. Take an hour, a night or a week to start them or come back when you're ready, and we'll let the rawkin' raw journey begin. Onward and upward, let's move from health to health, success to success, joy to joy, love to love, abundance to abundance.

Raw Bites

- *Sit down to eat.*
- *Bless and put love in the food you prepare.*
- *Sing to the food you prepare. (My mother always did. Madam Butterfly was also the secret to the sauce.)*
- *Eat less, live more.*
- *Take on a creative hobby—paint, sing, garden, knit, write, decorate, dance, play an instrument, skate or draw, write poetry or make a treasure map.*

Chapter 3

Peeling the Onion

"Nothing is particularly hard if you divide it into small jobs."
—Henry Ford

Have you taken a trip down the aisles of the self-help section of your local bookstore lately? It's an enlightening experience, with plenty to choose from: *5 Easy Steps to Losing Weight, Six-Pack Abs Made Simple, Get Rich Quick, The Fast and Easy Road to Personal Success* and hundreds more. It seems if you want to sell a self-help book these days, you need to put the word "easy" on the cover. "Simple" and "fast" will also work, along with any plan that advocates results in less than 30 days. I don't know about you, but I'm personally waiting for *Instamatic Weight loss, Washboard Abs, Get Richer Quicker,* and *A Wrinkle Free Life.* I'll buy one of those. But the way I was living my life, I seemed to be on the path to *The Incredibly Long, Winding, Lonely and Painful Road to Misery.* It took me the first 28 years to get to the life I wanted to lead.

Of course, I understand the need to encourage and inspire. I love an optimistic book title as much as the next person. In fact, I hope *The Raw Truth To The Fountain of Youth* will be that for you. We all need to feel as if there is light at the end of our own tunnels.

We need hope. What we don't need is false hope. We don't need to believe something is easier than it really is. We don't need to con ourselves into believing that we can start something today and see life-changing results tomorrow. Ha! Wishful thinking. Wishing and hoping never got anybody anywhere. We don't need a wishbone, we need a backbone!

Unfortunately, that's easier said than done. While we may have been told as kids that we should be patient because anything worth having is worth waiting for, as soon as we became adults we threw such nonsense out the door. After spending a lifetime waiting for recess, weekends, vacations, marriage, kids, birthdays and holidays; not to mention, waiting to date, drink, drive, see "R" rated movies and have sex, we decided that (once we were out of our parent's house) we wanted it all—and fast. In spite of what we tell our kids, we tell ourselves that anything worth having is worth having immediately. As a society, we want an immediate return on our minimal investment. We want fast food, instant relationships, immediate health, overnight success and a quick way to make money, lose weight, skate great, be a star athlete, gain power and achieve fame. Our unhealthy obsession with instant gratification ("I want what I want, when I want it") is really your inner three-year old having a tantrum. Most of us are resistant to any personal growth that rejects the theory that we can have it all, right this very second.

> *"Anything worth doing is worth doing slowly."*
> —Mae West

Oftentimes, when we decide to stretch ourselves and pursue some higher calling, we quit in the early stages because we're not getting results fast enough, often choosing a solution that is quicker and less painful. That's why the drug industry is a multi-billion dollar enterprise. It's easier to take a pill to dull the pain than it is to deal with the real issues and do the work; the same way it's easier to smoke and caffeinate your way to weight loss than it is to eat less, give up unhealthy foods, exercise more and deal with your feelings and fears. Shortcuts may work for a while, but usually at the expense of longer lasting and permanent ill health. There is no easy way to remedy this: we have to stop the destructive reliance on the quick fix. We must come to realize that the "no pain," "I can get something for nothing," and the belief that we can "get what we want while never having to pay the price" is a big fat lie. We need to heal ourselves for good, bringing ourselves back to health, joy and vitality in a slow and steady manner.

I call it **Peeling the Onion.**

Merrillism #5: "Hail to the Snail and the Kale."

Peeling the Onion is a philosophy that is the cornerstone of all great achievement. It is an idea that is as simple as it is powerful: *Do one thing at a time, master it, and then move on.* You wouldn't try to run a marathon without first being able to walk around the block, anymore than you should go completely raw without first cutting back from four burgers a week to three. To get to the core of who we are and what we want to achieve, we MUST peel one layer at a time, to see what's underneath it, and get to the cause and the core, allowing each layer to make us stronger than the one before, bringing us closer to who we really are—to the strength that comes from the center of our being, which is perfect, whole, complete, always and forever.

Think about it. It's impossible to get straight to the center of an onion without destroying the onion in the process. It's the same with people. We can't immediately get to the core of who we are without unbalancing and potentially hurting ourselves in the process. We have to do the groundwork first. Humans are meant to develop in stages. We transition from childhood to adulthood to our senior years; each time of our life is built upon the years and lessons that came before it. This gives us the foundation that allows us to plant our feet firmly on the ground, while allowing us to truly own each step of our journey. Be where your feet are. If we want to preserve the integrity of our health, we need to peel our onion one layer at a time. Peeling is a process, not an event. This is true with the food we eat, the exercise regimens we adopt, as well as all the goals we set for ourselves. Going raw is a process, not an event as well. Start with being a weekend "Rawarrior" then a monthly "Veggie-Vegan Diva" to a full time "Rawk-star."

Merrillism #6: "The Slower You Go, The Faster You'll Grow."

So, wherever you are on your journey, commit yourself to mastering one lesson at a time. Part of the reason these chapters are so short is to insure focused attention on one thing. Let it stay in your heart, mind, psyche and consciousness for longer than a fleeting moment. And once we can do one thing well, we will then move on to the next, *always quitting from a point of achievement*. This is critically important and, for long-term success, non-negotiable. It's just like skating—you need to learn to go forward before you can go backwards. People always ask me to teach them to skate backwards before they know how to go forward or stop. Quitting from the point of achievement is recognizing that *completion is perfection*. If we finish one thing well, it's perfect. As we peel our own onions, that's the only instant gratification we're after. Addicts are fanatics—if it's not perfect, they quit. To win, you have to stay in the game and keep playing, no matter what.

Merrillism #7: "Completion Is Perfection; Complete Everything You Start."

Mind you, this is not just practical reality, it's also liberating. This take it slow, "Peeling the Onion" philosophy doesn't ask you to be perfect today, it asks only that, for today, have a beginning, a middle and an end. And that tomorrow, you are just a little better than you were today. That doesn't seem so overwhelming does it? You don't need to run 26 miles; just walk one minute longer than you did the day before. You don't need to lose 150 pounds, only to eat a little healthier today than you did yesterday. Let go of one slice of bread. And certainly nobody is asking you to turn raw overnight, just consider eating a salad with your steak, or throwing in a few sprigs of parsley to give you the enzymes you need to help you digest that porterhouse. By peeling the onion slowly, there are no artificially high bars to hurdle, just slow steady progress like the beat of your heart. Keep going, you may not feel like you're where you want to be, but you're a lot further along than you were. Let's all be bright, bold and beautiful. You already are who you want to be, it's time to find it, bring it on and turn the lights on. Shine your light and be brighter than bright NOW!

Once you have begun the process of peeling your onion— drinking more water, exercising regularly, adding more raw organic foods to your diet and finding a creative and spiritual outlet—you'll find that giving up things like alcohol, drugs, coffee, carbs, preservatives, meat, sugar and bread will be a lot easier. You'll find all those negative habits you once had becoming easier to shed. Over time, you will develop the discipline, commitment, and willingness with ease that will allow you to overcome any resistance—effortlessly and easily becoming a powerful ball of motion that is unstoppable. You will have cooked up self love, the only cooked dish worthy of enjoying.

What happens next is another miracle of the Universe. You will suddenly find yourself succeeding, and with each success, you'll be building your power and self-esteem, which will make it easier to do the next thing you have to do—to peel the next layer and the one after that. It's like the Olympic champion who wins a gold medal, then comes right back and does it again. Having already tasted victory, proving to herself that she knows how to win, it becomes easier to win a second, third or fourth time. Just ask Lance Armstrong who won the Tour de France seven times in a row before he retired from cycling. Talk about quitting from a place of achievement! The mystique of winning is erased or transformed into a self-fulfilling prophecy of possibility. If you know you can succeed, it's more likely you'll do it again. Donald Trump once said, "If you can make it once, you can make it again." Kristi Yamaguchi won four world championships and one Olympic championship in figure skating. It wasn't about winning; it was about the joy of self-expression and skating.

I certainly didn't get into raw overnight. It took me 28 years, all of it using the Peel the Onion philosophy. I let go of processed foods, and then I let go of preservatives. I let go of coffee, then alcohol, cigarettes and drugs. I let go of meat, then fish, dairy, white flour, sugar substitutes and carbs and, finally, when I was ready, sugar. I didn't do it all at once. I did it in stages. In fact, I'm sure if I began my journey thinking that I had to give up sugar, I never would have started in the first place. You would have had to pry the sugar out of my hands and dragged me away from the candy, cookies and ice cream aisle kicking and screaming. Instead, I allowed myself the luxury of moving in stages. I never thought of my growth as an all or nothing proposition. I found out I was an extremist; it was all or nothing for me, black or white. I didn't know how to live in the grey areas of life. And when I did learn, my goals were never that overwhelming, which allowed me to enjoy success after success—not big ones—but enough to give me the strength to keep moving, to keep peeling, until one day I woke up and realized that I could do anything I set my mind to. I now move from success to success, health to health, abundance to abundance, joy to joy, love to love, and so on and so on.

So, for the remainder of our journey, I'm asking you to peel the onion slowly. Be kind to yourself as you take each small step, slowly and flowingly. Know that with each success you enjoy, you will gather momentum, and your power will begin to build until your journey is taking a life of its own, moving you in the exact direction you want to go, toward the dream you so richly deserve. You'll find the force is behind you, with you and working it out. Thoreau said, "If one advances confidently in the direction of their dreams, and endeavors to live the life which they have imagined, they will meet with a success unexpected in common hours." So commit with confidence and the Universe will help you achieve the success you imagine.

Remember, the joy we find is not just at the end of the tunnel, but in the day to day power we give to ourselves each time we peel away another layer, moving closer and closer to who we are meant to be. The world gets more out of me when I eat something vital and alive because I become more vital and alive. I am able to offer that energy as a contribution to the world around me.

Raw Bites

- *If you insist on eating animals, and their by-products, buy and eat only certified organic, free-range meat, poultry, dairy and eggs; they are healthier and taste better too. However, I suggest eliminating all animal products from your diet, slowly but surely.*

- *Move your body an hour every day. Walk, run, do yoga, dance, skate, ride a bike, play tennis, volleyball, garden, stretch, skip, jump rope, bounce on a mini trampoline, take the stairs two at a time. Move your body.*
- *Spend time in the good outdoors. Nature heals. That's why they call her Mother Nature.*
- *When insanity and cravings strike, raw fruits and vegetables help defend the urge.*

Chapter 4

Lessons from the 4th Grade

"The only thing that interferes with my learning is my education."
—Albert Einstein

"…along with my ego, stubbornness and defiance."
—Debbie Merrill

Robert Fulghum wrote the best selling book *All I Really Need to Know I Learned in Kindergarten*. Kindergarten is where you learn the basics: sharing, fair play, self-expression, and the importance of cleaning up your own mess. You learn how to count, print your name and are taught not to hit, bite or scratch your classmates. Your school day is spent learning, singing, thinking, playing, dancing, drawing, working, painting, napping, sharing and communicating with others. You are living a truly balanced life. You are encouraged to ask for help when you need it and give help when you are able. You are encouraged to express yourself creatively, and taught that it's okay to color outside the lines and make a mess, as long as you clean it up afterwards. You learn to be in a community of "we" and not just "me."

Unfortunately, kindergarten is the last time balance is taught in school. As soon as you enter the first grade, naps go out the window, followed closely by creative expression and coloring outside the lines. Next thing you know, you've traded your finger paints for a #2 pencil and are hard at work learning the rules of grammar, memorizing multiplication tables and mastering long division. You are busy memorizing facts and dates and learning about history. You remember who discovered America but you begin to forget yourself—the raw, unprocessed self you were born to be, allowed to get dirty, play in the mud and run naked and free. It's not your fault, it's not your parents' fault, nor does blame fall to your teachers or even the school boards. They simply taught you what they knew. Don't get me wrong; I'm not down on education. Quite the contrary—life is all about learning. Learn to listen, and listen to learn.

I just advocate a more balanced approach. Who decided that it is more important to memorize the capital of Italy than it is to paint from your heart, write from your soul or sing like no one is listening? One of my main purposes in life, and the reason I wrote this book, is so that I can be the fertilizer for the garden of intelligence and help heal my fellow man back to health, fitness, creativity and spirituality with the wisdom and experience given to me. In other words, I am here to inspire, motivate, share and serve. It's not *about* me, it's *through* me. If, when you read this, you're thinking, "Debbie, that's just a load of crap!" You're right! That's exactly what fertilizer is, is it not? And having lived the raw life for more than 18 years means that I am chock full of nutrients, knowledge, experience and wisdom guaranteed to help you grow, glow and flow in this direction and lifestyle.

Health is achieved by stepping up to the buffet table of life with courage, conviction and commitment, taking what you need and not overloading your plate. Health is wanting what you have and not wanting what you don't have. Don't be average and ordinary with your health, creativity and fitness. Be extraordinary! Whatever you can't let go of has you. Whatever you forgive and accept brings your freedom and peace. Release what is not working for you in health, fitness, spirit and creativity so that you can embrace what is and be free, fulfilled, deserving and receptive.

I have fond memories of my mother, Elvira; she was enthusiastic, caring, creative and sincerely interested in motivating me to achieve success. One method she used was a system most parents use called "Rapid Rewards." Whenever I shined, for wearing clothes she purchased (that I hated), skating well, getting good grades in school, making my parents proud and dancing well, I received a food reward like McDonald's or Carvel Ice Cream with colored sprinkles, or a school reward, like skipping class and going skating, or delaying homework to go out on a Friday night. It was manipulative, and it worked like a charm. I learned that food was love, and I was loved; doing well meant rewards, and doing poorly meant punishment, shame, unworthiness and guilt. I internalized that to mean that my performance determined whether I was a good or bad person and that I always had to shine and be perfect and perform to be loved and accepted. I wanted my parents to be happy, love me, and look good and love one another. I thought that was my responsibility so I became an overachiever and perfectionist. I was the conduit for keeping them together; it was a full time, exhausting job for me along with my skating and school schedule.

My mother expressed her love through food as well. If you didn't love her food, you didn't love her. My father was the same. If I did well at practice, he brought home pizza, ice cream, donuts and toys; then he was in a good mood and he was nice to my mom. It was important to me to be the best, but I wasn't. I wanted to be the best, the first and the only. I learned that sugar, clothing, days off from school and toys were the ultimate reward.

"What's right isn't always popular.
What's popular isn't always right."
—Howard Cosell

Like many of you, I didn't grow up with enlightened parents. I came from a loud, lovable Italian family who used food as a cure all and a weapon. A tomato across the table and banging pots and pans was common music and activity in my house. Feeling sad? Have some gnocchi. Bad day at school? Nothing a little macaroni and meatballs wouldn't cure. My mom was a great cook and an excellent baker and, as I said, she infused the food she prepared with love—so forks full of pasta dripping with her famous sauce really did ease the pain. My mom used food to soothe, celebrate, compensate, manipulate and satiate. "Mangiare!" she'd proclaim as she set down a steaming hot plate of homemade Parmesan noodles. We ate everything, and in the process we learned that food was the way to de-stress, express and suppress our emotions and communicate with one another. If I didn't eat it, it meant I was angry. If Dad left the table, he was upset. If Mom banged the pots and pans, she was angry, emotional and needy. It was like mind reading. No one said what they really felt; it was all unexpressed emotion without intention and communication through sound, food and unclear body language. There was an elephant at the kitchen table and no one said anything. That's how I learned to communicate the first 28 years of my growing up. You don't communicate what you are really feeling, you hide it or stuff it down. I was a good student and I learned it and it took years of hard work to unlearn those lessons. The sad part was, I made it mean something terrible about me and them and I carried that around for another 28 years. That was a heavy burden for me for all that time.

"The great aim of education is not knowledge, but action."
—Herbert Spencer

This chapter is about *un*learning those childhood lessons. Not the math and grammar, those come in handy from time to time, but the pressure to be perfect, the suppression of your creativity and using food as a reward and substitution for self-expression. Using food, alcohol, substances, cigarettes, compulsive spending and spending beyond our means are escape mechanisms designed to numb out and avoid anything and everything—that is not the answer. These unhealthful substances are not a reward for a job well done. Overeating and overindulging offers temporary relief of permanent pain. Food will not heal or comfort your emotional pain. It just blinds you from the real pain. Don't you want permanent relief of temporary pain? I know I do. Food and fear go together. It's our "go to" for everything and by breaking that association you are breaking the habit of using food, alcohol, cigarettes, money, spending and drugs to express yourself.

Addiction is a marker for a deeper problem. So stop it already. Please stop stuffing your anger. Stop stuffing it with butts, booze, bakeries, bad boys and compulsive spending. Stop drinking alcohol to forget that your wife, husband, boss or kid yelled at you or an agent rejected you today. Stop smoking your way to a "better body." Stop spending and accumulating debt to make up for a deeper inner lack of not feeling enough or that there is ever enough. It doesn't work and we both know it. I'm not telling you anything you don't already know. While you're at it, stop going out to eat every time you get a promotion, have a birthday, want to be with friends or celebrate an anniversary. I can think of a lot of ways to spend an anniversary with someone you love and not one of them involves food. You can get a massage, go for a walk and a talk in the park, skate or dance. What happened with just being with one another and talking? Before you start panicking and thinking that you have to give up celebratory dinners for the rest of eternity, relax.

Food is energy, fuel, and, when prepared with love, gives you the strength, power and energy you need to live. The nutrients feed your body and your brain so that you can think, create, act, breathe and dance your way through life.

Merrillism #8: "Eat For Need, Not For Greed."

This is where it gets interesting (and fun)! Now that you've decided to stop stuffing yourself, you will notice something interesting. You will start to feel—a lot. You may even become overwhelmed by how powerful your emotions can really be. It may scare you a little bit, or even a lot. Good! That means you are on the right path. It means you are alive and not walking dead anymore. Don't misunderstand; I am not suggesting you wallow in a big bowl of emotions. I'm simply pointing out that you will now need to find a way to direct your emotions in a new, healthy direction. Feelings pass. They come, go and flow. Be patient, don't act on them. Let them pass through you like your flowing blood. But it's important to replace your former bad habit with a new one. I suggest you have some fun with this one. Here are a few recommendations to get you started:

Express your *JOY* by: Dancing, twirling, turning, hopping, high kicking to music, making your own music, singing karaoke at the top of your voice, jumping for joy, laughing and giggling uncontrollably, calling your Mom, crying *happy* tears, shouting from the rooftops, playing an instrument, skating outdoors with nature and music.

Vent your *ANGER* by: Punching your pillow, jumping up and down, hitting a bataka bat or a tennis racquet into a pillow while screaming, crying, complaining, raging or adding sound; running, walking, raging, kick boxing or just kicking your feet and punching your fists up and down in bed.

Expend your GRIEF by: Crying, screaming at the ocean when no one's around, talking to your best friend, hugging your dog or teddy bear and talking to it or to the person you miss or have lost, writing, "write things right" (journaling), moaning, praying, walking, and most importantly—thanking the Universe for the opportunity to feel, express, release, uncover and grow.

Show your LOVE by: Embracing your honey, telling someone you love them and appreciating them for who they are to you; kissing a baby, your wife, husband, mother, father, child, pet, or yourself; giving yourself a hug with both arms, preparing a healthy meal, reading or watching a love story as it unfolds, writing a love note to someone, reading or writing poetry; really giving back and saying thank you, complimenting and acknowledging others, looking into the mirror and telling yourself, "I love you and I'm sorry for how I treated you all those years," and saying affirmations, such as "You are awesome, brilliant, extraordinary, loveable and deserving!" (Affirmations really start my day with self-love, worthiness and kindness.)

These are just a few ideas to get you started. If you like them, great! Use them and enjoy. If they don't speak to you, make up your own. Remember, this is *your* journey to take.

Finally, if you have children, pay attention to how you soothe them. Do you give your two-year-old a cookie when he cries? Do you let your little one suck on a lollipop after she gets her medical shots? Is chocolate ice cream the way you reward good grades? If you find yourself taking a trip to Pizza Italia to celebrate straight A's, stop and ask yourself, "Is food the only way we have fun, fellowship and communication?" Stop and think about what lessons you are teaching your kids that will have to be unlearned someday. I'm not preaching, just gently suggesting you think about it and follow your heart.

When you embark upon this wonderful and challenging road to transformation and miracles, remember to take it slow. Forgive yourself. Don't try to do everything at once and please, please, please don't try to be perfect. If you stop, stop from a point of achievement and then move on. Keep your foot on the gas, stop and start but lead with your heart.

Raw Bites

- *Your food is in one hand, your feelings are in the other and they don't mix. Please stop using food and substances to suppress your feelings.*
- *Give up that cocktail today or that one extra cigarette or sweet dessert*
- *Add one raw dish to every meal you eat. Here are some suggestions:*
  - **Breakfast**
    - *Top your cereal with seasonal berries or sliced banana, or just eat the fruit alone.*
    - *Eat half a grapefruit before your bacon and eggs (not only delicious, but helps you absorb iron). Or eliminate the pork, fat and cholesterol all together. Fruit is a meal.*
    - *Start your meal with sliced papaya, mango or melon or eat for dessert.*
    - *Eat your juice in the form of whole oranges, tangerines, tangelos and grapefruits. That's real fast food.*
    - *If you don't eat breakfast now, start. Fresh melon or berries are a great way to start your day. Most fruits are digested within 20 minutes when they are eaten with no other foods. (Always eat melons alone).*
  - *Lunch / Dinner*
    - *Make my Italian Stallion Salad with raw, fresh, seasonal organic produce. I like the "everything but the kitchen*

sink" approach: throw it all in. Use organic baby greens, romaine lettuce, kale, parsley, cilantro, celery, purple cabbage, juicy red tomatoes, red peppers, zucchinis, black Italian olives, avocado, sprouts, raw sprouted nuts. Finish it with a generous drizzle of organic olive oil or my Japanese Salad Dressing, Italian Stallion Dressing, Garlic the Great, Curry in a Hurry Sauce or my Spirulina Salad Dressing. (See recipe section).

○ Although I suggest leaving out all animal products, add chicken, shrimp, cheese, tofu, beans, yogurt or nuts if you're not quite ready to go totally raw, vegan or vegetarian.

○ Top your pizza with fresh vegetables or pineapple and skip the cheese, then there won't be much left of you to squeeze.

○ Eat fresh broccoli dipped in my Garlic the Great Curry in a Hurry Sauce. Or my Titillating Tomato Sauce Supreme, before your main course. (See recipe section).

○ Fresh veggies dressed with lemon juice make a great side dish. If you aren't ready to eat them raw, have them steamed or blanched. Try blending or pureeing a mixture of red or white cabbage, kale, celery, parsley, cauliflower, broccoli, zucchini, and beets into a soup or sauce. This is easier to digest if you have a hard time digesting raw vegetables. Blending is mending!

○ Start your meal with an arugula and cherry tomato salad dressed with lemon and olive oil.

○ Squeeze citrus in your water to sweeten, add a green leaf to make it come alive and to add live enzymes.

○ Two hours after your meal enjoy fresh berries, sliced pears, apples, persimmons, figs or mangos with some raw organic coconut butter to help digest the fructose in the fruit.

Chapter 5

Move It or Lose It– It's not Age, It's Rust!

"You're not getting old, you're getting old because you're eating old food."
—Debbie Merrill

"An object at rest will remain at rest unless acted on by an unbalanced force. An object in motion continues in motion with the same speed and in the same direction unless acted upon by an unbalanced force."
—Newton's 1st Law

"Nothing happens until something moves."
—Albert Einstein

Health should be a verb. You don't become a healthy person by sitting around and waiting for it to happen and you don't sit around and stay healthy forever. Health is not a destination; health is an action, it is now! Without it, all is lost. If you aren't where you want to be on the health scale right now, don't worry. You can get there. In fact, you are on your way right now. You picked up this book and now it's time to pick yourself up and take action. Sir Isaac Newton's First Law is commonly known as the "Law of Inertia" and, take it from me, *Inertia* is an okay place to visit every once in a while but you don't want to become a permanent resident. If you are living there now, or have stayed a bit too long, it's time to pack your bags and move out! Get up, get fit, get rolling, get raw and have some fun now. When you feel your worst, try your hardest. When you do good, you never know how much good you do!

Merrillism #9: "Move a Muscle, Change a Thought."

Have you ever noticed that when you have a difficult problem or issue that you just can't seem to wrap your head around and solve, that the simple act of taking a walk seems to clear your head? By letting go of the mind and tuning in to the body, your head clears and the perfect solution appears, seemingly out of the blue. Instead of banging your head against the wall trying to make a difficult decision, add a little movement and see where that takes you. The decision usually makes you. I know that when I am blocked creatively, when I can't figure out how to write a sentence, much less a page or a paragraph or make a decision in my life, I can

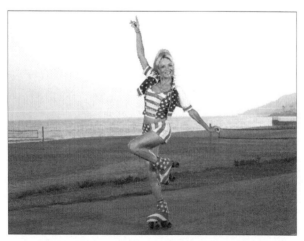

*Age is just a limit and a deadline we put on ourselves.
It's not age, it's rust, I am ageless and timeless!*

loosen my mind by moving my body. For me it's skating, dancing, yoga, walking, swimming or biking. For you it may be walking, running, ball games or gardening. Heck, if hula-hooping, vacuuming or cleaning revs you up, do that! It's not important *what* you do but *that* you move the body. If you have ever sat for hours stewing over the same old issue, brooding and blustering, then you know that sitting still stops the flow of productive thought. Moving your body frees your mind and your spirit, and relaxes you; the decision then takes form and comes to you effortlessly and easily. The body and the mind do not operate on separate channels. Sluggish bodies produce sluggish thoughts and when your body slows down or stops, your thoughts follow suit. Eating processed food creates processed thoughts that are overcooked, dead, unoriginal and mostly negative to your consciousness. When you stop moving, you speed up the aging process. Your metabolism slows down, your digestion slows down, your ambition, motivation and mind slow down and you look and feel older. Mind you, I'm not saying you can't rest every once in a while, just be careful not to live at the rest stop. When people tell me they are tired and old, I say, "It's not age, it's rust." So, get off your tired butt and use it or, I guarantee you, you *will* lose it. If you tell your body it doesn't need to move, it won't, it'll get stuck and ache.

One of the most important ingredients to good health is exercise. I'm sure you have read much about the benefits of exercise. You already know there are all sorts of machines, fat burners, weight loss programs and gurus out there. I'm equally sure you have watched hours of prime time programming dedicated to the promotion of working out. I don't like to call it exercise or working out. I like to call it playing or playing out. When a drummer goes to do a gig, he doesn't say I'm going to work, he says I'm going to play. We need to turn work and exercise into play. We need to play our way to movement and make our work and exercise our play. Do what you love, and not what you *have* to do or what you *think* you have to do or what you hate to do, or you won't do it, so you won't receive the benefit from it. Do movement that you enjoy and that makes your heart sing. And move your body an hour every day. If you truly enjoy it, you'll do it longer, burn more calories and it won't feel like exercise to you because you enjoy it. You will receive the benefits of a fit body, a healthy mind and a happy spirit.

Exercise is good for you and, especially if you are trying to lose or maintain weight, it is essential. If you choose to do it even just a little bit, you know that exercising releases "feel good" endorphins, gets oxygen pumping through your blood and to your brain, and decreases your appetite. If you are consistent, it strengthens your heart and bones, relieves compulsive thinking and behavior, keeps your carriage and posture upright, relieves constipation in mind and bowels, and keeps you feeling and looking younger and less stressed. Most people exercise to get and stay thin but I believe the best reason to exercise is to keep moving and stay mobile, agile and alive. You don't have to believe me. In fact, I secretly hope that you don't because then you'll be doubly amazed at the results you achieve. I am not about to try to change your mind because I don't have to. I am asking you to change it yourself by getting your body moving. You see, you don't have to *want* to move; you just have to move. As a matter of fact, the times when you don't feel like moving are the best times to get up and *get* moving. You don't have to like it, you just have to do it. You'll fall so in love with yourself and how you feel, you'll want to ask yourself out.

When I was skating, I would skate every day. It wasn't because my parents made me or because I was itching to get out of my warm cozy bed at four a.m. in the dead of winter at 19 degrees to skate outdoors while smelling Stella Dora home baked biscuits (this bakery was next to the ice skating rink in Riverdale, NY where I trained) - that's what I had to look forward to. In fact, my dad used to say, "Debbie, are you sure you want to go? You don't have to." The truth is I didn't want to go but I didn't want to get behind either, so I went. I got up, suited up and showed up. That's the secret to working out every day, showing up. That's actually the secret to success at anything, just showing up. I used to start my practice half asleep, and most of the time my top didn't match my tights, I had my pants on inside out and my skate laces were all crooked and not tucked in, but I skated anyway and ten minutes in, I was completely involved and sweating. I loved it and didn't ever want to stop. Time flew by. You see, I didn't wait to feel inspired to skate; I skated my way to inspiration. The trick is, you don't have to *feel* like working out, you just have to dress up, show up and play out. Inspiration follows movement, not the other way around. It works with everything. Trust me, I don't always feel like writing but I write anyway. I put pen to paper, show up, and pray for inspiration, commit to someone, and then I take action. That's what I'm asking you to do. Show up, go through the motions, play and pray your way to inspiration. You don't have to like it at first; you just have to do it. The Universe likes and rewards action and movement.

Merrillism #10: "Getting Up And Getting Going, Keeps You Growing, Glowing and Flowing."

I promise you, you will never regret playing out. You will never finish a "play out" session panting, sweating, feeling energized and say, "Boy, that was a waste of time! I wish I had eaten a jelly donut instead." It simply won't happen. You may struggle with getting out of bed, you may hate it while you're doing it but you will always, always be glad you did. How many things in life can you say that about? If you think about how you will feel at the end of your "play out," it will make the beginning easier to do and get to. You don't only feel better after a "play out," you feel better about yourself. Keep your eyes on the finish line, not on the starting line. Act your way into right thinking, not the other way around.

So, here's the deal. Starting right now, exercise is non-negotiable. At this very minute I want you to stop, put the book down and grab a piece of paper and something to write with. Are you back? Good. You are about to enter into a very simple and very important agreement—with yourself.

Easy Flow and Glow to Go Contract

I, _____, agree to commit myself to daily, playful movement. This means that I will exercise and move my body *doing something I enjoy*, at least six days a week for at least 45 minutes to an hour. I will allow myself one day of rest and recovery. I understand that this is a life long commitment to my own health and well-being. I further understand that I will face challenges along the way. I agree to be kind to myself and forgive myself when I fall down, backslide or fail. I agree to get right back up and start again. I understand that from this day forward, exercise is non-negotiable, that it is an integral part of my life (even if it's only thirty minutes a day). I understand that this contract is binding and fully enforceable by me. I understand I am accountable for this and declare this is a commitment and loving promise to make for myself, my family, friends and the world around me.

_____   _____

(Signature)   (Date)

Now, take these 5 easy steps:

#1. I want you to sign the contract.

#2. Make three copies.

#3. Post one copy somewhere you can see it every day; your bathroom mirror, your night stand, the refrigerator, any place you'd like to remind yourself that exercise is not an activity you complete. It's an on-going process like brushing your teeth, washing your face and eating nutritious, healthy foods.

#4. Put one in your treasure box and turn the box physically and spiritually over to the Universe.

#5. Give the third copy to a close friend or family member so you can keep the contract alive and accountable between you and another person and your higher spirit. Where two or more are gathered, the higher spirit can work through.

Remember, like all forms of growth, making exercise a daily habit is work, so go easy on yourself at first. Start from where you are and, here comes the disclaimer, get a thorough check-up from your nutritionist or homeopathic MD before beginning any exercise program. I can't see you, I don't know where you are on the fitness scale but *you* do. So, take responsibility for your health and get up, get fit, get moving, get going, get rolling, get raw now!

If you are a certified couch potato whose idea of exercise involves the remote control, a spoon, and a pint of ice cream, then I don't recommend you start off by training for a marathon—at least not yet. It's important to set yourself up for success by taking baby steps toward your goal. If you reach the end of your rope, tie a knot and hang on—you are in for a rawsome, awesome ride and a great backside!

Start Stepping

Walking is easy, free and almost anyone can do it. Get outside and walk. Get a walking partner. If it's too cold or too hot then get yourself to the nearest mall, beach or park, and walk there. You'll get a fantastic workout and save money by walking past the stores instead of exercising your wallet inside. Dancing, either alone or with a partner, is a fun, creative way to increase your joy and decrease your waistline. I dance three times a week. It lifts my spirits, sensuality, creativity, improves my posture and is fun. I believe dancing and skating revives lives and raw foods save lives. So dance through your life now. If you prefer to roll, then strap on skates (ice, in-line or quads), jump on a bike (10-speed, mountain or beach cruiser) and hit the road. Don't forget a helmet and full protective gear. If you have trouble getting motivated, then join a gym, take a swimming class, yoga class, tai chi, chi gong or dance class, find a workout partner or hire a trainer. Support is out there; you just have to look for it and accept it. Find the exercise you love to do and you will never workout a day in your life!

If you are disabled, sit and get fit. Yes, you can obtain quite a workout while sitting in your chair or wheelchair. Move your arms and legs, turn your torso, move your neck and head, wiggle your ankles, your toes and fingers, and circulate your hands and wrists. Tighten and release your buns, press your palms together to improve your pecs and bust line. I taught a class at the Salvation Army for women over seventy called "Sit and Get Fit." When my dad was dying of Alzheimer's, I would go to the nursing facility and entertain the patients with music while I encouraged them to exercise. My Dad and the seniors moved their arms, hips, torsos, legs, fingers, toes, wrists and neck to music while sitting in a chair or wheelchair. We all had a ball. We even played pass the ball for right and left brain integration, coordination and to keep their reflexes alive and alert. They had smiles on their faces; they were breathing, glowing, enjoying, and actually getting some exercise.

My dad lived five years longer than expected because I spent this precious, creative time playing with him and loving him. There are always other options for moving your body. Get creative. Get fit. Get going. Get moving. Get rolling.

You only get one body, folks, this is it. Take care of it and it will take care of you. Aging is a state of mind. I focus on living, not age. A warped body leads to a warped mind and a warped spirit. A creaky body leads to a creaky mind and a creaky spirit. Circular, negative thoughts create negative energy, negative actions, and behavior. I'm not saying this will be easy or that negative thinking won't creep up on you at times. As you begin to exercise, you will have doubts and fears. You may think, "This is too hard," or "It will never work, why bother." Pride says, "You don't have to do it" and Fear says, "Why bother?" Stop! You can't get indigestion from swallowing your pride. It's okay to have those thoughts, feel the feeling, and do it anyway. Action is the law of attraction. Let me repeat myself: It's okay to have a negative thought now and then, just don't invite it to stay overnight and live rent free in your head with the rest of your negative committee. Have the thought, feel the feeling and do it anyway, and the results will amaze you.

Merrillism #11: "The Chatter Doesn't Matter."

A funny thing happens when you start to get into the exercise flow, you begin to crave healthier food and more exercise. You are less likely to reach for a cheeseburger, and more likely to desire the satisfying crunch of broccoli or my leafy Serenity Salad. You begin to replace candy corn with nature's candy: fruit. You begin to entertain the idea of eating pesticide free and organic with no panic. Moving your body really does move your mind and your spirit—all the parts of you working together to create the very best **you** you can be. Remember, growth is not easy but with continuity, commitment and consistency, you build confidence, gain courage, exercise control and eventually you achieve, conquer and succeed!

*"People underestimate their capacity for change.
There is never a right time to do a difficult thing. A leader's job
is to help people have vision of their potential."*
—John Porter

When you give and energize yourself in the form of movement in the world, this will help you get into your exercise or "play out." Look at it as giving to the world and others. You are giving the gift of health, and you get to keep it for yourself by giving it away. Be an attraction, rather than a promotion of health in your life. People always want what I have and I do no promoting. They come to me in line at the supermarket, the gym, the movies, the post office or just parked in traffic, like bees to honey. When I stand for health for myself, I stand for health for the world. When I do it for me, I do it for we. My personal commitment to a healthful life is actually helpful to others, because I am a living example of what is possible and empowering others to be like me too. It makes it easier to do it for me, by doing it for you. You can do the same. If you don't believe in miracles, this book will help you be one.

How Do I Do It For Me?
by Debbie Merrill

I was taught they need to like me
I'm here to bring joy and please them all
I thought if only this one time I'd really absorb their call

"Hey Baby, you're great, we love you", "Oh please just do
  it again."

It all became just one loud sound and only lasted about
    five or ten
Then there I was alone with me feeling high—in doubt
    and curious
Good or bad? Why can't I perform like one grand
    Stradivarius

I'm supposed to be a channel of expression, not a show off
    frightened or taunted
I only get one chance to do all the things I've dreamed
    and wanted

My desire is to be myself and do what I'm capable of
Coming from my heart and joy, which really means it's love

It's about time I do it for me, accept what I have, make
    a shift
For I am God's creation, and my talent but the gift!

Go For It!

Raw Bites

- ***Move your body.*** *Wake up and give me twenty. Do twenty push-ups before you start your day. Exercise before you eat. Give yourself oxygen, fresh air, then breakfast. You'll eat less, live more, look and feel better and your day will be great.*
- ***Move your feet.*** *Sign up for a dance class with your partner. Learn to cha cha, salsa, pole dance, tap, disco or tango. Dancing is great exercise, it promotes closeness and non-verbal, sensual*

creative communication and brings joy to your relationships. Don't have a partner? Sign up anyway. Most dance studios offer lessons with or without a partner and it's a fun way to meet new people and express your creativity and inner dancer.

- ***Move your spirit.*** *As suggested in Chapter 1, create a visual treasure map of the life you imagine for yourself. You are only limited by your imagination, so dream big.*

- ***Move and expand your mind.*** *Learn one new thing today. Look up a word in the dictionary or Thesaurus and incorporate it into your vocabulary. Sign up for language or writing classes at your local community college. Write poetry, journal, write a book (I did!), screenplay, love letter, thank you card or love note. Share your mind, body and spirit with the world, and the world will respond back to you in the form of health, wealth, prosperity and love.*

- ***Practice meditation for relaxation and inspiration.*** *The memory of God comes to the quiet mind.*

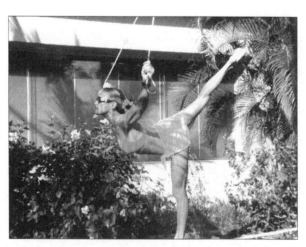

Move a muscle, change a thought.

Chapter 6

Instant Gratification

"Instant gratification takes too long."
—Carrie Fisher

As children, we couldn't wait—for recess, our next birthday, summer vacation, Christmas, to lose our first tooth, to lick the spoon, to turn 18 and to go to college. Big or small, we were always in a hurry to get to the next thing. Every car trip was punctuated with multiple choruses of our favorite song, the "Are We There Yet?" blues. As adults, not much has changed. We can't wait to graduate, get our first job, be promoted, get married, buy our first, second or third house, get thin, and get rich and famous. And now we are in a rush to get healthy, get young, get a facelift or get liposuction. (Not for my life would I go under the knife.) We all want it and we all want it now in sitcom timing. I'll bet you can't wait to finish this chapter so you can move on to the next one.

Like Veruca Salt in *Willy Wonka and the Chocolate Factory*, we "Want it—NOW!" And now spelled backwards is won. If we get it now, it means we've won, we've conquered, we've achieved, and that is truly backwards thinking. We have fallen in to the trap of chasing instant gratification, buying into the idea that we can have it all—right this very second. TiVo lets us skip past the commercials and fast-forward through the slow parts; MTV sells sex, drugs and rock 'n roll in under three minutes and it only takes 0.13 seconds to

Google "instant gratification." Society tells us that faster is better and we believe it. We are even dying faster. We are having more heart attacks, strokes, car accidents, suicides and homicides in less time. I call it sitcom timing: the idea that it is possible to solve any problem, change any situation and improve our lives in 22 minutes flat. There are still only 60 seconds in a minute and that cannot be changed.

I hate to be the one to break it to you, but sitcom timing is not reality and life does not come with a built-in laugh track. The truth is, the great obstacle in achieving awareness is the need for instant gratification. We are constantly rushing, and our efforts to achieve health are no exception. You know the truth: *nothing happens instantly*. It didn't take you a day to get sick. It took a lifetime. So it's not going to take a day to get better. Remember—recovery, healing, losing weight, getting fit, spiritual growth, giving up addictions and becoming healthy is a process, not an event. It's not "Here today, gone to Maui." It's not instant. Anything you get instantly you never keep. If you lose weight fast, you gain it back faster. But, if you lose it slowly, while developing a new way of eating and fitness, it will stay off. Take time with transitioning your food plan and changing to a healthier lifestyle, and you will be rewarded with a fit body, a healthy mind and a happy spirit for the rest of your life. The irony is, the more time you take, the more time you *have* to take. You don't have time *not* to take time, time is your friend. Remember, weeds grow fast; flowers take time to bloom.

Merrillism #12: "There Is More to Life Than Making it Go Faster."

Think about it. Is instant coffee just as good as the real thing? How about fast food, quick bread, instant oatmeal, or a quick workout? Can you get it right now? Sure. But will it satisfy you? Maybe for an instant, but I guarantee you, in an hour you'll be looking for your next quick fix. There is no quick minute. A minute has always been, and will always be, exactly 60 seconds—no more, no less. There are 30 days to a month, three months to a season, 12 months to a year, it is what it is.

As much as you want to change and grow, it won't happen in three minutes, three hours or even three days. Give it three weeks, three months or three seasons. Does this mean you won't see *any* shift in three days? Of course not. It simply means that you cannot expect to see lasting results in only a few days or months. To see (and feel) real results takes time. Contrary to what all the advertisements for anti-aging products tell us, time is not your enemy. Time is a gift and your friend. Show your appreciation by taking time with yourself and letting time work *for* you. Let time be your friend, not your enemy. Trying to do more in less time is one of life's toughest challenges. We need to do less in more time instead. Give time, time.

There is a little Veruca Salt in all of us. Trust me, there are times when I just want to get there already! I am suggesting that you remind your inner spoiled child to practice patience, because practicing patience and persistence equals permanence. If it were easy, everyone would be doing it. It's not easy, but it's not impossible either. I was able to turn my life around, and I have a gift for turning other people's lives around too, both on and off skates. They call me the skating therapist and spinning top. I love to turn. I've been turning others and myself around my entire life. I discovered that if I could turn on skates, I could turn my life and health around, and that it's actually much easier than doing a double axel! I did it and so can you—in fact, you're already doing it. You are reading this book.

Raw Bites

- **Stop and smell the roses**, *literally. Slow down and live. "You're not livin' if you're driven."*

- **Drink More Water.** *It prevents dehydration, cleans out the body, and promotes the natural healing process. Substituting water for beverages high in calories can also help control weight. You don't need to drown yourself with 8-10 glasses a day, just start by drinking more than you do currently. Listen to your body. It will tell you when you've had enough. Most of the time when you think you are hungry, you're actually thirsty. You're craving water and oxygen and natural sugar. Drink before you eat, or eat fruit (which is 80% water) one half hour before your meal. Believe me, you will see how satisfied you feel, and you will probably eat less of your meal. Try it, it works.*

- **Take an emergency five-minute vacation.** *Vacate the mind. Give yourself a break. Create five minutes in your day to do nothing. Find a quiet spot, kick off your shoes (or skates), and pull over in your car in an area by nature, a forest of trees, a park, the ocean, the mountains, a sunset or horizon. Sit or lie down, close your eyes and just breathe for five full minutes. That's it. That's all you have to do. Breathe. Don't think, plan, strategize, worry, or fret. It's harder than it sounds, but you'll be glad you did. Worry is an ironic form of hope.*

Chapter 7

Lessons from
the (B)rink

*"I've come to believe that all my past failures and frustrations
were actually laying the foundation for the understandings
that have created the new level of living I now enjoy."*
—Anthony Robbins

The very first time I performed I was five years old and it was in front of an audience of 500 people. I had stage fright so bad I almost couldn't do it. I stood there, dressed in pink sequins, rhinestones and ruffles, my tap shoes glued to the floor, frozen with fear. It was hearing my mother's voice from the front row that finally got me through it, "Go on Debbie. Keep going!" she whispered loudly. And, at the age of five, I became alive and I did it. You could say the performance bug bit me that day in the school gymnasium in Yonkers, New York. I started out with tap dancing and ballet, then when it came time to put on toe shoes, I swapped them out for blades—figure skating blades that is—and I never looked back. The moment I strapped on those skates, I knew. I was home. The ice rink was my refuge—from being ordinary, and from the fighting at home—and it would be my salvation—and my escape from the never-ending fighting between my parents. They

61

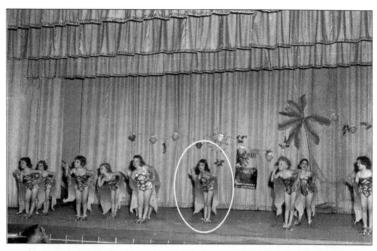

My first performance on stage dancing and singing as little Miss Muffit at age 5. That's when I got the performance bug.

argued over everything from money to how the house should look. My mother took great pains keeping it museum-quality sterile. My dad and I wanted to live in a home but every impeccably cleaned object was considered hands-off. Not only did she try to maintain total control over the house and everything in it she tried to control me, too. We battled all the time. If she said black, I said blue. We were two strong willed Italian women who wanted to be validated and accepted by everyone and, more important, we both craved my dad's attention and love. I soon grew to despise her controlling and over protectiveness and as a result, became very rebellious, feisty and argumentative. Even though my mother was a beautiful woman (an Elizabeth Taylor look alike) with vibrant green eyes, lustrous black hair and peaches and cream complexion, I tried my best never to look like her. Even as a young girl, I was terrified of being overweight and out of shape like my mom. Both my parents were overweight and short, and no matter how well dressed and perfectly coifed they were, it didn't stop people from staring, or making fun of them. I was determined to be different, and on the ice, I was. Plus, I could wear chiffon, sequins, rhinestones and glitter to my heart's content.

I was self-taught for many years until my mom decided to enroll me in figure skating lessons. I wanted to be Peggy Fleming, Barbie, Queen of the Ice Rink, so I practiced all the time. At twelve, I started my real training. I had the same coach as Dorothy Hamill, who was a few years younger than me, and I was determined to improve. When I wasn't in school, I was on the ice. I was determined to be an Olympic champion and show the world that Debbie DiGiacomo was indeed *special* and a one of a kind talent. I also got a lot of praise from my parents for skating. They were proud of me and I craved their approval almost as much as I craved sugar.

My love affair with figure skating and all that accompanied it (being thin, being pretty and being the best) was matched in intensity by only one thing, my addiction to sugar. My body and my mind began fighting an internal war that would last almost half a lifetime. I was under enormous pressure to be thin, beautiful, sexy, and to be an obliging daughter and athlete all at the same time. They all wanted me to be a super star, the next Olympic champion or star of the Ice Capades as much as I did. So much I had to live up to! But even though I knew I couldn't live up to their expectations, I also knew that I couldn't let them down. I assumed they wouldn't accept me if I didn't live up to their dreams, and felt they wouldn't love me and would one day abandon me. As a matter of fact, I felt that if I ever failed at anything, I would have to leave the planet because I couldn't face them. The pressure from my own internal dialogue was, "I'll never be a champion or a star so why bother; if I can't be Dorothy Hamill or Peggy Fleming, I won't try or participate. So I'll quit, give up and resign, and do something else. I'll show them." But I cut off my nose to spite my face. I did this for the next 10 years, until I found guidance, health, vegetarianism, fitness and spirituality.

I was also older than most of my competitors and too old to be a competitive skater, so I struggled to keep my weight down and hide my age. It's the same thing every female figure skater, gymnast and ballerina goes through today. I was a puppet of protocol. But I was living a lie. I also began to develop breasts and a bootie, and for a figure skater, that was a real handicap. I was competing against young girls and I wanted to look like them. So, at age 12, I began dieting—living on cottage cheese, cantaloupe and Melba toast. All that deprivation would eventually lead me to overindulge in my craving for sugar and so I overate cookies, ice cream, peanut butter and cake. I was entering a vicious and dangerous cycle of dieting and over exercising to compensate for my sugar cravings. I was perplexed, confused and ashamed, so I told no one. I craved the zing, the bling, and to be a "Miss Thing." There was one missing spring, how do I get rid of this sugar fling? How do I juggle it all?

Ice Rage in a Cage

All of this affected my skating. When I was eating all that sugar, I couldn't perform to the best of my ability. I got irritable and cranky when I couldn't land a jump. I lacked patience, I couldn't stay in the process, my timing was off and I had a very short attention span. I couldn't take direction from my coach. I was very stubborn, I was not coachable and I got angry, really angry and combative. I was filled with rage and I took it out on the ice. I would skate around and make big holes in the ice, cursing God and everyone (including myself), kicking and complaining. After my lessons, the Zamboni guy would come by and hand me a big bucket of snow ice and make me fill up the holes. But I could never fill up the holes inside myself. There was a hole in my soul that no amount of food, validation or standing ovation could fill. I had the feeling and belief that I wasn't good enough, and there was something wrong with me and there wasn't enough in the world for me. I had a poverty consciousness, a pauper mentality. I got temporary relief from food, sugar, skating and by spending money. Then that would pass and I would need more of something...anything...just more, more, more galore! I held the belief that if some is good, more must be better. Inevitably, my anger was followed closely by a case of the *Oh Friggits*. "Oh friggit, I quit! I'm never skating again. I give up! I can't learn." I know now that "I can't" really means, "I don't want to." My parents tried to help. They got me an Olympic coach. They spent more money. But it's what they *didn't* do that really mattered. They didn't take me to a nutritionist. They didn't get me proper health education. Why? Because they didn't know any better. In those days, the focus was on making your jumps higher, bigger and cleaner; being thin, beautiful and sexy and wearing gorgeous costumes and getting through a four minute routine without stopping or making any mistakes; and, of course, passing all your skating tests. It wasn't about proper nutrition, balance and rest. When offered the best, what I really needed was rest. Overskating, overworking, overstressing, sleeping less, skating and eating more. What I didn't know then was that my diet wasn't allowing me to do those things—to focus, to concentrate, have patience, stamina, joy, and rest and to accept myself and my craft's process. I hated the learning process. I wanted to just have it done. I was eating more and more sugar, more and more carbs, and gaining weight. I couldn't perform my skating skills to the best of my ability. I didn't like myself, my craft or anyone else. I wanted to be free of worries, and just have wings on my feet and soar. I probably had low blood sugar, but all I knew was that I was miserable and that eating sugar gave me a temporary lift. I was burning the candle at both ends; I was at war with myself. I had it all backwards: *war* spelled backwards is *raw*. Little did I know that eating raw would end the war.

I was a perfectionist involved in a sport where you have to

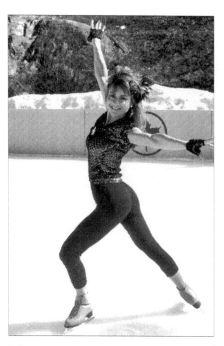

My years training as an amateur and professional figure skater gave me discipline and commitment. Not reaching my Olympic goal taught me one great lesson, " You only lose when you quit."

fall fifty times to succeed once; needless to say on a 1/8th of an inch of a blade. It was a slippery road and I was slipping and sliding all the way. But I was committed. In figure skating, there were eight tests you had to pass in order to qualify for the Olympics and World Competitions back then. Most people fail twice before achieving a passing score, but I passed each of the first seven tests all the on the first try. I didn't know it then, but failing every once in a while would have been a gift. It would have taught me that failing isn't losing. Falling didn't bother me, it was the failing I couldn't take. The greatest successes often follow the most difficult failures. Today, I teach my students to see their failures as stepping-stones, rather than stumbling blocks. I remind them that it's the breakdowns that allow the breakthroughs to occur. Back then, I learned that it's perfection, or nothing. It's 10.0, or why bother. Black and white, rigid, dogmatic thinking was my way of life. For this reason, passing my final test was a Herculean task. I began training with Gus Lussi, who trained all the greats, including Dorothy Hamill and Robin Cousins, and he told me I was jumping in the wrong direction. All those years of skating and training with top notch coaches and Gus was the only one to tell me the truth. If that isn't a metaphor for my life, I don't know what is. No one told me the truth and I wasn't telling myself the truth either.

As a figure skater, I had to relearn everything I thought I knew. I was still eating sugar but had begun to recognize that it wasn't good for me and tried to cut back. When it came time to take my final test, I was practicing eight hours a day, working on double axels, lots of jumping, and my show routine, then at the eleventh hour I tore all the ligaments and cartilage in my right knee. I was just 17. It took years to heal but when I finally was able to skate again, I took just the compulsory figure portion of the test. I was thrilled with my performance, elated in fact, and then I learned that I had failed by 1/8 of a point from one out of three judges. You need all three judges to pass you, in order to pass the 8th test. That was it for me. I was through. I quit right then and there. My inability to be less than perfect, accept failure and face it, bounce back with resilience and follow-through led me to throw in the towel and just leave everything behind. I gave up my dream of competitive and show skating on an international level—letting my rage, pride, hurt and ego win out. Eventually, I found it easier to drown my sorrows in substances, preservatives and junk food, partying and suppressing my feelings of loss and rejection until I was 27 years old. Then I found help in 12-step programs, therapy, health gurus, a vegetarian diet, plus a new-found regimen of fitness and self-expression which led me to a connection of truth in myself and with my higher spirit. This all brought me to my true wealth, health and creative expression.

Work Addiction
by Debbie Merrill

Universal order of a higher presence
Has to become part of my internal essence
In order to be decisive and secure with inner peace
The enormity and chaos of my work must change or cease

When frustrated and overwhelmed with problems of another
I let this power have me become controlling, like a mother
I'm not a guru but catalyst helping others to recover
It's not my job to give answers, only to uncover

I believe in the inherent beauty and wisdom of all beings
When I display the same they're attracted without seeing
It's people pleasing, care taking, overextending myself
The feeling of less than, I've put myself on the shelf

I feel like a supporting player in my life
Everything else comes first in spite of my strife

Try to channel your energies with a purposeful connection
You have something special to contribute in the world that
    will give you direction
Flipping from one activity to another, accomplishing
    only motion
Flying like a butterfly, becoming scattered without notion

Pressure and frustration while being inconsistent
This addiction is forceful, determined and persistent
When not happy with what you are doing and not giving it
    your best
It's time to slow down, balance and discipline, the key—get
    some rest

Find out exactly what you offer, have fun and where you fit
The gift you give to the world is yourself, yes, that's it!
You're Not Livin' If You're Driven!

Do what you love and you'll never work a day in your life

I was angry with myself for not being perfect, angry with my coaches for not correcting me earlier and angry with the judges for failing me. I felt abandoned, discounted, and ripped off. It was not a happy time. So, at the age of 18, I picked myself up, moved to Miami to attend college and traded my skates for disco shoes, and my sequins for bikinis and boas. And, I was back on the sugar. I ate fried chicken with honey to quell the slush fund of hurt and rage inside me. And it worked for a while; seven years in fact. Besides, money was tight and popcorn and cookies were cheaper than carrots. I went to parties, drank Dom Perignon, smoked *Kools*, ate caviar and stone crabs and danced until 6am—all for the first time in my life. I stopped skating, and started dancing, smoking and swimming and dropped down to 98 pounds. I was a jockaholic, and wanted to be fit and healthy. Instead, I was a thin, sexy, disco queen "making the scene," but detouring to destruction. I was ashamed of myself, remorseful and full of guilt for quitting skating so I sabotaged myself with food, drink, tobacco, constant partying and an unhealthy living style. I felt like a quitter. This feeling drove me to be driven for the rest of my life. I know today that when I'm driven, I'm not livin'. My lifestyle was insane. Something had to stop.

> *"The definition of insanity is doing the same thing over and over and expecting different results."*
> —Benjamin Franklin

Finally I realized that *I* was the something that needed to change, shift, know and grow. I had to stop what I was doing and acknowledge that it wasn't working. I had to stop doing the things that were making me sick and start doing the things that made me better. It sure *looked* like my lifestyle was working—to everyone else. After all, I was living my dream, wasn't I? Actually, I just thought I was. From the age of 18 to 27, I bounced back and forth between college and professional ice shows, performing all over the world and teaching skating; I was thin, tan, pretty and profoundly unhappy. The choices I was making in my life were not working for me. You know, in the end, my athletic ability was both my barometer, and my messenger. I found that if I overate, I didn't want to exercise and that eating an abundance of certain foods like sugar, carbs and fats made me not want to skate or dance. My thinking was foggy and mocus (mind out of focus). I struggled with depression and self-hatred, and my self-esteem was in the toilet. What was once my strength, was now my weakness.

That is when I learned that discontent, demoralization and desperation could be a great teacher, and that the road to health often begins with pain. Pain was my motivator. It pushed me forward. No pain, no gain. I made the choice to turn my weakness into strength. The saying, "the pain pushes you until the vision pulls you" is a great truth. I knew the truth would set me free, but it angered me at first. I was finally in enough pain to ask for help. I was ready to do, be, and live differently. So I got support, got educated and stepped forward into my own life. It wasn't instant. There was no thunderbolt that made me turn things around. Rather, it was a series of thunderbolts, miracles, divine interventions, synchronicities, people, events and the willingness to let change and growth into my life. Now, I live a visionary life. I am pulled, motivated and inspired by my vision every day and it is a beautiful, happy, rewarding place to be.

Merrillism #13: "First it Gets Worse, Then it Gets Different, Then it Gets Better, Then it Gets Real."

The reason I am here, sharing my story with you, is not because I think my story is so extraordinary, but to be of service, to make a contribution and to let my life (and my mistakes) be an inspiration, lesson and motivation for you. If my experiences can help you realize *your* goals and live *your* life to its fullest potential, without detouring into destruction and taking the shortcut to awareness and power while you overcome your demons, blind spots and unhappiness, then it's worth telling.

Assignment to be in Alignment

By now you know that growth is messy and uncomfortable, but unless it's messy and uncomfortable, it's not growth. You also know that real, lasting success comes from having the willingness and the courage to change, transform and let go. Today, we are going to begin working out, on the inside. I want you to start keeping a food journal. You don't have to do it forever, but you should commit to a week. If that's too daunting right now, then give yourself at least a day.

Step 1. Write down everything you eat during the day and how much you eat of it. I mean everything. Every donut, hamburger, salad and curly fry you put in your mouth. Write it down. Every breath mint, finger full of frosting, kernel of popcorn, pint of beer, stick of gum, glass of OJ, and frappuccino. It all goes in your journal. Don't forget to include the number of cigarettes you smoked, cocktails you drank and the chips you snacked on, even if it was just one. If you don't know exactly what you're eating, it makes it much harder to transition. Denial sneaks in.

So get educated and gain clarity. It's time. Clarity and knowledge are power.

Sidebar To The Rawbar
Food Facts

- Did you know that a banana has 100 calories, but 80% of it is water? My favorite fast food also contains lots of fiber, about 10 % protein and only 3% fat and is loaded with potassium and is easily digested.
- A snack of raw cacao is a great energy booster and is one of my favorite "pick me ups." Try mixing it with raw goji berries for sweetness, amino acids and vitamin C. Raw cacao contains nearly 20 times the antioxidant levels of red wine and has up to 30 times the antioxidants found in green tea. It also diminishes appetite, aids in weight loss, opens the heart shocker, nourishes the brain for increased alertness and intellectual stimulation.
- Organic goji berries build strength and increase vitality. They contain 18 kinds of amino acids and are a complete protein source known to stimulate the production of human growth hormone associated with longevity.
- Have a fruit smoothie with spirulina loaded with B12 for healthy nerves and tissues. It's a great digestible protein source rich in iron and magnesium, without fat and cholesterol, great for transitioning to a raw veggie vegan diet.
- Try some of these easy simple quick snack attacks to the future, they will not leave you dull and fatigued after eating, you will be extremely satisfied, mentally alert and physically energized. You will be raw on the roll!

Step 2. Next, write down how you felt while you ate it. I want you to really think about this. How hungry were you before you ate? Were you mildly hungry, starving, thirsty, bored, depressed, angry or emotional? Or were you eating because the clock said it was time for lunch? Did you want to eat? Were you rushing, gulping it down, standing, breathing, and thinking negative thoughts and resentment? Were you sad, anxious, happy or excited? How did you feel afterwards? Did you eat until you were stuffed? Or did you stop when you felt satisfied? Or maybe you don't know how you felt. Now, dig deeper. Did the food you ate satisfy something beyond hunger? Did it relieve your blues, give you more energy, or calm your rage? Or did you stuff your emotions, numb out, or dull them with the food you ate? How about an hour afterwards? Two hours? Did it give you energy, joy, creative expression, inspiration and contentment? Or, did it make you feel tired, lazy and lethargic? Answering these questions slowly over the course of time and researching this knowledge about yourself will help you with your relationship with food, health and your life. This will help you discover which foods work and don't work for you, and what foods are your triggers, "NO" foods or comfort foods?

Merrillism #14: "You Can't Heal What You Can't Feel and Can't Deal With."

I know this may seem like a lot of work at first, but nobody said this was going to be a piece of cake. After you have kept your journal for a week, I want you to look for patterns. What do you eat the most of? Was it healthy? Are you eating late at night, or in the middle of the night? How much are you eating? Are you scarfing down salads? Are you breathing and tasting your food in a calm relaxed setting? Or are you bingeing on sugary snacks or potato chips, eating standing up? What food can you not get enough of? What's your trigger food? (Trigger foods are foods that, once you taste them, cause an insatiable craving for more and you can't stop. Ice cream, cookies, popcorn and all corn products are my trigger foods.) It's very important to recognize what your trigger food is so you can avoid it. You probably have a food sensitivity, allergy or addiction to the food you cannot let go of. I ate tofu three times a day every day for seven years when I was a vegetarian/vegan, before I went raw. It was the hardest food I had to give up, along with corn. That's how I knew I was addicted and allergic to soy and corn. When I gave it up after going raw vegan, I felt and looked better while going through the withdrawals. So I kept going. However, tofu is a good transition food while giving up meat and dairy and going vegetarian/vegan. Moderation is the key with all food.

Discovering your trigger food is, as they say, half the battle. Because when you uncover what the block is, you can get busy discarding it. This is a tough one, I know. So, as I have said, take your time. It may take you a day, a week, a month, a year, or a lifetime, and that's okay. This is a way of life, not a diet. Once you discover what is running you in your food and life, you will be that much closer to being powerful in your life and attaining true, lasting health, happiness, creativity, freedom and spirituality. Remember, whatever you give power to has you. Whatever you surrender to sets you free. The truth always sets you free, but it makes you angry first. To thine own self be true, or blue? Which is for you?

Raw Bites

- *Let go of one food that you think you cannot live without. The one food that if you were stranded on a desert island, you would pick as your only sustenance. Let it go, **just for today**. If you feel like it, let it go tomorrow too.*

- *"Substitution is the solution." Substitute your bad food for one that tastes just like it that you enjoy and is healthy, preferably fresh, ripe, whole, raw and organic.*
- *Have patience, seek education, do the diligence.*
- *Share your successes and failures.*
- *Admit your lack of integrity and honesty.*
- *Ask your higher power for help, guidance, and willingness.*

Chapter 8

Road to Raw:

How to Become a Raw Veggie Vegan
Viva Las Vegan!

*"Food is a love note from God; its letters are written
by the rays of the sun. It says, 'I love you and I shall take care
of you with the offerings of my earth'."*
—Gabriel Cousens, M.D. (H), Conscious Eating

My journey on the road to becoming a Raw Veggie Vegan began when what I saw reflected in the mirror didn't match the vision of what I knew my life could be. Sure, I looked good on the outside; but I saw right through the tanned, fragile woman with the nice figure and pretty face—and into the truth of who I had become: an unhealthy, sugar addicted, workaholic, jocka-holic who was falling apart from the inside out. I was a vegetarian who ate more crap than vegetables. Instead, I ate tortilla chips, ice cream, cookies, peanut butter, muffins, cake, granola, homemade butter cookies, onion rings, "nutrition" bars, popcorn with loads of butter and sundaes topped with butterscotch, chocolate sauce, chocolate chips, colored sprinkles and nuts. I ate some veggies like french fries, carrots, and the parsley on my plate, and I justified eating all this excessive amount of sugar and high fatty foods with the mantra, "Well, at least I'm not eating meat!" Since I didn't eat meat, I thought I was better than most people, and doing well. I talked the talk, but I didn't always walk the walk. I was not doing what I believed in and knew I could do.

I was a lacto-ovo for many years, which means I let go of meat and fish, but I still ate dairy and eggs, and I still cooked my food. The next step was becoming macrobiotic, which meant eating primarily steamed vegetables, beans, brown rice, seaweed, some fish, small amounts of seasonal fruit and only when they were in season. Since I had already stopped eating meat, the transition to macro was a bit easier for me—except the part where I couldn't eat sugar. I'm not going to lie; it was difficult in the beginning. Giving up bacon was a million times easier than giving up Entenmanns's Crumb Cakes. Entenmann's and me, we went way back. I had a joke in my circle that I majored in the study of Entenmannology. I had every variety of Entenmann's cakes or cookies ever made. That was one relationship I didn't want to let go of. But the transition was easier when I started seeing benefits: I lost weight, felt good, had more energy and I stopped getting sick. My skin cleared up, my blood sugar improved and I experienced greater clarity of mind.

Despite myself, I had stumbled upon the right road. I wasn't sure how I got there but I was going to stay on it until something else came along. Living in New York City did something miraculous for me, I was at the right place at the right time. This is where I discovered vegetarianism, veganism, macrobiotics and healthy food. After sticking to a macro diet for several years, I decided it was time to let go of fish for good. It was becoming clear that my road was leading me to becoming a vegan. I was consuming no animals or animal by-products, no flour, sugar, dairy or salt, and giving up alcohol, tobacco and prescription drugs. All the while I was incorporating more raw foods into my diet on an unconscious level. I was transitioning myself to a raw lifestyle without realizing it, so it took some time. I was probably 70% raw without even knowing it or trying to be, by just being a vegan. When I started, as a sugarholic vegetarian, I was maybe 2% raw. I slowly built on that number becoming 10%, then 25%, 50% and so on. Today I am a 100% raw veggie vegan diva and I have never felt more alive, ageless, energized, clear headed, and comfortable in my body. And do you know what else? I lost my cravings for sugars, carbohydrates and bad fats. I love, crave and substitute fruit in its natural state for sugar today, but in moderation. I didn't do this overnight but over time. I'll say it again, if I can do it, *so can you.*

> *"I do not try to dance better than anyone else.*
> *I only try to dance better than myself."*
> —Mikhail Baryshnikov

I recognize that our stories, and the roads we choose, may be very different. That's a good thing. After all, if we all chose the same road, there would be an awful lot of traffic. You may already be well on your way. Or, you may be wondering how to get on *your* road. Some of you may even be thinking, "There's a road?" As I have said, where you begin depends on where you are right now. Perhaps you have already made the transition to vegetarianism. Good for you. Your journey has already begun. Or, you may be lost on a side street somewhere, wondering how you are going to find the highway without a map. The way to learn is to begin. Begin where you are. But you do need to begin now. You're not going to find the road unless you take that first step. Doing just a little helps a lot. I advise my clients to start by adding raw foods, and *then* eliminating unhealthy foods, like refined sugars, pre-packaged, processed foods and meats. Give up the pesticides, fumicides, fungicides, and herbicides so they all don't equal suicide. It is important to add first and eliminate second so you don't start your journey feeling deprived. Deprivation puts you in the fast lane to failure, overeating, and ill health. Moderation, not deprivation!

This is not about deprivation; this is about moderation, reju-venation, inspiration and innovation. This is a lifestyle that will keep you free from sickness, disease, disorder, depression, obesity, unconsciousness and drugs. This is, in my opinion, the raw truth to the fountain of youth. Some of the many benefits of the *raw on the roll* lifestyle are vitality, clarity, power, freedom, contentment, motivation, full creative expression and the transition from physi-cality to spirituality, while living in reality. Get out from under the sheets, give up being two sheets to the wind, give up the diet sheets and get rawkin' with your health and fitness. Viva Las Vegan!

"Get on the Rawkin' Raw Road of Happy Bliss"

Step 1. Start by eating organic. If you are still eating meat, make sure you choose organic, free-range meat and poultry. (I suggest giving up eating animals and their by-products all together.) Buy your vegetables at local farmer's markets or organic markets whenever possible and choose fresh, local, seasonal, pesti-cide-free organic vegetables. Organic local vegetables not only taste better, they are better for you. When it comes to produce, tailor your diet to eat whatever is in season and harvested as close to your home as possible. It not only ensures you will be eating fresher fruits and veggies with a higher vitamin and mineral content, it also helps save money at the checkout counter and supports local farmers and the environment. (Less carbon monoxide fumes due to the cost of flying or shipping the produce to your local grocery store.)

Step 2. Add one raw dish to each meal. This can be as simple as topping your pancakes with a sliced banana, eating salad with your burger, having an apple for dessert or adding sprouts to your salad. If you are the adventurous type, feel free to flip to the recipe section and try one of my Merrill Magic rawsome awesome recipes or two.

Step 3. I am 80% bling and 100% raw, but you don't have to eat exactly like me to learn from me. Just eat one completely raw meal every day. If that's too intense, make it every other day. Again, there are a lot of options. It can be as simple as eating melon for breakfast, or preparing a delicious, seasonal, organic salad for lunch or dinner, with sprouts, nuts or sprouted legumes. If you want to get acquainted with my favorite lover, buy a Vita-Mix® Blender. You can use it to whip up a quick and easy soup, (see my Green Keen Lean Machine Soup or Cocktail) or make a yummy fruit smoothie. Try some of my recipes in the recipe section of this book.

Step 4. Start making your main courses raw, and relegating cooked foods to side dishes. At this point, half your plate should be raw. You'll feel so satisfied, alive and satiated you won't want to eat the cooked side dish. When eating raw foods, especially raw super-foods, one needs to eat less because raw food is so nutrient dense. There is simply no need to overeat. How *much* you eat is just as important as *what* you eat. I see many "raw fooders" eat pounds of nuts, avocados, fruits and other fatty foods in one sitting, and then they wonder why they're gaining weight, have no energy and can't stay 100% raw! Consuming a high fat diet, whether it's cooked or raw, is not recommended. I say eat less, live more. Move more and lose more (if you need to). Keep the wisdom, lose the weight.

Step 5. If you haven't already started letting go of meat, you can do it all at once, or one at a time. Bless the cow for now and let it go. Bless the chicken and get busy kickin' the animal habit. If you want to fast track this part, I suggest visiting a slaughterhouse, checking out a documentary or DVD, (I like the DVD "Eating" produced and directed by Michael Anderson) or try reading one of the many books on the subject (I like *Diet for a New America*) by John Robbins. And before you even think of picking up a jumbo size of anything, watch the film "Supersize Me" by filmmaker Morgan Spurlock; this irreverent look at obesity, and the link to fast food corporations will really get the message in your face. And you'll no longer want to eat anything with a face.

Merrillism #15: "Food Without Fire Takes Your Knowledge, Energy and Power Even Higher."

Step 6. Let go of processed foods, refined sugars, prepackaged meals, instant foods and cooked foods. Eliminate white flour, dairy products and sugar, including high fructose corn syrup (hfcs). Sugar comes in many different forms and names, watch out for them. When you read the labels look for names such as barley malt, maltodextrin, evaporated cane juice, fructose, caramel, date sugar, dextrose, fruit juice concentrate, malt syrup, mannitol, molasses and brown rice syrup. Avoid them at all costs.. Choose your foods wisely. This one is hard for a lot of people, so take it easy. Remember, it's okay to fall—as long as you get back up. It's not what you do once in awhile; it's what you do every day that counts.

Step 7. Continue adding raw meals to your monthly, weekly and daily routine. You may start out, as I did, at 2% and slowly work your way up to 100%. Or you may not. You may choose to stay at 80%, 50% or even 20% and that's fine. It's your rawkin' raw road of happy bliss.

Merrillism #16: "Do it The Way You Can Do it, Until YOU Can Do it the Way You Want to Do it, But Do it!"

My first drug of choice was fear; the rest evolved from that. As you continue down the rawkin' *road to raw bliss*, there will be speed bumps, fears, potholes, hills and other obstacles to impede your progress. That's why I'm here, to help you stay the course. The road I was on was not called "Easy Street," and I took the occasional detour. I was impatient with myself. I wanted to get on the right road and get there already. I know first hand that making the transition is not easy, giving up addictions is difficult and painful;

choosing health is sometimes hard. I ate because I was upset, and I was upset because I ate. The raw lifestyle helped me to overcome emotional eating, food cravings, binging, dieting and peaks and valleys with my mood swings and health. I'm here to help you find an easier, softer, quicker road. As the famous book, *The Secret*, tells us, "Incurable is curable from within." Or, as I like to say, true health is an inside job. In the chapters to come, I will offer more tips, tricks and suggestions to help you get over the bumps in the road, like giving up sugar, caffeine and cooked carbs. Stop asking "Why?" Why-ing is dying. Just ask *how?*

Raw Bites

- *You've made it this far, so I know you have been working very hard. I'm proud of you. So, pat yourself on the back. Give yourself a break. Do something today that is just for you. Take a bubble or salt bath, talk to a friend on the phone, walk on the beach, squish your toes in the mud or sand, get a massage, sing karaoke, ride a roller coaster, take your favorite class, watch the sun rise or set, spend time in nature, see a funny movie and laugh, dance naked in your living room, play on the swings, read a trashy novel, buy yourself some flowers, buy new shoes (or skates), go to a concert, let loose, let go, be playful and have some fun!*

- *Give up white table salt. Use Celtic sea salt or pink Himalayan crystal sea salt.*

- *Give up white bread, pasta, potatoes, and sugar, as well as dairy, which includes milk, cheese, butter, yogurt, ice cream, sour cream, and cottage cheese.*

- *Shop at your local farmer's market. Choose local fresh and organic seasonal fruits and vegetables.*

Debbie Merrill's
Raw on the Roll Success System

"Body and mind, and spirit, all combine,
to make the Creature, human and divine."
—Ella Wheeler Wilcox

Eating more live, raw foods will offer you a fit body, a healthy mind and a happy spirit. Too many of us spend too much time looking forward to our next meal, rather than our next moment. We need to "Eat to live," not "Live to eat." The raw lifestyle is ubiquitous—we don't become healthy by what we eat alone. True health is achieved by what and how we think, the way we move our body, the richness of our spiritual life and our creative expression. We are made up of more than just flesh and blood; and my *Raw on the Roll Success System* is about integrating and honoring our whole selves. It is not a fad, but a way of living. It's a holistic, majestic approach to life (we are all Kings and Queens here to glorify the inner and outer spirit), recognizing that your **mind**, **body** and **spirit** are all equally important in creating a whole, balanced self. Nurturing your mind and spirit is as important as nurturing your body. When you accept yourself fully—your idiosyncrasies and faults, as well as your talents—your negative self-perceptions disappear and you become free to love yourself, others and life. That is the gift of health, and nothing tastes as good as health feels. My system works for me and it works for countless others. If you are willing, it can work for you too. It works if you want it, if you are willing, if you work it, and if you let it. Just do it for the health of it— *your* health of it!

Good luck and good health to you!

The Power of the Mind

"He who masters his mind masters himself"
—Author Unknown

Your mind can be a powerful ally, or a fierce enemy. The choice is yours. In other words, you make the choice to use the power of your own thoughts to do good in the world, or to cause harm to yourself or others. I don't know about you, but I choose to do good. Meaning, I make a conscious decision every day to think positively, rather than negatively. I won't lie to you; it's not easy at first. Negative thinking is easier and you'll find an unlimited supply of "friends" to support your *stinking thinking*. However, you can't have two thoughts at the same time, a negative and a positive. So if you switch to thinking positive, and not negative, this will add to your health, well-being and joy.

Next time you are in the break room at work, listen to the conversations around you. Are they positive and nurturing, or filled with complaints and criticisms? More often than not, you will hear conversations about how annoyed your fellow co-workers are with the boss, which body parts they hate the most, or how their kids, husband or in-laws are driving them up a wall. As negative as we are when it comes to others, we are even harsher on ourselves. How many times a day do you look in the mirror and think, "Wow, I look fantastic! My thighs are perfect and I really am enough!"

Conversely, how many times a day do you complain about being tired, overworked, overweight, unattractive, lonely, stressed or broke? My guess is that you're probably more negative than positive. At first the transition to healthier thinking may be painful, because you will have to acknowledge the negativity you have been living with and holding onto before you can transform it. But at least it is conscious pain, rather than unconscious pain. Your pain will now be out in the open, where you can deal with it. Accept it, name it, claim it and dump it, forever, an eyelash at a time.

I am a big believer in the power of positive thinking. My belief comes from my failures in positive thinking, as much as in my successes. As I mentioned earlier, I sabotaged my career with negative thinking and negative behavior. It talked me out of the rink and into fear, doubt and self-destruction. In order to perform double axles (two and a half revolutions in the air, landing backwards on one foot), I had to believe that it was possible for me and that I was capable to perform such a difficult move. I had to believe that I could train my body, spirit and mind to do this, and that I was worthy of this. I had to own it for myself first. Sadly, I chose to tell myself that I wasn't good enough; I wasn't worthy of doing a double axel and it would never happen for me. It was my interpretation of what I was telling myself that made me fail. It doesn't matter that what I was telling myself was not the truth. What matters is that I believed it. Athletic ability alone was not enough, stinking thinking created doubt in my mind, body and spirit as well as in my performance. A lack of confidence and courage swelled within me, purging me of the little self-esteem I had. It created a drastic, life long, irrevocable change in my professional ice skating career, my demeanor and in my attitude toward myself and my life.

Merrillism #17: "Think it, Ink it and Thank it."

It is not enough to simply turn off the negative noise machine in our heads; we need to change the channel and listen to a different station. I have found that the most effective way to do that is through positive affirmations. By practicing positive affirmations on a daily basis, you can change the direction of your life. I know this to be true because I have done it and so have countless others. The reason I wasn't healthy in my mind and body had nothing to do with reality, but rather with the stories I told myself about my habits, beliefs, fears and poor food choices from my past. I had to free myself from these negative thoughts, and put them behind me to get on with the positive actions of today. I can hear some of you raising objections already, "Debbie, that's B.S.!" or "It will never work." Well, I'm here to tell you that it doesn't matter that you don't believe it right now, try it anyway. I am asking you to take a leap of faith and just do it. This will bring you peace during the storm of life, not peace from the storm.

Here's a few important points regarding making effective affirmations. **Affirmations must be stated in the present tense.** The future is just that, the future. If you say, "I will soon be rich and in love!" you are setting yourself up to be rich and in love—*someday*. You want to be rich and in love right now, so state your affirmation in the present tense, "I am now rich and in love!" or, "I choose to be rich and in love, now!" Additionally, **affirmations must be framed as positive statements**, as the subconscious does not recognize negative words. For example, the statement "I am *not* fat," is understood by your subconscious as "I am fat." Frame your statements carefully in the affirmative: "My body is thin, healthy, firm, fit, clean and beautiful!" **Affirmations should be spoken aloud**, preferably throughout the day and with enthusiasm. And finally, **impress your subconscious mind with your affirmations by writing them down.** Ink it and think it, or think it and ink it. Either way works. I suggest you say and write five affirmations every day. Create new ones in whatever areas you have trouble or breakdowns. You will increase the benefits you receive by saying your affirmations to yourself in the mirror. Look yourself straight in the eye and repeat your affirmations with energy and excitement every day. Doing this daily is crucial. You have been pouring negative thoughts into your brain and out of your mouth for years—transforming your thinking will not happen overnight. If only it were that easy! You need to practice affirmations every single day. Think of it like exercise for your brain. Drain your brain of the old terrain and retrain your brain and body with the new. Take note of how you speak about yourself and life as well. Let only positive words exit your mouth. As an ex-native New Yorker, I really work hard at giving up using foul language; it is fowl food for me, and I do not eat fowl or recommend eating or speaking it, for you as well. Once I retrained my brain, I stopped *enduring* my health and started *enjoying* my health. Like your body, your mind needs to be trained on a daily basis. He who masters his mind masters his body. What the mind can conceive, believe and receive, one can achieve.

Your Body

"A fit body and a healthy mind equal a happy spirit."

I love the expression "Food is life," because, particularly when speaking of raw food, it is true. Cooking kills. Yes, it kills bacteria and other diseases but it also destroys the spirit of the food, the life force and the enzymes; so when you eat cooked food, you are essentially eating dead food. It is food that contains no oxygen, water, enzymes and no live energy. The energy and spirit of the food is gone, there is no life. When you consume raw foods, you are literally eating life! The vitality of the food is preserved, and its love, spirit and high vibration remain intact, which is why raw food is so completely nourishing. It feeds your brain, body and cells as well as your soul. Now that's real soul food.

Eating a raw, organic, animal-free diet is a self-nurturing way to treat your temple. Raw foods retain 100% of their nutritional value, nothing added and nothing taken away. Cooking food can take away as much as 85% of its nutritional value, which means you need to eat more of it to reap the benefits. The process of heating food also destroys enzymes, which aid in digestion and allow energy and nutrition to be delivered to the body at a faster rate. The number one, life enhancing benefit of eating a raw diet is abundant energy, clarity of mind, and alert sensitivity. Since the body is not working overtime, trying to digest cooked foods, you feel more energized, sleep less yet feel more rested, experience greater clarity of thinking, and are more focused. That's why I say I discovered the fountain of youth. I have the same energy and enthusiasm, the same lust for life that I had when I was a teenager. Do you ever marvel at the pure unbridled energy of a four year old—how they run around for hours on end, finding joy in the simplest exchanges, laughing, loving and living every moment to the utmost? Never wanting to go to bed, they perceive the next moment is going to be the biggest miracle of their lives. Waiting, wanting and expecting miracles, magic and believing in them, this is the childlike essence we need to return to. That is how I feel most of the time—from raw to awe! That is the gift of living raw. I even have my 18-year-old "figure eight" back.

Merrillism #18: "The Food You Eat Affects the Moods You Greet."

Another major benefit of a raw lifestyle is weight management. Perhaps you were drawn to this book for just that reason. I have to be honest, looking hot was what first attracted me to the raw lifestyle. As I learned more about raw food and the raw lifestyle, I quickly realized that I didn't know many raw vegans who were overweight. I still don't. Raw foods not only contain less fat and starches than cooked foods, they are richer in nutrients. Logically, the more nourishing, healthy food you consume, the cleaner and more efficient your body becomes and the less you need to eat. In other words, the higher the quality of the food you eat, the lower the quantity you need to eat, which allows for weight loss, maintaining weight and higher energy levels. What a concept: eat less and live more! I came into the raw lifestyle for the vanity, but I stayed for the vitality and the sanity. I went from physicality to originality to spirituality while being able to live and deal in reality. Basically, I went from raw to awe.

Your Spirit

"I have been driven many times upon my knees by the overwhelming conviction that I had nowhere else to go."
—Abraham Lincoln

When I started out on the *road to raw*, I didn't know where the road would lead, or even what road I was on. All I knew was that I needed help. I needed something to save me because I simply could not, or would not, save myself. So I prayed. I prayed for a miracle and waited. Then I prayed some more. That was my routine, praying and waiting, praying and waiting. And you know what, my prayers were answered—not in the way that I expected—but in the way that I needed them. I stopped fighting and started listening, and eventually the answers came. I was sent to the right people, places, and things, events, bookstores, lectures, etc. I began my journey one step at a time, convinced that all foods should be eaten from the Garden of Vegan. That was my miracle. Where's yours? Act as if your life depended on you, and pray as if it depended on a higher force for the answers.

"There are only two ways to live your life. One is as though nothing is a miracle. The other is as though everything is a miracle."
—Albert Einstein

I realize that there are a lot of different core beliefs out there in the world. I have my faith, and you have yours. Far be it from me to tell you what to believe. The only thing I will say is that it is important *to* believe in something. It may be God, Jesus, Buddha, the Ocean, Allah, the Universe, a rock, your Higher Power or your

Higher Self. Prayer is a powerful healer. If you have trouble with the word, think of prayer as a conversation with yourself—your highest, most evolved self. To pray is to ask, and to meditate is to listen. Both are essential. The first thing I do when I wake up in the morning is say *thank you* and *please;* and the last thing I do before I go to bed is say *thank you.* I begin each day with gratitude by asking for help, guidance and acceptance, where I can be of service in my community and the world. I end each day with gratitude as well. I encourage you to do the same. Don't quit before the miracle. As the saying goes, "When the going gets tough, the tough get going." If you feel like giving up, "Fake it 'til you make it." It will happen, I promise you. Be grateful for everything you have in your life, on your plate and in the world. With gratitude you can turn a meal into a feast, a house into a home, despair into hope and sickness into recovery. Recovery is to take back, recover, retrieve. It's time to take back what you were born with, which is great health, fitness, spirituality and creativity. It's your birthright. May today be a beautiful and auspicious commencement to a new, fabulously magical, miraculous lifestyle.

My **Raw Truth to the Fountain of Youth Food-for-Life Plan** de-stresses the body, impresses the mind and expresses the spirit so that you have a fit body, a healthy mind and a happy spirit. Some people tell me that it's impossible to eat an entirely raw diet. I get that. Eating how our parents and ancestors ate is simply their belief system, society's training, corporate advertising and our own habit hunger. If you were to close your eyes and hold your nose, and a friend fed you one of my fabulous persimmon or mamay smoothies with shredded coconut and cacao butter, your mind, body and tummy would have the same satiation, contentment and joy as if you were eating ice cream or your mom's homemade butter cookies. You really wouldn't know the difference. I suggest you recreate what you love in the cooked, junk food world, into the raw food/vegetarian/vegan world. For example, when I crave sweets I eat sweet fruits such as bananas, dates, persimmons, papaya, mamay, goji, mulberries and Incan berries with raw coconut butter or coconut oil. When I crave ice cream, I drink my favorite smoothie and sometimes I freeze it. Now you can even purchase raw ice cream or make your own. It's thick, rich, creamy and sweet, just like real ice cream. In fact it *is* real ice cream, the other is fake. In my cooked vegetarian days, when I craved carbs, I made a kabocha squash casserole with brown rice, tofu, flax seed oil, bananas or plantains. I also made sweet potatoes with soy margarine, shredded coconut and toasted sunflower seeds. These substitutes helped me to transition to a meatless lifestyle and satisfied my sugar, fat and carb craving. Find your substitutes that help you let go of your unhealthy trigger foods. Transition and move forward to a healthier lifestyle now. What are you waiting for?

Be honest about it and you'll improve, but, if you lie about it, you'll be inauthentic with yourself. Try just one meal without animals, or one organic meal. Have one less cigarette a day, don't drink cocktails every day, give up that extra cup of coffee, or take an extra lap around the block and start where you are. Do one thing about the issue each day, and that issue will disappear. Doing something to overcome your weakness each day will strengthen you. Eventually what was once your weakness will become your strength. It will also motivate you to keep doing more and more and more. It's a ripple effect that will take you on a roll. A roll from your sole to your soul. Staying in action restores inspiration and motivation. Again, it's peeling the onion. It's a transformational domino effect; one thing pushes another thing and it keeps pushing you forward, until one day you wake up, and find yourself an enlightened master—a healthy, happy, and fit enlightened master! Practice positive thinking and goal setting, be honest, stay in action, ask for help, meditate, pray and accept, and be ready to receive miracles. If you do those things every day, there is nothing you cannot accomplish. You will *be* the miracle you seek.

Raw Bites

- **Create one affirmation.** *Write it down on a piece of paper and post it where you can see it every day—tape it to your mirror or say it into the mirror, stick it in your purse or wallet, put it on the fridge, on the bedroom ceiling, your computer, dashboard or write it on your hand. Repeat it as often as you can throughout the day—while you get ready in the morning, while you exercise, when the sun is rising or setting, in the car and before you go to sleep. Share it with others. Giving it away and announcing it to the Universe makes it a real conviction, commitment and allows it manifest.*

- **Make today a raw day.** *Make a choice to consume only raw organic, vegan foods today for the whole day. Put love and joy in your food. Tomorrow you can make a different choice. The garden of vegan contains many options.*

- **Pray before you eat.** *Prayer is medicine; your higher force is your doctor. Remember to bless and give thanks for your food before you eat it. Hippocrates said, "Let food be thy medicine and let medicine be thy food."*

- **Be honest in all areas of your life.** *(With yourself and everyone in your life.)*

- **Be willing to receive** *without earning it or deserving it.*

- **Tell yourself there is a miracle** *in your life today and everyday.*

- **Bless you = BE-LESS-YOU**

- **Be willing to own who you are and the gifts you've been given.**

Chapter 9

Over the Hump Lesson #1

*"Live life on life's terms and conditions.
Ours will never be right, ready or good enough...
so we will never live. We will only survive."*
—Author Unknown

Congratulations! As the old advertisement says, "You've come a long way, baby." Right about now, you may be experiencing a bump in the road, or even a few bumps and a doughnut hole or two. This is actually a good thing. You're feeling it and not eating it. It means you are ready for the next step in your personal evolution. You are ready to get *over the hump*. Don't worry; you don't have to go it alone—I'll be there every step of the way. Think of me as your own personal coach, guru or angel. Imagine that I am writing this book just for you, to help you reveal the power that you have inside until you can find it on your own. Focus on what you want your health to be, rather than what you don't want it to be. By getting our health back, we get our power, brilliance, beauty and intelligence back. Let's get healthy, America, let's create a healthy world.

Commitment

Merrillism #19: "Continuity Plus Commitment Enhances Learning and Success."

This is a turning point. You have been preparing your mind, body and spirit to make the transition to a new, healthy you. You've dipped your big toe in the pool and discovered that the water is fine—now it's time to jump in! Take the plunge. You are suited up and ready for action; now it's time to commit. Does this mean you are going to be perfect from here on out, that you won't make mistakes, stumble and fall? No. It simply means that when you do fall, you will get right back up like the blow-up doll at the fair. It bounces quickly back up again. You may find that you need to stay on this chapter for a while. It may take some time to absorb the lessons and put them into action. That's okay. Remember, whatever is stopping you from achieving your health and fitness goals is what's stopping you in your life. How we do anything is how we do everything. Stay as long as you need to, and remember, quit from a point of achievement. What would your life be like with great health? Focus on that and not how hard it is and your pitfalls. Now, draw that into your life with action and the tools I've given you. Wow! What a healthy happy life that would be for you and me. Your health affects the world around you as well. Please know that your great health is not only for you, but for your loved ones, family, friends, community and the world. One of my favorite affirmations is, "As you give the gift of health to the world, the world will give the gift of health back to you." So radiate health, revel in it, and share your easy "flow and glow to go." Be bold, bright, brilliant, beautiful and your best. Do the best you can and forget the rest.

1. Commit to eating one raw meal a day, every day. Up until now, you have been slowly integrating raw foods into your diet—eating one or more raw dishes with each meal. Now it's time to put down the fork and pick up the pen. Start journaling your feelings every day. If you are feeling angry, sad, anxious, resentful, procrastinating, shameful, irritable, tired, bored, lonely or hungry just write it all out, instead of stuffing it all down. "Writing things right" takes it out of compulsivity, the going in circles in your mind, and directly into a straight line of clarity on the page. The hand is closest to the heart, so when you write, you come from the heart of your desires and thoughts. Get it out, shout it out, write it out, jog it out, sing it out, skate it out, knit it out, or dance it out, but get it out. We are stuffing it down, getting big and round, and the truth of why we are eating can never be found. Get to the truth of why you are destroying yourself with your fork, foods, and unhealthy lifestyle and habits. Remember what I said, "The truth shall set you free." But, first it will tick you off. It will. And it will set your *fat* free as well. Feel the frustration and do it anyway. Write down your commitment to this new way of eating and post it on your refrigerator, mirror, computer or car—somewhere you can see it every day. Tell people about your commitment; affirm it, so you can hold yourself accountable. For example, "I eat for need, not for greed," or "My body is keen, clean, lean and serene."

2. Commit to daily exercise. If you haven't already done so, it's time to start an exercise routine. You should aim for six days a week, but if you are currently at zero, you need to work up to it. Start with 30 minutes, three days a week and build from there. Make sure you check with your homeopathic MD or specialist of your choice before you begin, but as soon as you do—JUMP IN! There are a myriad of exercise options available to you; I encourage you to try them all and find things to do that you enjoy. Try taking a dance class—it doesn't matter what kind—hip-hop, ballroom, belly, tap, jazz, ballet, burlesque, or pole—as long as you do it, it counts. Completion is perfection. Fitness classes, either at a gym, private studio or local community college, are a wonderful way to get started. Exercising in a group is fun and you will meet like-minded individuals who share your commitment to health. If you prefer solitary exercise, try hiking, biking, inline skating, ice skating, yoga, weight lifting or brisk walking (I take "prayer walks" three times a week while praying and saying my affirmations and sun gazing). If you live where it snows, try cross-country or downhill skiing, snowboarding or ice skating. If you are fortunate enough to live near the ocean, start swimming, surfing, or walking in the sand. Join a gym—most have treadmills, stationary bikes, elliptical machines and stair-masters along with free weights and exercise machines. Lifting weights builds muscle and burns calories and helps combat osteoporosis. Exercise is a personal triumph over laziness and procrastination, as well as a wise use of time and is an investment in excellence. Increasing your exercise may decrease the risk of Alzheimer's disease as well as giving up alcohol and smoking. A lot of people fail to stick with an exercise program because of one thing—boredom. That's why I suggest you find activities you actually enjoy doing. You will also benefit from varying your routine; your body is very adaptable and gets used to doing the same old thing. I do a different exercise everyday so that I don't look like a dancer or a swimmer or a weight lifter or a yogi or a skater—I look like all of them. I have shape, strength, grace, fitness, flexibility, agility, mobility, stamina and aliveness in my physical body. Remember, you don't have to *always* enjoy it; you just have to do it. Doing it is easy once you get started. A workout (or playout, as I call it) is 25% perspiration and 75% determination. You will not only feel better, you will feel better about yourself.

Exercise makes you better today than you were yesterday. If you are too busy to work on your health and body, then you are too busy. How sad is that? Jack LaLanne once told me, "Fitness is the king, nutrition is the queen, and if you practice both you will live in the kingdom." According to Center of Disease Control, some of the leading causes of death in the US per year are:

- Heart disease—over 685,000
- Cancer—over 500,00
- Stroke—245,000
- Tobacco—approximately 400,000
- Unhealthy diet and lack of regular exercise—approximately 300,000
- Alcohol abuse—approximately 100,000
- Illegal drugs—approximately 20,000

Create an affirmation about your new attitude toward working out such as:

- *My body is fit, healthy, firm and beautiful!*
- *I love to exercise—and it shows!*
- *I exercise every day and every way!*
- *I now skate, dance, hike, walk, jog, and play effortlessly and easily.*
- *My body loves to soar and roar to the core with my exercise!*
- *I now spend as much time as possible in the good outdoors; nature heals me.*
- *I love myself exactly the way I am.*
- *I am enough, I have enough, I do enough, there is enough.*
- *When I play out regularly, my problems diminish and my confidence soars.*

I know you won't always feel like exercising and to that I say, so what? Join the club. I don't feel like it every day either, but I am committed. So I do it whether I feel like it our not. Comfort yourself with care, and care enough to give comfort. We teach others how to treat us. If we don't treat ourselves well, others and the world will not respond to us well. Don't be a supporting player in your life. Be the leading role in your life and you'll be able to lead and help others in their quest for health and happiness while you keep yours. I've learned that winners are the people who do what has to be done when it needs to be done. Winners do what losers won't. You will keep your health longer the more you give it away. Every person has the ability to transform their relationship with their health and their body, especially with the information and resources available to us in the world today. The time is ripe right now. Think of it like any other commitment; marriage, job, raising kids. I am sure there are some days you wake up, roll over and think about calling in sick to work or staying in bed and not dealing with getting the kids off to school, cleaning the house, making dinner for your family or taking that class. But you are committed, so you do it anyway. It's the same with your health. You exercise and eat right because you make a commitment to yourself. I believe that the promises you make to yourself should be at least as important as the promises you make to your spouse, your children, to your boss and your friends. Don't you?

3. Blend. Many people find the task of preparing food in a whole new way overwhelming at first. So I say, don't do it. At least not at first. While you are incorporating vegetarian, organic, raw foods into your diet, you may find the transition easier to make without the added pressure of learning new techniques and recipes in the kitchen. Don't worry, when you do get there, you will find that *un*cooking is significantly easier than cooking, but for now keep it simple. Let someone else do it if you want. You can buy prepared vegetarian, vegan and raw dishes at any natural or health food store. If you have a Whole Foods Market, or Mother's

Market in your town or if you live near Erewhon Natural Foods Market in Hollywood, California, I suggest shopping there. If you have a natural foods or farmer's market in your neighborhood, go shop there. You will find a plethora of already prepared, delicious vegetarian or vegan dishes that you can eat at home. These days, you can even find these items at your regular grocery store; just look for the label that says, "raw, certified organic" or "vegan." You can even hire raw/vegan/vegetarian chefs to deliver to your home for a day, a week or a month. If you prefer to eat out, look for organic, vegetarian, vegan and raw restaurants in your city. If you live in a large city like Los Angeles, San Francisco, New York, Atlanta, Chicago or Miami, you will find no shortage of restaurants that will cater to your every dietary need. Many cities even have eateries dedicated to the raw lifestyle. If you are fortunate to live near a raw restaurant, I encourage you to try it. You will be amazed at the variety and complexity of tasty dishes on the menu. Never be too shy to ask for a doggy bag either. You can even try takeout. Ask questions about the ingredients and duplicate your own versions at home. Create new plates with your mate. It's fun! If you live in a smaller town, you may have fewer options available to you, but you can usually ask your favorite restaurant to prepare a meat-free dish for you. You can get a salad anywhere in the world. Even fast food drive-thrus have them if you're really stuck.

It's so easy to pack a brown bag lunch. I usually take fruits and veggies, nuts, avocado and green leaves with me every day for lunch and/or dinner if I'm on the roll for many hours. No work's involved, I just grab, eat and go.

Read books on vegetarianism, veganism and raw foods. You'll get educated and inspired to find the courage, confidence and control to transition your behaviors towards a healthier lifestyle now. You may have to do a bit of research to find what you are looking for, so use the internet and talk to people. It may take a bit of extra effort on your part in the beginning, but later it will be effortless and easy. It's worth it. Anything worth doing is worth doing well.

4. Let go and let in. If you haven't already done so, choose one food to let go of today. Just one. This is important. Pick one food to say goodbye to and add something you like to replace it. This is not about deprivation and denial. It's about letting go and letting flow. Then, after you have successfully made the replacement, choose one more, and so on. This is called the transition process. For many people, eliminating foods from their diet is hard, so give yourself the best opportunity to succeed by going at it slowly. Remember, doing a little helps a lot. We all love to crunch and munch, which is why we eat chips, popcorn and crackers. Try fresh veggies instead. I love the crunch of cucumbers, red cabbage, broccoli, snow peas, radishes, zucchini, celery and lacinato kale. This crunch is better to me than any dry corn chip, which I would probably eat with salsa and guacamole and end up polishing off the entire bag. The water, oxygen and fiber in my crunch and munch of veggies has much more comfort than any cooked junk snack I used to eat. Try it. It's a great habit to get into. It replaces bread for me and it's a great tip and trick. When you eat bread, there is danger ahead. Stock your refrigerator with fresh, ripe, whole, raw, organic foods, fruits and veggies. They are nature's fast food and they give us fast energy. Like many people, I used to live for caffeine: my nectar of the gods was eight ounces of black, Cuban Bustelo espresso. Now, it's wheatgrass and green juice. I call it my Raw On The Roll Green Keen Lean Machine Energy Cocktail. (See my recipe in back of book.) The important thing is that you don't have to try to do everything all at once. You'll end up feeling deprived, cranky and more likely to overeat the foods you are trying to give up. Let go one by one, and you'll get it done. Eat slowly, walk slowly, talk slowly, and think quickly. Remember to chew your liquids and drink your solids.

Transitioning to a new, healthy lifestyle isn't always easy. Letting go of old, bad habits may bring up a lot of issues for you, but in order to fit in you've got to stand out. Please don't be afraid to be different and unique with what you eat and do. Take a stand for who you are and what you do. If you don't stand for something, you'll fall for anything. Be a pioneer and a leader in the health movement and your health will move in the direction you want it to move. You will find others following you and asking you for help, and your own health problems will slip away. When you fear less you fail less. Fear less, fail less, fear less, fall less. Or, you may be going along just fine, exercising, eating lots of veggies and—Boom! You suddenly have the urge to wolf down a double cheeseburger and chase it with a bottle of cola and a bag of Oreos®. Obviously, I don't recommend you do this, but if you do give in to your inner junkie by having a tantrum and eating a Chunky®, it's important to forgive yourself, bounce back, try again and move on. The darkest hour is only 60 minutes long. You can endure it, this craving will eventually pass. Forgiveness is part of compassionate eating, just like being a vegan and refraining from killing and eating animals is. This healthy lifestyle need never be a chore, it needs be your choice. You may have to do this deliberately at first, until it comes naturally. Dwelling on your transgression and punishing yourself will not move you further along the road of happy bliss. Once again seek progression, not perfection. Keep it fun and exciting every day.

The good news is, once you start getting over the hump, you're going to start feeling better. The better you feel, the more you do; and the more you do, the more you are able to do. And on and on until you achieve the goal you set out to achieve. Action breeds action, restores integrity and motivation. You will have more energy, your thoughts will become clearer and more focused, and your body will begin to change. Nothing motivates action like seeing results and feeling good. There is nothing quite like doing

something you didn't know you could do. You will feel more energized and experience more excitement about life. When you are
energized and excited about life every day, you are truly happy
and healthy. After a while, you won't miss the foods you thought
you couldn't live with out. You will love all the great feelings that
avoiding them brings about. What you don't eat, you don't crave.
I always tell myself, "When in doubt, leave it out. And when
in doubt, don't." I got over the hump, and now I'm picking up
speed and so will you, as long as you keep rolling and moving.

Raw Bites

- **Expand.** *Try something new today. A new sport, activity or meet new people. Do something you have always wanted to do or go somewhere you have always wanted to go. It can be a new restaurant, neighborhood, city or class to enroll in. Strike up a conversation with a stranger in line at the post office, visit a museum or fly a kite. It doesn't matter what you choose, as long as it's new to you. Stepping outside your comfort zone is an excellent way to stretch your imagination, gain education and inspiration and prove to yourself that you can do more than you know.*

- *Follow your Bliss, and where there were once walls the Universe will open doors.*

- *Let's get wicked, kick it, lick it, and get rid of the gunk and junk in the trunk.*

- *Let raw food open the gates of Heaven to the Fountain of Youth for you.*

- *The only time success comes before work is in the dictionary.*

- *It will work if you work at it.*

- *Be generous everyday to yourself and others.*

- *"He who finds himself loses his misery" —Matthew Arnold*

Chapter 10

Fake It
'Til You Make It

"If you only do what you know you can do—
you never do very much."
—Tom Krause

Think big. Act big. Be big. And, if the *big thing* you want to do doesn't scare you, it's not big enough. I started my inline skating school over twenty years ago with two things: the dream of bringing the grace and artistry of figure skating to the bike paths of Southern California and the belief that I had something unique, special and different to offer. I did not have any experience in running a business, or even the proven ability to teach others inline skating; I was a figure ice skater. I had absolutely no proof that I could do it, but I knew I had the talent to do it, and I believed in myself, so I decided to "fake it 'til I made it," until I made my dream a reality. I simply refused to believe that it was *not* possible. It never occurred to me that I *couldn't* do it. I knew that I had something to share, so I created a way to accomplish my dream. I acted "as if" I was a successful teacher with a booming business doing what I loved and helping others. It worked because it wasn't *about* me, it was *through* me. Today, I have successfully taught my program to thousands of students all over the world.

My clients range from young children to A-list celebrities, from absolute beginners to advanced skaters. I teach stars, starters and die harders. I also teach the physically challenged, as well as blind and disabled children and adults. As a young girl, I imagined myself dressed in a sparkly get-up, skating with the stars and champions, and today I do just that. I literally dreamt my life into action by acting "as if" I already had what I knew I wanted. In other words, I just had to do it, so I faked it until I made it come true.

"Fake it 'til you make it" was my mantra. In fact, it still is. When I am teaching my students to skate and when I teach health education, I say, "fake it 'til you make it." You see, if you fake it long enough, acting as if you are a confident, fluid skater or a person infused with radiant health and richness, it eventually becomes the truth. The key is to act your way into right thinking and behavior. You don't get self-esteem at the store. You can't buy it prepackaged or ready to wear, and you can't get it from others. You must create it. You must create doing esteemable things that will bring you self-esteem.

By acting "as if" you are healthy, beautiful, energetic, talented and enough, you will realize the truth—that you already are all of those things, and more. It's not enough to think it, you have to *be* it, *do* it, *share* it, *act* upon it and then you have it. And then a funny thing will happen; the Universe will rush to support you. The right people will magically appear to help you accomplish your goals. Everything will line up like the solar system. Synchronicity will be in your favor. You'll stumble upon the perfect book, or the perfect person at the perfect time, and that will help you get to the next level. The walls you used to bang in to will suddenly have doors that swing open at the precise moment you arrive. Some people call it "The Law of Attraction," "Good Luck," "Coincidence," synchronicity, miracles, magic or timing. Call it all of the above, I call it acting your way into right thinking and behavior. Draw it to you by who you are being and believing. The truth is, it doesn't matter what you call it, as long as you do it, it will work for you.

So, in your journey to becoming healthy and whole, create and be who you already are. Ask yourself, how would I be and behave if I had true, complete health? What action would I take right now? And then, take that action. This is key. You must act upon it. Thinking alone will not get you there. If you are thinking without acting, you will stay on the couch, procrastinat<u>ing</u>, wait<u>ing</u>, deny<u>ing</u> and delay<u>ing</u>; do<u>ing</u> the "ing" thing, which is noth<u>ing</u>. If you want to learn how to skate, you've got to put on your skates, stand up and push yourself forward. Maybe you want to become a raw fooder so you can look and feel great, have more energy and live life fully alive. Ask yourself, if I were a raw food vegan, how would I behave today? What would I eat? How would I feel? Then *be* and *do* as if you feel that and have it now. Fake it, don't forsake it. It's your life we're talking about here, so embellish, cherish and relish in it. The only way out is through it. The power that is within you will draw it to you. Look within to begin.

> *"Everybody should do at least two things each day*
> *that he hates to do, just for practice."*
> —William James

Raw Bites

- *Take Contrary Action. I understand that it's not always easy to dress up, show up and "just do it" with a smile on your face and a song in your heart. Sometimes you want to stomp your feet, flail your fists and shout, "I don't wanna!" Have your tantrum, that's okay. But do the thing anyway. Do something you don't want to do once a day. You can complain and moan about it, but do it anyway. I call it contrary action. It works miracles. Take things in increments. You don't have to become a raw fooder all at once. Eat meat once a week. Eat one raw meal a day. Do it the way you can do it, until you can do it the way you want to do it, but do it. Remember, you get where you want to go by staying in action, instead of detouring into destruction. When I complete a contrary action and see the results, I automatically feel better about myself. This is a food-free esteemable act; a reward for me, not like the rapid rewards my mother gave me. I love this exercise and money can't buy this one.*

- *When I eat raw, it's easy on me and I'm easy on you.*
- *Just pop the nuts, drink the grass, and snack on fruit. That's how you'll keep in shape and stay so cute.*
- *Count your joys instead of your tears. Count your courages instead of your fears.*
- *Misery and poor health are decisions you make. Choose great health.*

Section 2

First Course: Understanding

Chapter 11

Introduction: Planting the Seed

"The first step toward change is awareness.
The second step is acceptance."
—Nathaniel Branden

N ow that you are awake, aware, alive and alert it's time to get
to work and begin to understand how to sow the small seeds
of change that will eventually reap big rewards. Remember,
"Inch by inch it's a cinch, and yard by yard it's very hard," so we
will take it slow. If you can forgive yourself for your past mistakes
and accept yourself as you are now, then you have already taken the
first important step toward living your best, most fulfilling life.

I have found that, when you think you have lost yourself, you
are really just in the process of rediscovering the real you. In order
to find yourself, you have to lose yourself. Selflessness is the way
to health. This section is all about realizing the truth of where you
are—how your actions and mindset are affecting your health, your
spirit and your creativity—and how you can get to an extraordinary
place. As actress Shirley MacLaine says, "The only way to get the
fruit off the tree is to go out on a limb." The more you risk, the
more you succeed. I don't know more than you, I just know more
than I did, and through this lifestyle, you will too. Only you can

take responsibility for your health. It's time to wake up, get up, get rolling, get healthy, get fit, and get raw. Look at how you breathe, feel, act and experience your day. The simple truth is, you hold the key to your health and happiness in your hands. There is no ledge to know-ledge. You can become whatever you want to become, you can create your life however you want it to be. You only have to take that first, brave step toward continuing action, and the life you desire is yours.

> *"Do not die with your music still inside you."*
> —Author Unknown

It works if you want it, if you let it and if you work it. It's already working because you found this book. You found me and I found you. There is a saying that, when the student is ready the teacher appears and when the teacher is ready, the student appears. Please don't think less of yourself, think about yourself less. Everything begins and ends with you—*starting right now*. Let your heart's desire become on fire. Let's go from raw to awe, or from awe to raw.

> *"I once was lost but now am found, Was blind but now I see."*
> —lyrics from *Amazing Grace*

I once thought that the more you ate, the more you lived, when, in fact, eating less is living more. The truth is, I wasn't craving a full belly, I was craving a full life. The problem was, I didn't have the tools to create the life I wanted; the life I knew, deep down, I deserved and could create. I felt powerless, hopeless, worthless, lost, alone and blind. I didn't have anyone to point me in the right direction, so I stumbled along in the dark, grasping on to familiar objects, looking for landmarks and trying to avoid land mines while I found my own way. I kept going, putting one foot in front of the other and, eventually, I did find my way. By moving forward, persisting and having faith, I found people, places and things to help me along my journey. They were my beacons of light and gurus until I was strong enough to carry my own torch, be my own leader and follow my own intuition, inner guidance and desire. Now that I am able, I hope you will allow me to light *your* way. Not forever, but until you are strong enough to carry your own torch and love yourself back to health and fitness. Please allow me to teach you how to teach yourself, allow me to teach you to think on your own feet, be light on your feet and then be the light for someone else and teach others what you have learned. I said it, I meant it, and now I represent it. You can represent it too. Represent it in your life and in the lives of those around you who you love, inspire and encourage. Be an attraction, rather than a promotion with regard to your health, because as you give to the world, so the world will give back to you the gift of health and fitness. Great health is making time for you, taking time for friends and family, and giving time to others.

"Whatever we plant in our subconscious mind and nourish with repetition and emotion will one day become a reality."
—Earl Nightingale

I'm not afraid of hard work, or of a little sweat, but I believe that achieving one's goals really comes down to 90% inspiration and 10% perspiration. A lot of people think it's the other way around, but I believe that a little inspiration goes a long way. Let some of this seep into your heart, spirit and consciousness for a fleeting moment. If none of it works for you, if my story doesn't resonate with you, then give the book away. It may not be the beacon you are seekin'. But if even one line speaks to you in a calm clear voice that you recognize as truth, then let that mustard seed be planted. Then water it and let it grow and you will get that easy flow and glow to go, *for good*. Take some risks, take contrary action, think outside the box, get out of your comfort zone, find your blind spots, and find out what you don't know you don't know. It's all great food for thought. How you do anything is how you do everything. I'm suggesting that you please don't quit before the miracle.

Raw Bites

- *Think about, thank about, bring about.*
- *Get raw now. I just showed you how.*
- *Live a life that's uncut and uncooked, or be cooked.*
- *Disorder causes disease in the body, a lack of law and order.*
- *Raw food is Mother Nature's law, bringing order to the body, mind and spirit.*
- *Live in the raw Law and Order theme and you'll improve your self-esteem.*
- *Success is when opportunity meets readiness.*
- *Seize the moment.*
- *Say yes to life. Stay in action. Be where your feet are.*
- *Dress up and show up, and life will rush in to meet your every need.*
- *Fruit is raw, fast food. Fruit is a dessert.*

Chapter 12

Paralysis of Perfectionism

"It is better to do something imperfectly than nothing flawlessly."
—Robert Schuller

My 20's and 30's were dominated by the three "P's"—Perfectionism, Procrastination and Paralysis. I sometimes think that being a perfectionist is something I was born with, that it is imbedded in my DNA. As long as I can remember, I have been obsessed with the idea of being perfect. I tried to be the perfect daughter, the perfect student and the perfect performer with a perfect body, and it nearly turned me into the perfect nothing. I think one of the reasons I loved wearing my "getups" so much was because the sequins, feathers and rhinestones made me feel closer to my ideal. I wanted to be Ann Margaret, Peggy Fleming, Madonna, or the Virgin Mary, instead of just Debbie. In my mind, being Debbie from Yonkers, N.Y. was not good enough. Regular me was as far from perfect as one could get, and I wanted nothing to do with me.

When it came to skating, my obsession with being perfect was both a help and a hindrance. The athlete in me understood that I was going to have to pick myself up off the ice every time I failed to land a jump, but the perfectionist in me thought not landing a jump

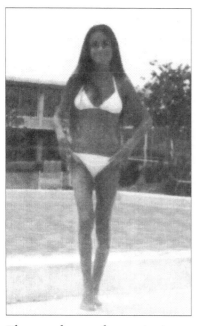

The second stage of my eating issues, I was either overweight or underweight, always trying to find the perfect weight. I let the worst in me sabotage the best in me, but that was then.

the first time and falling meant I was defective or inadequate. I also felt the need to have a perfect skater's body—with a flat chest, narrow hips and no bottom—like all the other kids. The problem was, they *were* kids. The skaters I was competing against were 8, 9 and 10 and I was 12-16. Well, like I said, I wanted to be like everyone else but myself. I felt as though it was not OK to be me, that I was supposed to be someone else. What a conundrum this was for a 12-year- old. I'm of Italian descent, and I developed curves and breasts at a pretty early age. Most people thought I had a cute figure, but all I could see was what I was *not*. So I tried dieting my way to perfection and I think you know how that turned out. Yes, I was thin, but I was also not well. (Thin is not always healthy.) Even as I began to evolve into becoming vegetarian, then macrobiotic, vegan and a raw vegan, I was afraid to mess up. I was dogmatic, rigid and myopic in my thinking, and eating—causing me to rebel a lot and beat myself up for my perceived failures. I made myself wrong with guilt and perfectionism, and that made it all worse.

Eventually I learned that perfectionism is a disorder and, if I didn't want to let it kill me, I'd have to let it go and give it up. I wasted a lot of years and tears paralyzed by my pathological need to be perfect. Don't get caught in the same trap. The truth is, you can't make a mistake. When you realize you made a mistake, take immediate steps to correct it. If you eat one more vegetable or one less processed food today than you ate yesterday, you have succeeded. There are no failures, only slow successes. Self-nurturing or well-being is being well and in good health. Yesterday is history and tomorrow is a mystery. Yesterday is gone and tomorrow has not arrived yet, all we have is the present, that's why they call it a gift. Forgive yourself and everyone else. Please don't hold grudges. It eats at you and you eat at it. In case you didn't know, life came without instructions. So seek education, enthusiasm, instruction and encouragement in your life. Forgive yourself and others. That's the road to health.

The Present

> *"What matters is to live in the present, live now,*
> *for every moment is now. It is your thoughts and*
> *acts of the moment that create your future."*
> —Sai Baba

Don't get me wrong, it's okay to strive for perfection. In fact, I encourage you to shoot for the moon, go for the gold and do the very best you can. If you don't make it, at least you'll wind up among the stars, on your way to becoming your own shining star. Just don't let the pursuit of perfection stop you from acting in the moment. Look, as I said before, I think being a perfectionist is a part of who I am—what has made the difference for me is not letting it stop me from being, living, completing and setting goals and acting in the moment. Perfectionism can be a dangerous trap, if you let it. So, don't. Don't wait for the perfect moment, perfect conditions or the perfect mate, job, house or body to begin living the life of your dreams. Don't wait for *x, y and z* to begin your journey to health. Be the change you want to have in your life now, because now is all we have. Redefine perfection for yourself. For me, the perfect moment is right now. This is the perfect moment to begin, to be happy, to be healthy and to be free. Now is the perfect time to say yes to life. Complete everything you start. Completion is perfection. Look folks, none of us knows how many more moments we have to spend and the best way to ensure we get more of them is to take care of our whole selves: mind, body and spirit everyday. None of us is getting out of here alive, and while we are still vertical and above ground, please enjoy everything you've got; be grateful, loving, forgiving, happy, generous, optimistic and healthy, and you will have the best life ever. The present is a gift; I suggest you open it. Be fulfilled and deserving, not full and unworthy. These suggestions are guidelines for progression, not perfection.

Merrillism 20#: "Do Your Best and Forget the Rest."

As you know by now, I am big on completion. I believe that it is important to finish what you start and as I have said many times before, only quit from a point of achievement. I have come to recognize that completion is perfection. Perfection is not performing perfectly—executing the perfect jump, writing the perfect sentence or eating the perfect foods. Perfection is, quite simply, dancing, writing, exercising, painting and eating as many good and eliminating as many bad foods as you can *right now, and completing it to the best of your ability*. The thing is, you don't have to do it right the first time, you just have to do it. You can always go back and fix your mistakes. The more you do, the more you are able to do, so just do it now. Do it now, do it over, do it differently, do it again later, but just do it.

That was a huge concept for me. I thought everything had to be done perfectly right the first time, and that I only got one shot. That may have been true when I was a competitive figure skater; you get one time in a four-minute routine to prove yourself perfect and wait for the perfect score of 10. But my life is not a figure skating competition—and I'm not going out for the Olympic Gold now—it's my life. No one is scoring me but me. I had to train myself to get off my case, lighten up in all areas of my life, and wear life loosely. I learned to play the game of life and enjoy the playing just for play. This is a very loving tool, and it really works, so try it now. I didn't learn it until late in life. Practice makes progress and I'm satisfied with progress today. I used to use perfectionism as an excuse—if I couldn't do it perfectly the first time, I didn't want to do it all. Well, I can tell you, as a skater, that doesn't work very well. You have to attempt a lot of jumps and suffer a lot of falls to make your first good one. If you know baseball, then you know that the greatest hitters of all time, on average, fail seven out of ten times at bat. But you also know that it's the three hits they did make that count. I can guess that the great players didn't always wait for the perfect pitch to hit the ball. So why should you?

Are you paralyzed by perfection? Do you put things off, waiting for conditions to be just right before you begin a new project? If you find yourself waiting for the stars to align, to get to your goal weight, or to get to be an expert at something before you start something new (or finish something old), you might be a perfectionist. It's like when people call me for a skating lesson and say they want to get proficient at skating first, before they come for the lesson. (How ridiculous! Let someone coach you, accept the help.) So, quit it already! Be willing to accept help and guidance. I know, easier said than done but it is possible. Break the cycle. Take a step. I don't even care if it's in the right direction—you can take a step sideways, cross ways or even backwards (just like skating) if you want, just take the step. Go in the direction you want to go. Direction is more important than speed. Don't let prideful perfectionism and artistic avoidance stop you in your creativity or your health. Do it imperfectly, it's such a relief to know that!

I want you to try something right now. Think of something

you've wanted to do, or that you need to do, or think you should do, but have been putting off. You know, that "thing" that you want to accomplish but you have been waiting for the right time, the right amount of money to come in, the perfect person to do it with, the right season or a sign from the Universe to do it. It can be large or small—a business call you've been putting off, cleaning the closet, starting an exercise regime, signing up for a class, seeing a nutritionist, preparing or shopping for a new (raw) dish—whatever. Got it? Good. This is the right time, the weather is fine and you've received the sign you've been waiting for (this book and this knowledge) so go do it! Right now. I believe how you do anything is how you do everything. Put the book down, and take action. Look up the phone number and make the call, open the closet door and start cleaning, go for a walk, do sit ups and lunges, open your refrigerator, sharpen your knives, buy the juicer. *It's time.* Start your raw on the roll and get in control. The good news is that you only have to do it for five minutes. If you want to do more, great, but you only have to commit to five minutes. Now go ahead and "bookend it" by calling someone right now and telling them what you are about to do. Then call them again when you finish it. (We'll talk more about this later but for now, just make the call!) Ready, set, go! You can't do right wrong and you can't do wrong right. Whatever you think the reason is why you can't do it, it's probably just fear—and it's not age, it's rust. So put the book down and come back when you are done.

Now, don't you feel better? Did you do it perfectly? Probably not. Guess what? It doesn't matter. What matters is that you stepped up to the plate and took a swing. It doesn't really matter if you whiffed it and missed the ball completely or if you hit a home run—either way, you did it. Congratulations. Now don't you feel better about yourself? You're now building self-esteem, confidence, dignity and momentum. Thank you for accepting my support. I believe in you. Now you believe in you, too.

Raw Bites

- *Feel the Fear. I have discovered that perfectionism is based in fear—fear of not looking good, fear of failure, of being ridiculed or shamed, fear of doing it wrong, fear of NO, fear of inadequacy. I love the title of one of my favorite books by Susan Jeffers,* Feel The Fear And Do It Anyway. *With the insights I gained from reading that book, I discovered that the best way to learn how to do a task I am afraid of doing is to just do it. By showing up and attempting it, it allowed me to discover, "Wow, that wasn't so scary after all." The fear of fear is more frightening than the activity or task itself. Once I got that, I was able to show up for many, many things in my life that I had been putting off because I was fearful of going through the fear and the feeling of fear and failure. But the only way out is through it. It's that ripple effect again. The more you do, the more you're able to do. I know I say this a lot, but it's important: "Don't deny it 'til you try it and apply it." Find that raw glow and flow to go. Bring the heart and the body will follow. Bring the body and the mind will follow.*

- *So do it imperfectly. Pick something, anything, you have been putting off and imagine doing it completely wrong. Imagine that, as you do it, everything that can possibly go wrong, does. Really get into it. Be specific, go into detail and don't leave anything out. Take it to the absolute extreme and visualize what's the worst that can happen? Can you live with that? If it helps you, write it down. I call it "horribilizing the experience." Writing things right. Now, stop. Take a breath. And do it anyway.*

- **When you lose, don't lose the lesson.**

- *Disease, disorder and sickness are markers for a deeper problem. Look within and you will win.*
- *Obstacles birth opportunities.*
- *Fear is false evidence appearing real.*
- *Prior proper planning prevents poor performance and problems.*

Chapter 13

Your Journey, Not Mine

*"The best day of your life is the one in which you decide
your life is your own. No apologies or excuses. No one to lean on,
rely on, or blame. The gift is yours—it is an amazing journey—
and you alone are responsible for the quality of it.
This is the day your life really begins."*
—Bob Moawad

Merrillism #21:
"Failure Is Fertilizer for Success."

I love the expression, "It's the journey, not the destination." Sure, it's a cliché but it also happens to be true, if a bit incomplete. In my version, the saying goes, "It's *your* journey and the destination may change." I share the story of my personal journey, not to tell you the road you *should* take, but to give you a map—filled with infinite possibilities. My own road has been bumpy at times, with lots of ditches, potholes and cracked ice. However, just as often, the ride has been as smooth as a cucumber, with long stretches of vast ocean, rolling hills and hairpin turns to keep me on my toes. My goal in writing this book is to help you avoid the detours so you can hit the highway at full speed—top down, hair blowing in the wind, music on full blast, singing at the top of your voice. I'm hoping to save you time, and help

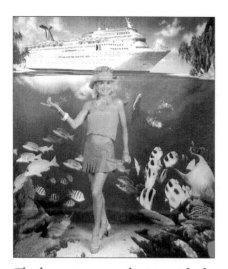

The longest journey begins with the first step. It's time to start your treasure map, and your journey. It's time to find out what you're really made of, so Bon Voyage, I'll see you on the rawkin' raw road of happy bliss!

you avoid pitfalls that I have encountered. I have taken this path before you, so you can bypass the detours to destruction and obstruction that I took. Take the highway with miles of smiles. While editing this book, I realized that I was forgetting to do some of the things I am telling you to do, and it reminded me to walk my talk again. If you think I am helping you with this book, well then, yes, I am, and you are helping *me*. So, I ask you again, please help others by sharing your own journey and staying in action. This allows you to keep your integrity, motivation and to stay on that rawkin' raw road of happy bliss.

Merrillism #22: "Share Everything You Know with Others; You Can't Keep it Until You Give it Away."

I marvel at where my journey has taken me; I am enjoying this stretch of highway and look forward to the road ahead, knowing it will lead me exactly where I need to be, at exactly the right time. When I was young, my dream was to be an Olympic medalist—to stand on the center block, proudly wearing the gold and singing the National Anthem as my Mom and Dad looked on, beaming with pride. For me, that was the ultimate validation, my way of proving to the world (and myself) that I was worthy of love, acceptance, adulation and that I was somebody. I tried so hard to make that dream come true—by being the perfect figure skater—so that my parents, my teachers and my coaches would be proud and look good. I wanted them to sit up and take notice, and give me what I could not give myself—love, acceptance, validation and admiration. Ultimately, my attempts to mold myself into what I thought others wanted me to be failed. All that driving and striving for perfection led to injuries and ill health. What I didn't realize at the time was that, as Mick Jagger says, "You can't always get what you want, but if you try sometimes, you might find you get what you need." I really needed to love myself in order to nourish and find myself. Raw foods help me do that. That's why I tell everyone, eating raw helps me go from raw to richness and from raw to awe. That's what the raw lifestyle has done for me. It was an inside job, not an outside destination.

My competitive skating career may have been sidelined, but it was the fork in the road that eventually led me to my true heart's desire. I combined my athletic ability with my dancing and acting skills, and turned myself into a performer—working in professional ice shows all over the world, performing on Broadway in *The Marriage of Figaro* with Christopher Reeves, and finally landing in Los Angeles, and working in television and film; teaching Steve Martin to skate for the movie *L.A. Story*, (with a skating role of my own in the film). For me, being a performer has led to a much richer and more fulfilling life than I could have ever imagined—and that's

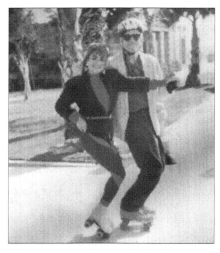

Here I am skating in L.A. Story, *and teaching Steve to skate for the movie. What a great athlete, actor and human being Steve Martin is.*

coming from someone with a big imagination! As Einstein said, "Imagination is everything. It is the preview of life's coming attractions." (By the way, Einstein was a vegetarian.) Eventually my dream expanded and I began to teach skating and health education, which has been a remarkable, uplifting gift in my life. I am able to impart my knowledge of skating with the love and understanding I wish I had received when I was learning. I have triumphed over my painful past by offering my students empathy, patience, acceptance, fun, motivation and inspiration, along with instruction. I didn't know it when I was dreaming of the gold, but those were the things I needed myself as a competitive figure skater (and as a daughter), and did not receive.

For me, right now is the most exciting time in my life because my career path and my health path have come together to form one big beautiful open road—lined with green grass and tall, fruit bearing trees. My dream of living a healthy, energetic, spiritual, creative, integrated life has been realized in the most wonderful way and it keeps opening up abundantly and with that, my goal has once again expanded. I have been fortunate to have had the opportunity to introduce my rawsome lifestyle to the world, my students, my clients, friends, family, and fellow enthusiasts. I run a successful skating school in Santa Monica, teaching 1000's of students from all over the world, and that experience led me to produce a wonderful DVD, *Learn To In-Line Skate to Look and Feel Great*, which reached even more people. And now, with this book, I hope to share with an even larger audience. By finally allowing true, complete health into my life, I am able to share it with the world in work that is so rewarding and fun. I had to treat the disorder of not loving myself in order to cause wellness. I had to love myself back to health, not the other way around. It's the ripple effect—I am nurturing the world back to health and fitness, radiating the raw truth from myself directly to you, in ever expanding three turns and figure eights. I believe that the opportunity to share what you know is true divinity and purpose, and the surest path to spiritual growth and health. Knowledge is power. Clarity is powerful. Action is excellence. Keep the law of attraction alive with regard to your health—be health, do health, and you will have health. Share your health with others and let it be contagious. Share the message, not the mess.

"When we are sure that we are on the right road there is no need to plan our journey too far ahead. No need to burden ourselves with doubts and fears as to the obstacles that may bar our progress. We cannot take more than one step at a time."
—Orison Swett Marden

So, that is my journey. What is *yours*? And, if you don't know, how do you discover it? The answer is, you already have. By simply picking up this book and putting into practice the lessons you have learned so far, you have started rolling on down the road of happy bliss. I encourage you to continue your journey by remaining open to what the world is offering you: whether it is this book, or other books that speak to you, a course, a teacher, or simply a person you admire, you are entitled to receive the gift. By opening your heart and mind to new information, you will continue to grow. Be Honest, Open and Willing. That is the "HOW" of it. We do not need to know the "why" of it. Remember, "why-ing is dying." By getting our health back, we get our power, brilliance, beauty and intelligence back.

Merrillism #23: "Stop Doing the Things that Make You Sick, and Start Doing the Things that Make You Better."

The important thing to remember is that you must honor your own uniqueness and do what is right for you. If what you learn from me and find that applying the principles outlined in this book enrich your life, great! I will have accomplished what I set out to do. After trying and applying what you have learned, you find that it's not your thing, that's fine too. Take what you like and what works for you, and leave the rest or save it for later or when you are ready. Remember, it's *your* journey, it's *your* life and only *you* can decide what is best for you. All health is an inside job. The foods you eat affect the moods you greet. As Socrates once said, "An unexamined life is a life not worth living." Uncover, discover, discard and recover your health and life now!

Merrillism #24: Follow Your Heart's Desire and You Will Be on Fire."

Goethe once said, "Until one is committed, there is hesitancy, the chance to draw back, always ineffectiveness concerning all acts of initiative and creation. There is one elementary truth, the ignorance of which kills countless ideas and splendid plans: that the moment one defiantly commits oneself, then providence moves too. All sorts of things occur to help one that would never otherwise have occurred. A whole stream of events issues from the decision raising in one's favor all manner of unforeseen events, meetings and material assistance which no one could have dreamed would have come their way."

I have also learned a deep respect for one of **Goethe's couplets:** Whatever you can do or dream you can, begin it. Boldness has genius, power and magic in it.

Begin it now!

Raw Bites

- **Remember your beauty.** *We are all perfect just the way we are. If you have forgotten, take time out to remember this truth. Love, honor and celebrate yourself. Life can sometimes be a drag, so dress it up. Strut your stuff. Shake it 'til you break it, fake it 'til you make it and show me what your momma gave you.*

- **Accept yourself and bless others for being different.** *We are not all the same. Accept that fact and you will be 100% happier. I guarantee it. Look for ways to express your uniqueness and bless and acknowledge the uniqueness of others.*

- **These are the rules to never lose with your health:**

  - *Express yourself creatively and sensually in your work, your fitness and your fun. (Lack of expression equals depression.)*
  - *Believe in and spend time with a higher force everyday.*
  - *Spend time in the <u>G</u>ood <u>O</u>ut <u>D</u>oors = GOD*
  - *Exercise at least 30–60 minutes a day, everyday doing something you love that makes your heart sing. Not exercising is not an option.*
  - *Have fun and laugh everyday. Fun is limitless. Be more fun. Fun is health.*
  - *Slow down and live. You're not livin' if you're driven.*
  - *Surround yourself with loving, conscious, committed, healthy people.*
  - *To be perfectly satisfied and mentally poised, eat more of a plant based diet of fresh, ripe, whole, raw, organic fruits, vegetables, sprouted nuts, sprouted seeds and sprouted grains.*
  - *If you don't believe in miracles, come and be one.*

Chapter 14

Standard American Diet = Sad American Diet

"Trust yourself. You know more than you think you do."
—Benjamin Spock

The Standard American Diet is often referred to by its acronym, S.A.D. The SAD Diet and the pun, while unintended, is right on target. Although there are many deficiencies in the Standard American Diet, it's mainly what we are not eating (fruits and vegetables) that is killing us. Change your diet from SAD to GLAD, a diet rich in fresh, ripe, whole, raw, organic foods. Americans eat an excess of meat, fish, dairy, fat, sugar, and refined, processed foods, and not enough fruits, vegetables, nuts and seeds. Somewhere along the way, we stopped eating a diet consisting of natural foods and began loading up on CRAP (Cola/Cooked Food, Refined Foods, Alcohol/Aspirin, Preservatives/Processed Foods) instead. When the body adapts to the consumption of CRAP and gets used to overeating, it loses its built-in alarm system that tells the brain when to stop, which eventually causes food allergies, overeating and weight gain. The key is to stop *before* addictions and allergies set in. More people die in the kitchen than any other room in the house. My mother died of a stroke in the kitchen cooking organic chicken for the dog. The average American diet consists of less than 20% fresh, raw fruits, vegetables, sprouted nuts, seeds, grains and legumes—which means that over 80% of what we eat is cooked, processed foods that are high in meat, protein, fat, cholesterol, chemical and disease. These dietary imbalances are thought to cause, in full or in part, a plethora of diseases and disorders. All disease needs detoxification or it is a form of deficiency. According to the Surgeon General's 1988 report, "Dietary excesses or imbalances also contribute to other problems such as high blood pressure, obesity, dental diseases, osteoporosis and gastrointestinal disease, heart disease, diabetes and cancer. Together, these diet related conditions inflict a substantial burden of illness on Americans." The truly sad part is, not a lot has changed in twenty years. We are still a country that eats fast food, junk food and snack food at an alarming rate, and in gigantic proportions. We are becoming more unhealthy and bigger with each passing year and something has got to give. We are junk food hope fiends. We spend our days hoping and wishing we won't be affected by the damage we are doing to ourselves. But hoping and wishing never gets us anywhere. We're stuffing it down, getting bigger and round and the truth of why we are eating can never be found. We need to start letting go of old behaviors and start moving towards new ones. Instead of eating, try talking, walking, writing, mediating, doing yoga, breathing (oxygen is one of the best foods in life and it's right under your nose. It also fills you up.) Close your mouth and open your heart. Zip the lips and narrow the hips.

Merrillism #25: "Eat More Raw. That's Mother Nature's Law."

Raw foods are foods for life, foods for eternal life—and a gift of global goodness. I tell all my clients, when you are in the supermarket and are wondering whether or not to toss something in your cart remember the slogan, "When in doubt, leave it out." When in doubt, don't. I always apply this and it works. It immediately eliminates options I don't really need and helps me circumvent my addiction to CRAP food or raw junk food. The only aisle I'll ever walk down, at this stage of my life, is the fruit and vegetable aisle. Tell yourself you can have it tomorrow, then tomorrow comes and you won't want it, you will have overcome the craving. Another one to remember is, "What nature did not create, and the spirit has forgotten, man need not eat, for it is rotten." I live by this rule and it is my favorite tool. Vitamins are not food; they are used for gaps in the diet, not substitutes. Real food is the best thing you can do for your body. Eat more quality foods and you will eat less. Raw fruits and vegetables are the best snacks and they give you your rawsome, awesome energy back. Remember, disease is found in a non-oxygenated environment. Raw fruits, veggies, sprouted nuts and seeds create oxygen, enzymes and water for the body. Oxygen is a key factor in health, longevity, and preventing disease.

American cuisine has devolved from the simple preparation of perfect, whole foods containing all the nutrients needed to maintain good health to a diet consisting primarily of foods that are refined, processed, preserved and so thoroughly cooked that the finished product barely resembles anything found in nature. We are literally cooking our food to death, depleting it of vital minerals, vitamins and nutrients. Cooking, processing and pasteurizing food also destroys certain enzymes, which are essential components of sound health. Dead food creates dead energy and contributes to death and disease. Live food creates live energy and strengthens the life force and contributes to life. I am choosing life, what are you choosing? In his book, *Enzyme Nutrition*, Dr. Edward Howel explains, "I attest that the kitchen stove and its big brothers, the heat-treatment machinery in food factories, are responsible for destroying a whole category of food elements, namely the heat-sensitive, exogenous food enzymes. These nutritional supplements have always provided our endogenous (internal) enzymes with the enzymes reinforcements needed to check the disease-making process." I say the Bunsen burner was the culprit. In order to get the most nutritional bang for the buck, most foods are best consumed raw—as Mother Nature intended. The food is not devoid of enzymes, oxygen, water, vitamins and minerals that the body needs for well-being. Yet, despite the mountain of evidence to the contrary, we continue to cook, process and refine a large portion of the food we eat. We are a nation of anxious individuals, and we eat out of stress, and we eat out of boxes, bags, cans and jars—and it shows. Why do we continue to eat in a way that is so clearly detrimental to our health? Whether it is fettuccine Alfredo or Uncle Alfredo, Aunt Barbie or shrimp on the barbie, it's all cholesterol, fat, flesh, disease, poisons and it's making us fatter, angrier and sicker. To get rid of middle age spread, start by giving up bread, because with bread there is always danger ahead. Then move on from there. Like I said before, start with small, achievable goals without rigidity and self-blame. Rigid thoughts equal rigid beliefs. Less rigidity will bring more consistency for you with your health and well-being. It will give you longevity and vitality with your food plan achievement.

The truth is, the "health" industry doesn't want you to get healthy. And why should they? If you were to improve and take responsibility for your own health by becoming a more raw, natural being, then where would *they* be? Consider the pharmaceutical industry, for example—a multi billion-dollar business that *is* in business because of your ill health. Be your own doctor. You still have 100% of your time left. You are still here, alive and vital. Change your behavior towards a healthier lifestyle now, with this *Raw on the Roll Success System*. Think about it. If everyone simply cut the CRAP out of their diets and started to eat more raw fruits, vegetables and plants while moving their bodies for an hour each day, being creative and having a spiritual base, we would, as a world, collectively begin to heal—therefore eliminating the need for many of the drugs, diet pills, nutrition bars, energy drinks, mood elevators, sleep inducers, pain killers, cooked vitamins and nutritional supplements that make up the "health" industry. Perhaps we would be a peaceful, happy nation without wars if we were all happy, healthy, abundant and free. What would we have to fight over? Corporations have a lot invested in keeping us fat, unhappy and sick. How else are they going to sell all those pills for diet, depression, anxiety, and all that ails us? If you cannot pronounce it, don't eat it or take it. After all, it's not how you die; it's how you live. The raw lifestyle allows you to live pain-free, pill-free, and disease-free. Let yourself heal and be real, and you will end up being grateful, not hateful, happy, healthy and blissful.

I often say that we should call *health* insurance what it really is, *drug* insurance. Paying your monthly premiums doesn't insure that you will become (or stay) healthy; it only kicks in when you are sick—so you can pay to see the doctor who will undoubtedly send you away with a prescription that may or may not clear up your ailment, and may even require a second prescription to treat the side effects caused by the first. It's a merry-go-round of pill popping, poking, probing and cutting that never ends. You're paying for drugs that may never help you, and may hurt you in the long run. The raw lifestyle is like a certificate of deposit (CD); if you pull out too soon, you lose interest and pay a penalty. Stay on the *Raw on the Roll Success System* no matter what it takes. It works if you let it. Everyone is looking for a quick fix, a miracle drug to take away the pain, and get there faster and the drug companies are happy to oblige. They're lining their pockets with your weakness, your disorder, and your pain. Look at the recent drug overdoses by famous celebrities today. We now have a license to kill ourselves legally. This infuriates and saddens me very much.

Don't misunderstand, I'm not criticizing doctors; I love doctors! I have family members who are in the medical profession, and I was even in love with a doctor once. I realize their importance, and I know there are some diseases that only drugs can cure. While I believe that wheatgrass juice has remarkable healing properties, it's the nectar of the gods for me, I know that drinking it won't set a broken bone. I believe in seeing a doctor when it's absolutely necessary. I'm just here to offer an alternative, a way to jump off the merry-go-round, and prevent illness in the first place. As I said before, be your own doctor. If you are healthy, you don't need to see a doctor. They are overworked, and need to save their time for those who are really sick. I am suggesting you stop looking for the easy road—stop using drugs to solve your sickness—and empower yourself with real health. Health is wealth. You are the solution to your ailments, and through eating a plant-based diet, getting more exercise, reclaiming your creativity and spirituality, you can achieve it. Create, relate, mate and don't hesitate. The Universe loves and responds to now. Now is all we have. The power is in the now.

I find it the concept of "Whole Food Signatures" fascinating. The concept is based on the assumption that many whole foods have a shape or pattern that resembles a body organ of physiological function, and that this shape or pattern indicates the organ which will receive the most benefit upon consumption. Here is just a short list of examples of Whole Food Signatures:

- A *Tomato* has four chambers and is red. The heart is red and has four chambers. All of the research shows tomatoes are indeed pure heart and blood food.
- *Figs* are full of seeds and hang in twos when they grow. nutrients in figs increase both motility and counts of male sperm.
- *Sweet Potatoes* are shaped like the pancreas and actually balance the glycemic index of diabetes.

- *Olives* provide nutrients to support the function of the ovaries.
- *Grapefruits, oranges and other citrus fruits* are shaped like the female mammary glands and actually assist the movement of lymph in and out of the breasts to keep them healthy.
- *Onions* look like body cells. Today's research shows that onions help clear waste materials from all of the body cells. They even produce tears which wash the epithelial layers of the eyes.
- *Kidney Beans* actually heal and help maintain kidney function and yes, they look exactly like human kidneys.
- *Celery, Bok Choy, Rhubarb* resemble bones. These foods specifically target bone strength. Bones are 23% sodium and these foods are 23% sodium. If you don't have enough sodium in your diet the body pulls it from the bones, making them weak. These foods replenish the skeletal needs of the body.
- *Eggplant, Avocados and Pears* target the health and function of the womb and cervix. Today's research shows that when a woman eats one avocado a week, it balances hormones, sheds unwanted birth weight and prevents cervical cancers.

"People are dying because they are sick of living."

As I have said before, I haven't been sick in over 28 years—not even with a common cold. And it's not because I'm lucky or live in a bubble. Quite the contrary, I work with the public and kids every day, so there is no question that I am exposed to the same germs and viruses that you are. I have learned if you don't change your taste buds, habits and addictions, it will cost you your health; it did me. We are killing ourselves with our forks. Be at the cause of your actions and thoughts, and you will have a positive effect on your health now. Excess and ill health in children and teens is life threatening and can be reversed by consuming raw foods now. Excess and ill health for middle-aged people can shorten life and can be delayed by consuming raw foods now. Excess and ill health for seniors may have already set in, but consuming raw foods can contribute to a greater quality of life. The fact is, beginning to live the raw lifestyle in our youth and adulthood will help us be healthier seniors, with quality, mobility and longevity of life, with all our faculties in working order. Not planning is planning to fail. Plan your life by planning your meals, exercise, spiritual time, and creative time every day. Prioritize your priorities. We all know the saying, "You got to be in it to win it." We are responsible for what we do no matter what we feel.

Being sick isn't always about physical illness. Sick doesn't have to mean cancer. It can also mean being miserable, unhappy, tired, depressed, moody, irritable, overworked, under-loved, sleep deprived, constipated, creatively blocked, stagnated, sexually repressed, stifled, shut down and living in avoidance and denial. Practicing the same behavior over and over again and staying stuck, resentful, unhappy and unhealthy (emotionally and spiritually) can be causing your disorder and sickness. So, if you're wondering how you got sick, just take it backward. Look at your life backwards, live life forwards and you'll figure it all out. If you look, you will see that your thoughts, your behaviors, your actions, your eating, your lack of spiritual life, and your lack of creativity is how you got these setbacks. Lack of expression equals depression. It didn't just jump into your body one day. It gets created year after year—with stinking thinking, unhealthy eating, lack of exercise, lack of expression, and connection to a higher force. For me, it was fear that weakened my spirit and my body. Add to that all the cooked and processed food, prescription as well as recreational drugs, alcohol, nicotine, overworking, over-exercising and overspending, and I was heading downstream fast. When you absorb a lot of junk you have junk thoughts and actions. The less junk that goes in you, the less junk ends up in your trunk and less in the brain to drain. For me, the key to great health is living the raw lifestyle. And if you begin to transition from the SAD American Diet, which is full of CRAP, to the GLAD American diet of fresh ripe, whole, raw, organic fruits and vegetables, sprouted nuts, seeds and grains, you will begin to heal, deal and feel great. Simplify your diet, simplify your life. And you will begin to find clutter leaving you in all areas of your life.

Merrillism #26: "Let's Get Wicked and Kick it. Kick the CRAP Habit Now."

No one holds the key to change, the key to your happiness and health, but you. Nothing feels worse than a belly full of processed junk food and a brain full of knowledge—unless you decide to make yourself feel better by acting on that knowledge. Remember there is no ledge to knowledge. Once you know how to eat healthy and you begin to follow that healthier lifestyle, it's almost impossible to eat wrong and bad, because you know there is a real solution, and the guilt of ignoring the truth will eat at you, and you will eat at it. Once you know there is a solution, it's hard to practice the same old problematic behavior. Be humble, admit defeat, and get back on your feet. Ask for help, get strong, and out of your weaknesses you will gain strength. Are you eating at it or is it eating you? Please don't hold grudges—they also eat at you and you at them. Forgive to live. Eating junk food will not bring you the joy that it used to, because now you know there is an alternative solution that does work. You can't go back and use the old excuses and reasons anymore. Once I licked the junk food habit, I discovered that going backwards was almost impossible because eating a lot of sugar can do a lot of damage for me. My system is so clean that if I overload with unhealthy foods, I feel the negative effects much more intensely. So if you are fed up, messed up, shut up, and have *given* up, then get up, get fit, get rolling and get more raw now. Use that guilt and remorse to propel yourself forward and help you as you transition to a healthier lifestyle. It is time to stop living in denial and lying to yourself about the state of your health, and start getting real so you can begin to heal. See yourself living in health and in reality and you will be healthier. The highest frequency you can be on is love and health. When you are in health, you are in love. When you are in love you are in health. If you live this lifestyle, you will begin to finally understand what it is you have been missing—your vitality, spirit, energy, love and creativity will return and your life will change. You will find the self you lost. All you have to do is start. Try this affirmation today: *My health is phenomenal—I am healthy now.* You will be because you say so. Get your emotions out. Shout it out, write it out, sing it out, dance it out, talk it out, skate it out, jog it out, garden it out, yoga it out, golf it out, but get them out. Getting them out will not allow you to eat them down. Be interested in feeling good, not just looking good. As I say all the time, "Fear less fail less, fear less fall less," or "Feel the fear and do it anyway." Remember, FEAR stands for "Forget Everything And Run," and you've already done that. It's time to do things differently now. Let your fear knock at the door and faith will answer. Just knock and it will open. Start by eating better today than you did yesterday and by moving your body more today than you did the day before and you will begin to feel better. Then you will start to create the life you know you deserve today. How much lower do you want to go with your health? Your bottom may be six feet under! Go there in your mind and you will go there in the body. We are living in the most powerful time the world has ever seen. Everything is at our fingertips. We will now see the impossible become the possible. Remember to have fun doing this because the more fun you have, the more your health works. There is no thrill quite like doing something you didn't know you could do or would do if you could. Get healthy now just for the health of it. *You deserve it.*

Sidebar to the Rawbar

Become a label reader. Be on the lookout for "oses" (sugars) and the "cides" (chemicals). Many prepackaged, processed foods are loaded with sugar. Make sure sugar is at least fifth or lower on the list of ingredients—it may be disguised as dextrose, sucrose, lactose, fructose, maltodextrin, or barley malt but it's all sugar. Start reading labels and you'll find it in the most surprising places. I used to eat melba toast and graham crackers because they were considered "healthy" diet foods, but they were loaded with salt and sugar and my addiction to the sweet stuff wouldn't let me stop at just a few—I'd eat the whole box. I also say, "Eat no pesticides, vermicides, fungicides, herbicides and insecticides. They all equal suicide!" Now, I'm not saying that they will actually kill you, but they will slow you down. Over time, the toxicity builds up in your system and leaves you feeling sluggish, tired with poor bowel elimination, foggy thinking and slothfulness, to just name a few. So become a health detective, food police and read the labels. The life you save be your own. Eat more raw now while I am showing you how.

Raw Bites

- *Drink green cereal juices (I love wheatgrass), or algae supplements once a day. (For algae, I like E3Live® AFA blue-green algae, which provides 64 easily absorbed vitamins, minerals and enzymes and is loaded with chlorophyll.) Eating raw green living foods such as cereal grasses, chlorella, or blue-green algae provide an abundance of essential minerals, chlorophyll, B12, and anti-aging properties for the body, which helps conquer disease. My snack to the future is drinking two ounces of wheatgrass a day. I've been doing it for the past 28 years to keep sickness away, and I haven't had a cold, flu, virus or allergy in 28 years. Green is clean.*

- *Get rid of cooked, processed "nutritional" bars; they are loaded with sugar and fat. Try my* Raw on the Roll Energy Balls *or* Crunchy Cracklin' Crackers *instead.*
- *Incorporate these helpful, healthy tips in your day:*
  - ◆ *Eating animals is not an option. Please don't make your body a graveyard for dead animals.*
  - ◆ *Pledge to go veg.*
  - ◆ *Raw vegan food is your parachute for jumping into the world of well-being, fitness and vitality.*
  - ◆ *It's not age, it's rust. Stay active and in action.*
- *Don't be a helicopter healer with your health, hovering over every mistake you make. Be easy on yourself and let it happen like water flowing through your hand. It will flow effortlessly and easily if you don't try and hold onto it (you can't hold onto water).*
- *Once you are in action, know that it's all being done. Trust in the Universe to assist you.*
- *Meditate on your goals, and visions for your health.*
- *"Silence nourishes hope."*
- *Be a monument of the person you aspire to be like.*
- *Be a work in progress now.*
- *Nobility is humility and fertility for well-being.*
- *In the early 1800's, the average person consumed approximately 12 pounds per year of sugar. As of 2006, Americans ate and drank a whooping 180 pounds of sugar. (Get the Sugar Out by Ann Louise Gittleman, PhD, C.N.S., Three Rivers 2008)*

Chapter 15

Dreams and Goals

"You control your future, your destiny.
What you think about comes about. By recording
your dreams and goals on paper, you set in motion
the process of becoming the person you most want to be.
Put your future in good hands—your own."
—Mark Victor Hansen

I believe in goal setting and I practice it in every aspect of my life—always have. I didn't always do it correctly, setting achievable, healthy goals, but I did it. As a competitive figure skater, I had to set goals in order to improve. At first, my goals were simple: dress up, show up, and skate a little better than the day before. If I fell down, I'd get back up, and do it again. As I progressed in the sport, I continued to raise the bar: I learned to skate backwards, spin, jump, perform single then double jumps and on and on; goal after goal was set and reached. I had something to strive for, to complete and succeed at. I kept my eye on the prize, which back then, meant winning a gold medal, and I practiced every day. I passed test after test and kept on improving—getting my goals one by one, and then two by two. I did it by keeping my eye on the finish line, not on the starting line.

Merrillism #27: "There is Nothing to It but to Do It. Take a Stand for Your Health and Dreams and Those You Love, Now."

While I was successful in achieving my athletic goals (to a point), I was setting myself up to fail in other areas. When I was 15, I wanted to have the body of a 12 year old. Guess what? That's not a goal I could reasonably expect to achieve, no matter how much I dieted or tried to pretend my breasts didn't exist. I wanted to be thin and fit in with all the other kids I was competing against, but I *wasn't* a kid, I was a maturing woman trying to fit in to the figure skating world of young, mechanical, robotic machines. I was out of integrity with myself. I wanted to be what I was not. I ate nothing but cottage cheese, cantaloupe, carrots, apples and melba toast all week, only to end up overeating on ice cream, Entenmann's, choco-late chip cookies, and peanut butter by the tablespoonful when no one was looking. I thought if nobody was looking, it didn't count. Crazy as it sounds, I felt if I ate standing up, it didn't count either. By having unreasonable expectations and creating unrealistic goals, I continually fell short of my target. Naturally, I beat myself up for my perceived shortcomings and ended up feeling like a failure. It was a brutal cycle of self-abuse that eventually led me to quit my beloved sport altogether. It's a cycle that I would like to help you avoid, or at least recognize so that you don't repeat it. Give up eating for gratification, validation, recreation and on vacation.

Today I set goals, but with one important difference. I achieve the goals I create for myself because I make them with clarity and reasonable expectations. I take baby steps toward the goal and I get there, and you can too. I asked for help and support and asked people to hold my hand while I was taking difficult actions.

The **first** step in achieving your goals is to figure out what it is you want—what you *really* want. If you don't know what you are going after, you will never get it. How can you? If you can't name it, you can't claim it. So, if you don't know, go back to "Your Life" Recipe book and pull out your Treasure Map. Does it describe your true desires? If not, then you need to make a new treasure map for all areas of your life, and that's okay. Your goals, dreams, desires and plans for the future may have changed since you first created the map. That's OK. Make another one or add to the old one. Once you know what you want—optimum health, a new love, a fulfilling career, a new relationship, to learn to skate, sing, act, dance, paint, a new home—whatever it is, the next step is ask yourself what does it look like? Describe it; be specific in color, size, shape, place, name, age, time, amount, location etc.

This **second** step is important to ensure that your goal and your expectations surrounding that goal are realistic. Trying to go from being a 100% junk food eater your whole life to a 100% raw vegan in a day is a set up for disaster. Instead, you may want to reframe your goal as something that is challenging, but attainable—how about being 40% raw then 50%, then 60%? Think of losing five pounds in a month instead of 50. Be at the cause of your goals and you won't be at the effect of your negative thoughts. As the book, *The Secret* reveals, energy flows where attention goes. Follow your bliss, and where there were once walls, the Universe will open doors. ASAP for me means Always Say A Prayer first—it helps and works.

"You will achieve grand dreams, a day at a time, so set goals for each day / not long and difficult projects, but chores that will take you, step by step, toward your rainbow…Remember that you cannot build your pyramid in twenty-four hours. Be patient. Never allow your day to become so cluttered that you neglect your most important goal / to do the best you can, enjoy this day, and rest satisfied with what you have accomplished."
—Og Mandino

The **third** step is key; you need to form a plan by creating action steps that will move you toward your goal. You can take the elevator going down, but you have to take the steps to go up. What do you need to actually *do*, in order to successfully accomplish your goal? While affirmations, journaling, and reading books are all helpful tools, they will not get you to your goal all by themselves. Simply put, you need to take actions, on a daily basis, that bring you closer to accomplishing your goal. So, if your dream is to sing on stage, you need to sing every day. Take voice lessons, practice the scales, train your voice, listen to recordings of singers you admire and attend as many performances as you can. Then you need to seek out opportunities to sing and perform: join the church choir, sing karaoke, audition for a local theatre, or figure out how to produce your own show. You are not expected to do it perfectly, but you *are* expected to not give up when things don't go perfectly or your way. So, if your goal is to be a singer, then sing, sing and sing some more. Just keep singing. Follow your bliss and you will never miss!

Goals are dreams with deadlines.
—Diana Scharf Hunt

The **fourth** step is to set a time limit, a realistic time limit. Remember, if the only singing experience you have is by yourself, in the shower, you want to give yourself more than a week to make it to Broadway. I find deadlines to be extremely important; they give you that sense of urgency that is needed to motivate you toward your goals and forces you to honor your word and keep your commitments to yourself, others, and your goals. For instance, if you decide you want to sing on stage, set the date to make it happen. Trust me, if you know you have to sing a solo in front of your whole congregation or an audience full of paying strangers, you will practice your scales! When writing this book, I had to set a deadline on it or it would never have been completed. I would have finished it by the 1st of never. At one point, I realized I never wanted to finish it, that it meant I would have to risk putting it out there in the world. So, I set a goal, and now it is complete and imperfect and out in the world, instead of in my dreams, in my head, running in circles rent free, going nowhere but my bookshelf and helping no one. I figured it's better being in the world than on the shelf. I tell you, write a book. There is an inner writer in all of us. No one has had your experiences, trials and tribulations in the way you have had them. No one has traveled the road you have in the way you have. Uncovering the junk in your trunk may be the gift someone else needs to read. It's better to uncover, discard and share it than to put more in it. Your trash is someone else's treasure. Writing this book revealed me, healed me, and reminded me of my goals again and how to achieve them. This book wheeled me to contributing and being in the world again. Let the *raw richness and this book be your stepping stone, not your stumbling block. It rocketed me to the truth, The Raw Truth To The Fountain Of Youth.*

The **fifth** step is to persevere through the dark days. The darkest hour is only 60 minutes long. You can endure it. Whatever it is now, it will be different tomorrow. First it's hard, then it's easy, and then it's real. Stick with it and it will happen. Don't quit before the miracle. There is nothing quite like doing something you didn't know you could do. It's so self-rewarding and motivating. Get healthy now just for the health of it. We all want everything instantly—instant gratification and success. We have to be patient and know it is a process, not an event. It is a process not a verdict. Stay in the process of acceptance, stay in the process of patience and forgiveness. Bubble baths, massages and time-outs for yourself work great. It's the art of self-nurturing.

> *"Your goals are an excuse for the fun of the race."*
> —Debbie Merrill

The **sixth and final** step is of utmost importance and is very simple. Celebrate your accomplishments. It is imperative that you reward yourself for your hard work and acknowledge your triumphs. So, when you have achieved what you set out to do, relish the moment, enjoy it, celebrate it and share it. You deserve it. Then, you get to set a new goal! Throw yourself a positive party. Validate and applaud yourself or your mind will invite negativity. Allow yourself to see the impossible becoming the possible. Give yourself a hug, a high-five and an, "I love you" in the mirror. Remember my high school quote, "Let your dreams become your reality now."

These six steps will work with any goal you choose—be it a career goal, creative goal, financial goal, health goal or spiritual goal. If one of your goals is to become a raw foodist, you need to set smaller goals to get you there; but take baby steps towards the goal. Like eating raw once a week, then twice a week, then once a day, and so on. You don't go from being a meat and potatoes eater to vegan overnight, but if you set yourself up for success, you *will* get there, at exactly the right time. You can't change the wind, but you can adjust the sails.

Another way to look at goals is as commitments—to yourself. Successful people make commitments to themselves and others, and they keep them. And, when they don't, they are honest about it, make an apology and then do it differently the next time. If you don't yet have the willingness to honor your commitments to yourself, ask for help from others. Get a goal buddy, or two or three, and you can help each other through. I have a food buddy, an art buddy, a writing buddy and a goal buddy with whom I share on a daily basis. For instance, I call my writing buddy and say, "Today I am going to write a chapter on the book for one hour." I write the chapter and then I call again at the end of the task, after I have honored my commitment and completed the task. I call the process of calling before and after the specific action, book-ending.

It might sound a little silly at first, but it works. It's no fun having to call your writing buddy and say, "Uh, well, I almost completed the chapter but I had to pay some bills, answer emails, clean out the refrigerator and then well, my friend called and we got to talking about her deadbeat relationship…" To be quite honest, I just resisted honoring my word. If you have a good buddy, they will hold you to your commitments and not allow you to avoid them with excuses, circumstances and reasons, and you will do the same for them. We make and invent alibis so well it's become a fine art for us. Do the best you can and forget the rest. The act of completion and honoring your commitments builds integrity and momentum, which in turn builds true, long lasting self-esteem, progress and success. A master will always be a student, and a student will always need a teacher. Be a buddy, a helper, a teacher, and a coach for someone else. Champions coach champions.

Merrillism #28: "Prioritize Your Priorities."

You need to have a plan for you life and for recovering your health. Without one, you are just out there, flopping around without a net, wandering aimlessly, and living life haphazardly. Your plan is the net. Plan your meals, your exercise, your spirituality, your creativity, and your family time everyday. Prioritize your life. Prioritize your priorities. Most people get up in the morning, get themselves ready for work, get the kids off to school, work all day and just assume the rest will take care of itself—and then they are surprised when it doesn't. Family time doesn't just happen on its own; you've got to plan it out—otherwise you'll end up doing your own separate things, existing under the same roof, but living separate lives. That's not the same as spending time together. You've got to plan your exercise, and your eating too. If you wait until you have extra time to go for a walk, hit the gym or prepare a meal, it will never happen, and you'll end up frustrated with your lack of progress, eating in drive-thrus and from packaged foods; gaining weight, not feeling alive, energized, revitalized and fully self-expressed. It is important that you are focused on your true goals, rather than just keeping busy. Ask yourself these questions: Am I inventing things to do to avoid the important things (my goals and dreams)? Am I productive, or just active? Am I dressed for success going nowhere fast? Am I procrastinating out of fear? What are your crunch activities you use to fill time, to feel productive, yet avoid what you really need to do? Prioritize properly. There is no need for multi-tasking, trying to do more while accomplishing less. I suggest having at most, two high priority tasks or goals today. Do them specifically from start to finish without distractions. Please stop using drama, alibis, excuses and catastrophes to avoid achieving your dreams and goals. They are all great excuses. I love them and I use them too. Save your drama for your mama, save your drama for the page.

Merrillism #29: "Not Planning Is Planning to Fail. Proper Planning Prevents Poor Performance and Problems."

One of my favorite raw food mentors, David Wolfe, says, "People are dying because they are sick of living." When you are living a life without yourself, your dreams, your joys and your health, you are living a dead, dull life. So why live it? A diet devoid of oxygen, water, enzymes and nutrients is a diet of death. A life devoid of joy, love, self-expression, spirituality, peace, freedom, purpose, fulfillment and fitness is a dead life. We cannot live fully and healthfully without all of these ingredients. Give in to the pain in your health and your life, and you will find your joy in your health and your life where you did not expect it. When you feel you have lost it with your life and your health, don't lose the lesson. Remember the three "R's": Respect for yourself, Respect for others and Responsibility for all your actions. Ask yourself what is most important to you and focus on achieving those goals and taking daily action steps that will help you accomplish them. People make good company when they are doing what they love. If your health is a priority, then spend some time focusing on that. By going raw, we gain clarity to discover a chink in the walls that bad health has built. We then become well enough for the light of reason to shine through, we realize we are alive again. Read books, utilize the Internet, go to lectures, seek out like-minded people to partner with, and then get raw and get rolling!

"Learn from the past, set vivid, detailed goals for the future, and live in the only moment of time over which you have any control: now."
—Denis Waitley

There are 24 hours in a day, 60 seconds in a minute (there is no quick minute), three months in a season, and 12 months in a year. There is no such thing as microwave timing. We cannot force things to happen faster than they are supposed to, because life is a process, life happens on life's schedule. Practice patience and persistence and you will achieve extraordinary results. I am not saying that you must plan every moment of every day, leaving no room for spontaneity, interruptions, synchronicity or living in the moment. Quite the contrary, I am all about going with the flow, seizing and being in the moment and saying, "yes" to the exciting opportunities life tosses my way. Make room for the unexpected. Make room for miracles. Sometimes I chuck the plan out the window and go where the day takes me. Sometimes I just do what is in front of me to do. For example, a few years ago, I received a phone call from the producers of "Jimmy Kimmel Live!" at 6 pm, asking me if I could come perform on the show at 7pm! In one hour!? If you know anything about L.A. traffic, then you know it's virtually impossible to get anywhere during rush hour. And there I was at the natural food market buying broccoli and produce for my public TV show that I was shooting the next day, plus I had made plans to work on a million other projects that were in the works. And I had a head full of conditioner in my hair that I hadn't washed out yet because I was coming straight from the gym! But I couldn't turn down an offer like this! Thank God for ponytails and Pam Anderson's red skating outfit. Miraculously, I got there on time and performed my Merrill Magic skating routine. Then they asked me, "Oh, by the way, could you spend a week driving across country to be part of *The Road To The Super Bowl* show with Guillermo?" Wow! This is a definite example of when I make plans, the Universe laughs and interrupts. The beauty of having a plan is that it can change, so I

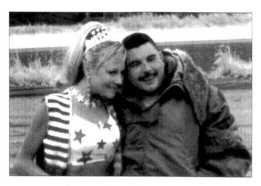

Raw on the road to the Super Bowl somewhere in Idaho with Guillermo Rodriguez, parking lot security guard on **Jimmy Kimmel Live!** *I even managed to get my raw* Dip in a Whip *on the trip, for dinner.*

reorganized my schedule and created a new plan so that I could "seize the moment." But if I didn't have a plan, if I wasn't already working on my goals, it's unlikely that the opportunity would have presented itself to me in the first place. If you want the phone to ring for work, get out of the house and get busy. If you want work, book a plane ticket out of town. Part of having goals and plans means you can deviate from them and change direction. Think of it as a life map—yes, you have your route planned out, but you can always decide to turn around, take a new road or even throw out the map and go wherever the road takes you. Shift your destination and journey. Direction and redirection is God's protection. I have found that *what* your goals are isn't nearly as important as having them. You can revise, amend, add to, or change your goals at any time, but you need a place from which to begin. That's why I suggest making the treasure map as well as a goal list, to spark your senses, desires and interests.

All my miracles, to my amazement, came through the back door when I was walking out the front door. While I was on my way to the dentist, I got a call to be on *Late Show with David Letterman*. I had to figure out how to fly a six-foot feather headdress, back piece, boa and myself to New York in 24 hours, while sitting in the dentist's chair, but I did it! After auditioning for my first Broadway play in New York City, "The Marriage of Figaro" with Christopher Reeve, I was weeping my way down Times Square ruminating over how horrible my audition went. Then the call came in and I got the role. My point is: expect the best and go for what you want. Worry less and enjoy more. Worrying is a rocking horse that never gets anywhere. Negative thinking is like a dark room where negatives are developed.

Sidebar to the Rawbar

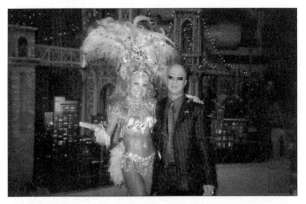

*It was great meeting Paul Shaffer for my skating perfor-mance on **The Late Show with David Letterman**. He played "Conga" for me while I skated the samba.*

Five To Keep You Alive—*And help you live a healthy, happy life.*
1. Exercise every day for at least one hour
2. Eat fresh, raw, organic, live foods (Non-organic soil is depleted of vitamins and minerals, and has chemicals and drugs saturating the soil, which comes in contact with your food. Please select organic only. You won't have to panic when it's organic. You'll be automatic, systematic, and instamatic.)
3. Write every day—Write things right
4. Pray and meditate daily
5. Creative expression—Do something creative that makes your heart sing at least once a day, every day.

Raw Bites

- *Pick your **goal**, make a **plan** and put it into action. My main goal is to be FAMOUS. Actually, it always has been, but I redefined it for myself, and now it means: FAMOUS= having <u>F</u>un <u>A</u>mong <u>M</u>any <u>O</u>ut in the <u>U</u>niverse <u>S</u>erving. It is a goal that I joyfully work on every day!*
- *Shop locally, eat sensibly, act locally, think globally.*
- *Eat great, exercise great, energy great.*
- *Set backs are set ups for success.*
- *Have fun every day—life is limiting, fun is limitless. Life can be more fun. Fun is healthy, fun is healthy food.*
- *Love and be kind to yourself and others everyday.*

Chapter 16

The Carrot and the Rabbit

*"Nothing will benefit human health
and increase chances for survival of life on Earth
as much as the evolution to a vegetarian diet."*
—Albert Einstein

T he idea of living a vegetarian or vegan lifestyle for moral, ethical or even health reasons is a touchy subject for some. People on both sides of the issue feel strongly about the choice they have made. Vegetarians cannot conceive of eating meat, and meat eaters can't conceive of eating "rabbit food." I choose to live a raw, vegan lifestyle, *now*. It wasn't always my choice, and I recognize that it may never be yours. And that's fine. Really. It is not my intention to judge you, condemn your choices or change them; nor is it my desire to shame you into making a different choice. I only wish to offer you an alternative, a way of looking at eating and at a lifestyle with different eyes. Perhaps after reading this chapter, you will decide to eliminate meat from your diet completely, or maybe you will simply cut down on how much, or the way in which you consume meat products. You may become committed to eating only "natural" meat, poultry and fish, or you may just shrug your shoulders and continue on your way. As I have said throughout, it's *your* journey, *your* choice and *your* life. Live it as you see fit. I only ask that you learn the facts. Be open-minded to doing things differently. There is always room for improvement. It's the largest room in the house and we all need to spend a lot more time there, myself included.

Merrillism #30: "Get the Raw WOW: Wake Up, Open Up and Be Willing."

There are a myriad of ways you can educate yourself: go to a slaughterhouse (that did it for me) or watch films like "Eating," "Diet For A New America," or "Super Size Me. " (Seeing is believing.) Think about what I have to say, and come to your own conclusion. After all, it is impossible to make an informed decision if you don't have the information, knowledge and visual on which to base it. Explore, expand, experiment and educate yourself on health.

Merrillism #31: "The More Meat We Eat, the More Disease We Treat. Not Eating Meat Is the Real Treat."

There are many reasons to abstain from eating meat, fish and poultry; for many people, it is simply a question of health. It is widely accepted by health experts—and this is entirely my opinion and personal belief based exclusively on my 28 years of experience—that a vegetarian diet is the best step human beings can take to protect themselves from heart disease, cancer and stroke. Eating meat, eggs and dairy has also been linked to osteoporosis, Alzheimer's (mad cow disease), asthma, obesity, heart disease, cholesterol, strokes, and other ailments. Fish flesh often contains bacteria and mercury (which can lead to brain damage) and other toxins like DDT, PCBs and dioxins (which are linked to cancer, fetal damage and nervous system disorders). Untreated ADD and depression can increase brain problems. Vegetarians have lower blood cholesterol levels, lower blood pressure and lower rates of hypertension, Type 2 diabetes and certain types of cancers than their meat-eating counterparts. Vegetarians are shown to have stronger immune systems, and are less susceptible to colds, flu and allergies. And having not had either for over 28 years, I can personally attest to that one! In short, refraining from meat, fish and dairy consumption means avoiding disease, embracing better health and having more energy to do the sports and activities that you love. As a professional athlete, that was reason enough for me to make the change. If better health is enough of a reason for you to make the change, then go for it, slowly. Take baby steps towards your goal. Take a leap of faith towards your goal of being a vegetarian, but take the leap and take it NOW (Now=N̲o O̲ther W̲ay). Great events are not done by impulse, but by small events all put together.

> *"If anyone wants to save the planet, all they have to do is just stop eating meat. That's the single most important thing you could do…Vegetarianism takes care of so many things in one shot: ecology, famine, cruelty."*
> —Sir Paul McCartney

If you need more, please consider the environmental impact of the meat industry. Did you know that livestock consumes 50% of our nation's water supply and 80% of our grain? 20 pounds of forage and grain and 2500 gallons of water are required to produce eleven pounds of meat. Multiply that by the half a million animals killed for meat every hour in the United States and it's clear what an enormous impact meat consumption has in this county alone. Farmed animals produce 130 times the excrement of the entire human population of the United States, and all that waste ends up in our water, topsoil and air, adding to contamination and pollution. There are waters in the Mississippi River (called the Dead

Zone), which are the size of New Jersey that are uninhabitable for marine life due to excessive amounts of animal excrement in the water. (See the DVD "Eating" by Michael Anderson). Are you living in a dead zone? Is there animal excrement in your food? Are you eating fried poop to disguise it? Our animals are eating dead fecal matter from other animals and we are eating them. We are eating diseased disease. Between the overuse of natural resources (water, crops and land) and the water and air pollution caused by animal waste and animal slaughter, it's no wonder that many environmental organizations believe that killing animals for food is one of the leading causes of environmental damage in this country. You may not like what I have to say, but please relate to this in a very heartfelt way.

For me, the most compelling reason to refrain from eating meat comes down to one very simple concept—compassion. Having compassion for animals means having compassion for another living soul, which, in turn, allows one to have self-compassion. And self-compassion leads directly back to having compassion for others and every living thing on the planet—it's a continuous circle. If we all practiced living compassionately, the world, I believe, would be a much happier, more peaceful, abundant and joyous-filled place to live. Compassion is the ultimate and most meaningful tool for emotional maturity because it helps us achieve our highest potential as human beings. Compassion allows us to live in harmony with nature and create a sustainable, viable future with our environment. As you become weaker in the ego, you become stronger in organic love and intelligence.

> *"Animals are my friends... and I don't eat my friends."*
> —George Bernard Shaw

Would you eat your dog, your horse, or your cat? In some parts of Asia they do, and here we eat cows, pigs and chickens. So where

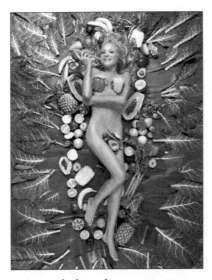

I ate and chased so many carrots in my life because of my sugar cravings that my palms and feet turned orange. I'm letting go of them for today and leaving them for the rabbits. Please choose your fruits and veggies wisely!

do we draw the line? We aren't born to be carnivores; we don't need to eat meat to survive and thrive. There is a saying, that if you put a carrot and a rabbit in a baby's crib, the child will eat the carrot and play with the rabbit. The rabbit, in turn, plays with the baby and eats the carrot. So, you see, that is really Mother Nature's Way. We can learn so much from animals. That is the natural order of things; it is our instinct to bond with, love and show kindness to our fellow living creatures. It is only once we grow up, trained by society and brainwashed by the meat, dairy and pharmaceutical industries that we decide to eat the rabbit and play with the carrot. Of course, we don't kill the rabbit (or the chicken or the cow) ourselves, that is done by someone else, out of our sight, so we don't have to think about what we are eating. Now I know some of you are thinking, "But I would never eat a cute, little cottontail bunny rabbit!" My question is, how can the same person who can't stomach the thought of eating Bugs Bunny for lunch have no problem eating an intelligent, inquisitive chicken, soulful cow or baby calf? The answer is simple. I personally believe that if everyone had to kill the meat they consume themselves, we'd have a lot more vegetarians in the world. It's just so easy to eat all kinds of meat that is literally served to us on a silver decorated platter, and we are completely oblivious to the unsavory acts that had to occur before that steak, chicken breast, fish filet or pork chop made it to our plates. You are what you eat, what you don't eat, what you eliminate, assimilate, and absorb. Persist, persevere and pursue, and the raw lifestyle will come to you. It's not hard to eat meat when it's wrapped in a fast food wrapper with a bright yellow star or when you call it a "Happy Meal" and call it a day. It is much harder to digest when you have all the facts, so I encourage you to get educated. Go to a chicken farm, and see how they are raised, treated, caged and killed for our food. The inhumane treatment of farm animals and pig gestation is horrifying and sad. After volunteering for the Humane Society to pass the bill for the Humane Treatment Of Farm Animals in California, I became more committed and compassionate to my raw vegan lifestyle. The cruel treatment of animals on factory farms makes them more susceptible to disease. It's bad for them and bad for us. Factory farms are among the most serious causes of resource depletion, pollution and global warming. After doing this I got a rude awakening and I felt better because I was doing something about the problem myself. Please take a stand for causes you believe in. (See resource section.)

My mother used to force me to eat my meat or I couldn't go out and play because she was fed the same lies that I needed more meat and animal flesh for protein. So, I did, even though I never wanted to. I spilled my milk at every meal. We couldn't salvage that, thank God. I hated milk as a kid and never drank it. Milk just smelled horrific to me; I couldn't get it past my nose and to my lips. The nose knows. It didn't go with food for me. It didn't combine well with anything for me. It tasted sour. I knew intuitively at a very young age that it was not good for me, and you can't smile with a sour stomach. Thank God for my intuition. I haven't had milk since I was six years old. If you are having a hard time letting go of milk, try my raw nut milks in the recipe section, or you can experiment with some of the soy milks on the market. (Soy milk is not raw, but can be a good choice while you are transitioning.)

There are many excellent resources for learning the truth about the meat production industry. *GoVeg.com*, for example, contains many well-researched articles about the brutal treatment of farmed animals who suffer so that humans can eat their flesh. I encourage you to take a moment and read the articles and watch the videos I suggested. Let go of your inner critic and learn to have more compassion for yourself, the animals, the environment, and generations to come. Exist in harmony with all, because the reality is, we are all one. One for all, and all for one. None of us is getting out of here alive, so now it is the time to thrive.

Please consider the following facts and statistics: (The following facts and figures I learned from watching the DVD "Eating, The RAVE Diet, 2nd Edition." Remember, I'm writing this from my point of view and my beliefs. I'm one among many who holds these beliefs as well. Please do your own research, do your own diligence.)

- Two out of three Americans die every year from eating related diseases. The biggest killer on the planet is our appetite for animals. Then we torture and kill other animals to find a cure for the diseases caused by eating animals in the first place. How insane. That is definitely the definition of insanity: doing the same thing and expecting different results.

- Cows start their abbreviated lives by being branded (suffering third degree burns), castrated and having their horns removed, all without any painkillers.

- Many cows die on their way to the slaughterhouse due to disease and the extreme cold or heat they experience in transit.

- Once the frightened cows arrive at the slaughterhouse, they are shot in the head with a bolt gun (to stun them), hung upside down, have their throat slit, and then they are skinned and taken apart piece by piece. That's probably your next steak dinner.

- Cows that are not sent to slaughterhouse are milked to death. Their bones become so brittle they can't support their own weight. After years and years of this they're exhausted and susceptible to many diseases. The animal equivalent to AIDS.
- Milk and meat come from cows being fed other dead, diseased cows, not grass, resulting in Mad Cow Disease.
- If the bolt gun misses the mark, and they often do, the cow remains fully conscious throughout the entire process and can feel everything.
- 80% of pigs have pneumonia.
- Veal calves are taken from their mothers at one day old, stuffed into small, dark crates to live out their short lives completely immobilized (they can't sit, lie down or move) and malnourished before being slaughtered.
- 99% of the nine billion chickens raised for meat spend their entire lives, from birth to death, in total confinement and most will never even see the sun until the day they are loaded on the truck to be slaughtered. Some chicks are thrown into crushers alive or smothered in trash bags then crushed.
- After having a large portion of their beaks cut off with a burning hot blade, without painkillers, many egg laying hens die from dehydration because eating and drinking is too painful. Every time you eat an egg you are supporting this practice of how they meet their death. 90% of chickens have cancer as they enter our food supply. Their bones are so brittle they break before they are killed or thrown into grinders and crushed.
- Hens have their beaks removed in order to prevent them from pecking each other to death due to the extreme stress

of living their entire lives in tiny wire cages with five to eleven other birds, unable to lift even one wing.

- Laying hens are subjected to "forced molting," a cruel procedure banned in some countries, where birds are starved for five to fourteen days to shock their bodies into entering an egg laying cycle in order to increase egg production.
- Chickens are transported to slaughter in all weather conditions, often traveling hundreds of miles in extreme cold or heat with no food or water. Many die along the way. This may be your Friday fried chicken dinner.
- Once birds arrive at the slaughterhouse, they are dumped from their crates, shackled and hung upside down by the ankles (many have their legs broken during this process), and they struggle to escape before being dragged through an electrical water bath that will paralyze, but not stun, them.
- Chickens are usually still conscious when their throats are slit.
- Millions of chickens miss the "cutter" and are fully conscious when they are dunked into the scalding hot water of the de-feathering tank.
- 87% of agricultural land is used to raise and feed animals that we eat.
- 260 million acres of land is used to raise cattle that we torture and eat.
- Countries with the highest amount of meat eaters have the highest rate of heart disease and cancer.
- Geese and ducks suffer the same cruel treatment as chickens: beak cutting, confinement and the pain of being inhumanely slaughtered.
- Foie gras literally translates to "fatty liver" and is arguably the cruelest example of animal torture for human gratification; it is obtained by force-feeding male ducks and geese enormous

amounts of grain until the liver grows up to ten times its normal size. That is your delicious liver pâté.

- These birds are force fed three to four pounds of grain by having a pipe shoved down their throats to deposit food directly into their stomachs two to three times per day for 12-21 days.
- Many birds experience additional suffering from puncture wounds to the neck caused by rough treatment.
- Stress sometimes causes the sick birds to cannibalize each other and tear out their own feathers. There will always be contrary beliefs, but I believe that diseases coming from central Asia are the direct result of Asians changing to an animal based diet (i.e. Bird flu).
- The procurement of foie gras is so cruel that Whole Foods Markets stopped selling it and, in 2004, the state of California banned the production and sale of products created by force-feeding. The practice is also outlawed in the city of Chicago and in many countries including the UK, Sweden and Germany.
- In America, our farms are corporate graveyards. We spend so much money and destroy our environment to feed, raise, torture and kill the animals we eat, then they kill us. Another insanity.
- We spend more money treating the sick animals we eat, than feeding the malnourished humans who are starving on the planet.

Many people say, "I'm a vegetarian—I only eat fish." Whether they fly, swim, trot or flap, the animals you eat are made of flesh, fat, cholesterol and disease. Rationalizing eating certain kinds of flesh, fish or hormone-free white meat because it contains some good oils and is labeled, "cage free, range free and organic," is like saying, "I'm eating an organic donut full of organic sugar and organic white flour because it contains some good organic oil." What you are doing is eating a lot of bad just to get a little bit of good. Does that really make sense? For me, eating animals is not an option. There are other vegetarian/vegan/raw vegan options. See my recipe section for new ideas on an old subject.

Consider the fish. *They are animals too.* Fish feel hunger and physical pain as well as emotional stress and fear.

- Farmed fish are routinely starved before slaughter to reduce water waste contamination.
- Salmon are starved for ten days before death. Some people say some of the oil is good for you so you should eat the whole flesh. I say, an animal diet clogs arteries, while a plant based diet opens them—and opens your heart as well. Eat some broccoli and my Sprouted Lentil Salad and open your heart. It's better for your love life, too. Have a steak, fries and a milkshake and close your heart. It's called a *heart attack.*
- Fish are killed with no regard to the pain they suffer. Their gills are slit and they bleed to death.
- Larger fish, like salmon, are clubbed over the head and killed or injured before being cut and left to die.
- Trout are often suffocated by having their water drained or simply packed in ice, while fully conscious, prolonging their suffering for at least 15 minutes before death.
- Commercial fishing hooks and nets injure and kill many other marine animals every day—sharks, sea turtles, seals, whales and even birds get caught up in nets and often die from their injuries.

Merrillism #32: "Eat Nothing With a Face: No Animals, That Means no Fish or Shellfish – Don't Be Selfish."

If, after reading this and knowing how the meat, eggs, dairy and fish you eat arrives on your plate, you still want to eat it, then please do so consciously. I'm suggesting you don't eat them at all because all the mounting evidence proves that the real cause of diabetes, cancer, heart and other diseases come from eating animals and animal by-products (eggs, dairy, cheese, milk, yogurt, ice cream. All of these foods weaken the immune system, and a plant-based diet strengthens the immune system. By eating a plant-based diet, these conditions can be strengthened, improved, and prevented. I feel that I've experienced it and know it to be true for me. What you do not eat, you do not crave. There are many ways to change your habit hungers. It really is just a bad habit, and bad habits can be broken. Would you rather be healthy, or right? Please try it for yourself. Get advice from doctors trained in plant-based diet and nutrition. They can help you reverse the problem. Once again, I suggest you be your own doctor first. No one else is living in your body and behind your eyeballs. You know your body better than anyone else because you're in it. You have to be in it to win it, so win it back.

There is a great deal of controversy on the subject of "compassionate" consumption but if you choose to consume meat and meat by-products (again, I don't suggest it), it is important to do so as humanely as possible, as minimally, and as infrequently as possible. Remember, it's just habit hunger, possibly laziness, and lack of facts and information about the issue. You can start by refraining from eating foie gras altogether. It is procured in a cruel, inhumane manner, and is incredibly unhealthy. The liver's primary purpose is to cleanse the body of toxins, so eating the diseased liver of another animal doesn't make sense for your conscience or your health. Eliminating veal from your diet is also a compassionate choice. Even if the veal you eat is not crated or tethered before being slaughtered, the baby calf is cruelly separated from its mother shortly after birth (causing pain to both mother and baby) and is underfed, then killed after living only a few short months. At the very least, if you choose meat, dairy and egg products, do it carefully. Natural food markets are the best place to shop for meat and meat by-products. Wherever you shop, make sure the meat you buy is certified organic, natural, pasture-fed, and is free from antibiotics and growth hormones. Poultry and egg products should also be antibiotic and hormone free as well as certified organic and cage free. This will ensure that the animals you eat have endured the least amount of suffering, and were treated humanely while they were alive. Of course, these products are more expensive, but I believe that spending a little extra to decrease the suffering of animals and yourself is the least we can do for our planet, our children, generations to come and ourselves. Otherwise you will be paying for it in drug insurance instead of health insurance, doctor and hospital bills. A raw vegan diet *is* your health insurance. You can also make it a priority to eat only in restaurants that serve certified organic, natural foods, and to avoid those who continue to sell veal, foie gras and non-organic meats or any animal products at all. Obviously, at the end of the day, it is up to you to decide how you want to live your life, and if you choose to eat meat, fish, eggs or dairy products, I hope you will choose to do so in the most compassionate, conscious, caring and organic way possible. My wish for you is to eliminate them slowly all together and feel better.

As you know, I'm not an advocate of eating animals or their by-products at all, and do not suggest it. Please abstain and save your brain. Brain torture in animals is due to animals eating other animals, not grass. They call it "animal cannibalism." Animals are eating cats, dogs, circus animals, road kill and pets. They are going brain dead. It's called mad-cow disease. I also believe we have a similar addiction to overeating meat—a disease in humans called Alzheimer's, the human form of mad-cow ("Eating, RAVE", diet DVD). 4 million people in the U.S. have Alzheimer's disease (1 million people in Japan have it). My dad died of it, my grandfather too. My mother died of a stroke. That's one of the reasons I wrote this book, so that you, your mom, dad and loved ones get the message, and not this mess told to us by the corporate graveyard leaders. My wish for you is that you let this knowledge and information seep in your consciousness, and know that when the answers come from something other than you, you will believe that there is something greater in you that can cure and help you. 85% of Americans are dying of hardening of the arteries, which is also called Alzheimer's. The arteries harden and oxygen cannot get to the brain so Alzheimer's, dementia and other degenerative diseases set in. In my opinion, all of these diseases and disorders come from an overindulgent appetite for animals. Eating a highly based animal diet after age 50 is like having one foot on the banana peel and one foot in the graveyard. Please do not spend your health chasing wealth and then your wealth chasing health.

Do not worry that not eating animal protein will compromise your health. While I believe that nothing can be further from the truth, please don't take my word for it. There are multitudes of resources and experts weighing in on the benefits of a plant-based diet and the protein it contains. It's easy to get enough protein from a variety of plants, vegetables, nut seeds and grains, as well as all the new super foods and green powders available to us today. (Please see Debbie Merrill's Top Ten Superfoods for Eternal Life). I am still thriving 28 years later, and going strong! I believe that corporations perpetuate the myth that we need to eat animal flesh and dairy to be healthy, so they can continue to sell more animal and dairy products. So, wake up and smell the truth, and nothing but the raw truth: *not* eating any kind of flesh and animal by-products is key to true health, happiness and longevity. Give yourself permission to let go, know and flow. Man cannot be content and healthy without his own approval.

Sidebar to the Rawbar

In my opinion and experience, vegetarians...

- live longer.
- have less disease and illness.
- have happier dispositions.
- have less heart attacks, cholesterol and obesity problems.
- are more active, maintain proper body weight.
- don't die of Alzheimer's, strokes, diabetes or heart attacks.

Did you know that convicts and murderers are rarely vegetarians? A survey I read stated that most rapists and murderers eat meat three times a day.

Celebrity Vegetarians

Albert Einstein
Leonardo Da Vinci
Billie Jean King
Mick Jagger
Ringo Star
Darryl Hannah
Dustin Hoffman
Pamela Anderson
Sir Isaac Newton
Martina Navratilova
Alicia Silverstone
David Bowie
Alec Baldwin

Plato
Andy Dick
Keenen Ivory Wayans
Woody Harrelson
Juliette Binoche
Anthony Hopkins
Patty Heffner
David Duchovny
Paul McCartney
Carl Lewis
Carol Alt
Ed Begley, Jr.
Forest Whitaker
Ryan Seacrest
Natalie Portman
Sting
Pierce Brosnan
Carrie Underwood

Raw Bites

- *Spend today as a vegan. Eat no meat, poultry, fish, eggs or dairy. Think of it as your gift to the animal kingdom, yourself and your heart.*
- *Volunteer in an animal shelter or for the Human Society of the United States.*
- *Change your diet and your pet's diet to a plant based diet and you will improve your health, be happier, freer, sexier and thinner. The less you carry around, the longer you are around.*
- *Visit a petting zoo and the next time you crave bacon, consider the source: a pig with pneumonia. Americans eat 225 pounds of meat a year.*

- *Ask your favorite restaurant to take veal and foie gras off the menu. Try eating in vegetarian, vegan and raw restaurants only. Ask your favorite grocery store for your favorite organic veggies and fruits. Supply equals demand. Ask and you shall receive. Remember, if you don't buy it, they won't supply it. Your dollar represents your voice.*

- *Buy a fish tank and make some new friends. Eating animals consumes 1/2 of our water supply and 130 tons more water than people. Feeding them, farming them, and disposing of their trash is such a waste of time and manual labor.*

- *Do not kill or play with your food. Pray with your food.*

- *Prayer is nourishment.*

- *Real wealth is real health from real food every day.*

- *You are what you think. You are what you eat. If you eat animals, you think like an animal, you become an animal, and you die like an animal.*

- *Eat more animals, have less feelings. Have more feelings; eat fewer animals.*

- *90% of chickens are drugged and have cancer as they enter our food supply.*

- *Our modern farm is a convalescent camp for animals.*

- *Grow your own food.*

- *Be a vegetarian and be a survivor. Survivors always win. When you survive one thing you survive everything.*

- *The more you risk, the more you succeed. Success is when opportunity meets readiness.*

- *Eat only vegan, raw, organic foods.*

- *Plant a fruit tree.*

- *Shop at local farmer's markets. Eat only locally grown, organic fruits and vegetables from your region in season. (For example, please don't eat berries from New Zealand in the middle of winter; they cost a fortune in cash, fuel and carbon monoxide to reach you. They are not even fresh or picked ripe and are probably frozen before they make it to market.) By eating more raw fruits and veggies, you will save on electric bills, appliances, cleaning up and money on groceries. You will also stop the contribution of carbon monoxide fumes and poisons in the environment from the airplanes, which is one of the causes of hundreds of thousands of people, including children, to suffer with asthma.*

- *Bike, skate or walk to work or to do your errands.*
- *Remember, be a label reader! My mother used to joke and say, "The only thing Debbie ever read as a kid was a menu." Now I read labels like crazy. The ingredient with the highest quantity in the product is usually the first ingredient listed. If the ingredient you want is not listed until fifth or lower, don't buy it. That means there isn't much of that ingredient in the product. If sugar or some chemical ingredient is listed first, second or third, that is what is making up most of the product. Please don't purchase it.*
- *Tell others about your new Raw on the Roll menu and lifestyle and inspire them.*
- *Fast food takes your money fast.*
- *Protein deficiency is very rare. Everything on the planet has protein in it.*
- *A plant-based diet mops up the mess the animal based diet leaves behind.*
- *Close your mouth, open your heart.*
- *Animals trust us. Every time we eat them we violate their trust.*
- *Change your food and you will change your health, your environment, and your world. You will live a life of longevity,*

fitness, beauty, compassion, tolerance and love.

- *There are 126 milligrams of calcium in five medium dried figs and only 1.3 grams of fat.*
- *1 ounce of almonds contains 66 milligrams of calcium and 16.2 grams of fat.*
- *2/3 cup of broccoli contains 88 milligrams of calcium and 0.3 grams of fat.*
- *2/3 cup of turnip greens contains 184 milligrams of calcium and 0.2 grams of fat.*
- *There are 195 milligrams of calcium and 8.4 grams of fat in 1 ounce of American cheese, which clogs the arteries, increases fat in the blood and circulatory system, causes weight gain, and mucus in the nose and throat. I call it choking throat coat. Want a coat for your throat? Eat some dairy like ice cream, milk, cheese, yogurt, and butter.*

As you can see, you can substitute "good" for "bad;" eating a vegan/vegetarian diet you can still get your basic nutritional needs met. Be healthy, live with more vitality, energy, health and beauty, and look like me and be a cutie with a tight little booty! Life already gave us the gift, the gift of life and the gift of desperation. Please don't throw it away for an operation!

Chapter 17

Over the Hump Lesson #2:
Do You Have Junk in the Trunk,
Or the Urgency for Plastic Surgery?

*"Any change, even a change for the better, is always
accompanied by drawbacks and discomforts."*
—Arnold Bennett

Let your setbacks be setups for success and see them for what
they truly are, opportunities for new growth. Today, I have
successfully made it over most of my humps. That doesn't
mean I am living my life perfectly, or that my eating is exactly what
it should be every single day, because I am not perfect. I am human.
It does mean that I work at forgiving myself for my mistakes and I
self-nurture. Health is my challenge and my gift and, most of the
time, I skate freely in the flow of life. I strive for that easy flow and
glow to go. One of the beautiful (and miraculous) things about
getting *over the hump* is that today, a mango tastes as good to me
as a hot fudge sundae did back in the days when I was putting junk
in my trunk. And that's not just a figure of speech. I was literally
putting junk food in the trunk. When I lived at home, I'd offer
to do the grocery shopping for my mom so I could secretly stock
up on sweets for myself. I would hide chocolate chip cookies and
crumb cakes in the trunk so my mother would not see my stash,

171

and then I'd tell her to go upstairs and I would carry the groceries for her so I could sneak the stuff out and hide it in my closet. I would act like the perfect daughter, but I was really just hiding my sugar fixes—just like my Mom did. When I was five, I would eat in bed under the covers when everyone was asleep, or no one was looking, in the schoolyard, even in the car—until the crumbs scattered about gave away my secret. I would eat the crumbs and leave the cake (you could say I was a finicky sugarholic), so I lost the grocery-shopping chore after that. I would eat anyplace I could find to feed my sugar addiction. It took me over 28 years to go from out of control to *Raw on the Roll*, but now I'm in control, I'm popping and I'm non-stopping. I got there, and so will you. There is nothing to it but to do it! If you don't change your taste buds, habits and addictions, it will cost you your health.

One of the biggest hurdles in changing your eating habits is what I call *habit hunger*. We are killing ourselves with our forks and at the dinner table, our habits and addictions to sugar, alcohol, drugs, dairy products, animals and prescription drugs. Like I said, eating unhealthy foods is nothing more than a bad habit, and bad habits can be broken. Addictions and bad habits have no barriers. They don't care who you are, how much money you make or how high your I.Q. is, they will take you prisoner. In order to rid yourself of an addiction, you need to name it, claim it and dump it. Dump the junk in your trunk and put some raw in your drawer now. What you don't eat or use you don't crave. For me, total abstinence is what got rid of my cravings. Raw foods were my savior. It took away my cravings for sugar, white flour, alcohol, tobacco, drugs and unhealthy foods. I haven't consumed sugar, white flour, alcohol, recreational or prescription drugs or coffee in 28 years. The way to start is to begin. Begin with my *Raw on the Roll Success System* now: Raw Foods, Fitness, Creativity, Spirituality and The Good Outdoors. It's *The Raw Truth To The Fountain Of Youth* lifestyle found in this book. Follow it, practice it everyday and give it away. Don't deny it 'til you try it and apply it and you don't even have to buy it because it's given to you free by Mother Nature. Leonardo Da Vinci said, "Beauty and vitality are a gift from nature for those who live by her laws."

I believe that the types of foods that most of us eat, and the way we eat them is simply a function of habit. If you grew up eating eggs, bacon and buttered toast for breakfast every day, then you will probably continue to do so. If your parents stocked the pantry with chips and cookies, then you will probably do the same. By now you should be familiar with your trigger foods—those favorites that you can't seem to stop yourself from eating—your "love" foods that remind you of mommy and daddy. Those are the foods that help you numb out to the alone zone of "Forget Everything And Run" (FEAR). The comfort foods that make you feel like everything is FINE, which really stands for Freaked-Out, Insecure, Neurotic and Emotional—the foods that cover up and stuff you up, and put you out of reality and clarity. For me, it was sugar. I'd eat it by the spoonful if I could. I found the best way to change my habit was to avoid temptation altogether. If you know a certain snack is a trigger for you, leave it on the shelf. Don't buy it or keep it in the house. When it doubt, leave it out. If that is not an option, then practice portion control. Eat a handful, rather than the whole box or bag, one cookie, not ten. Try counting, measuring, and weighing your food, that way you know how much you are eating. Get clarity with your portion sizes. One of the reasons that we eat such large quantities of junk food is that it lacks nutritional value. You need to eat more of it to feel full and satisfied. We are addicted to fat and sugar, and all junk foods have fat and/or sugar in them. If it contains sugar, it usually contains fat and vice-versa, and not always good fats. The only sugary food I can think of without fat is chewing gum. So I became compulsive with gum and sugarless mints. I substituted them for sugar. I could have bought a new car with the money I spent on those two things while I was kicking the sugar habit. It worked, because it got me over the hump. However, today I don't choose to chew gum or suck on Lifesavers. I haven't had them in 28 years either. Once I start I don't know if I'd be able to stop, and I don't need them anyway. They were a fix, a habit hunger to cover up and numb out what I was really feeling. Sugar destroyed my true feelings or smothered them all together. So, here's to giving up gum and mints to go numb. *Rawllelujah*, I'm over it and over that hump. The lesson is to abstain completely to get over the hump and get rid of the rump. Another great thing about the raw food lifestyle is that it limits my options. It's not a choice for me to indulge in junk food, cooked food, animals or processed foods, sugar, gum, candy etc.; they're not an option and they are not on my Raw Truth to the Fountain of Youth Food-for-Life plan, so I don't have them. It's a lot less work for me in the decision-making and purchasing process. Abstinence is the answer to all of my bad habits with food, CRAP, alcohol and drugs. If I eat something and it doesn't make me glow and want to go, the answer is no. If I eat sugar and CRAP, unfortunately, the result would be overeating which leads to feeling full, bloated and lethargic rather than satiated, energized and excited. So I don't, and won't.

Merrillism #33: "When in Doubt, Leave it Out."

When offered the best, what you really need is zest—the zest of raw foods. They will keep you fearless in flight, eating less, feeling light, sleeping through the night and your light will shine bright. The best place to start working on your habit hunger is at the grocery store. I hardly ever buy prepackaged foods anymore but I recognize that most people do, and that's perfectly fine—as long as you do so consciously. Unconscious buying leads to unconscious eating which leads to unconscious living, anxiety, depression, lethargy and frustration. You need to make conscious, informed decisions about what you are putting in your body. Think about what you are tossing in your cart and ask yourself if you really want to put that in your body. Ask, "Is it good for me? Will it give me energy, satisfy me, make me healthier, or make me feel good about myself? Or will I feel bad after I eat it?" Think it through until the end and don't pretend. Be true to yourself. If you cannot answer "yes" to the first 5 questions, leave it on the shelf. I find that simplicity is the answer to health. Keep it simple. Eat less, live more. When I asked Jack LaLanne, who's still fit and healthy at age 90+, to sum up the secret to longevity, he said, "I don't eat any man-made foods and I don't eat in between meals." Neither do I. I believe you will master this as you practice my Raw on the Roll Success System. You learn until you master, and mastery is sublime.

Merrillism #34: "Eating Bread Equals Danger Ahead and Then Your Energy Is Dead."

I have found one of the biggest habits Americans have is bread consumption. The average American eats 60 pounds of bread a year, and they wonder why they lack energy, and can't get their weight down. Eating bread slows down your brain as well as your body; it's called *grain drain*. I was addicted to bread like everybody else in the world. I loved all kinds of bread—Italian bread, crackers, muffins, rice cakes, pizza, bagels, and chips. I ate food with a cracker or a hunk of bread, instead of a fork. I learned that from my dad. Nothing goes better with bread than butter, cheese, gravy, sauce, meat and mayo so it's not only the bread that's bad for us; it's what we put on it. I think that bread is one of the most addictive foods you can put in your body and, when you eliminate it from your diet, you will realize that you have more energy, you'll lose weight and your thinking will become sharper and clearer. Put some bread in the pocket of your coat and add water. Let it sit overnight. In the morning, you will find that it's stuck to the coat pocket and you can't remove it easily. That's what it does in your colon. It sticks to the walls and lives there, making elimination difficult and constipation easy, especially if it's not whole grain bread. Please try my quinoa or buckwheat crackers in the recipe section. They are totally raw and a great way to get Essential Fatty Acids (EFA's), fiber and crunch into your system. Relax with flax for a healthier alternative.

It's important to note that many people are allergic to the yeast and gluten contained in grains (especially wheat), and don't even know it. If you are experiencing digestive problems, try eliminating wheat and gluten from your diet. There are numerous websites, resources, and organizations dedicated to educating consumers about gluten, which can cause celiac disease in the digestive system of susceptible individuals. Wheat and wheat products are found in many common food items for example, breads, flours and baking mixes, soups, soy sauce, mustards, and even in protein meals and protein drinks. So read labels, try avoiding wheat or gluten as well as yeast, another allergen, which can support the growth of Candida. Educate yourself on this topic if you are not feeling up to par. Try phasing bread out of your diet and see what happens. Start slowly by cutting down to one piece of toast instead of two, eating open-faced sandwiches, and switching to healthier breads that are made with whole grains. Flourless bread, sprouted essene breads, as well as live raw breads, are also available in stores now. The Raw Makery in Las Vegas has great breads, crackers and bread sticks and so do a lot of raw restaurants. Try making your own with my Crunchy Cracklin' Cracker recipes (see recipe section) which contain quinoa, oat groats or buckwheat. Just don't dehydrate them as long and they will be soft and thick like bread. You can also try all of the hundreds of raw crackers that are available to us now in the natural food markets and raw product websites. When I first went raw 18 years ago, there was no such thing as a raw cracker; I had to make all my own. Now, I can go to the store and buy a variety of sweet, savory, spicy, salty, Italian, Mexican, Indian or any kind of cracker I want. Take advantage of this sensational rawvolution of products available in the markets today. Then you can begin to discover other foods that are filling, and provide that chewy crunch you find in bread products. My transition foods to give you that crunch and to relieve the craving for bread are the following raw veggies—broccoli, red cabbage, kabocha squash, sweet potatoes, red peppers, radishes, jicama, celery and zucchini. I didn't make the switch consciously, I just started to eat more broccoli, red cabbage, kabocha squash, sweet potatoes and jicama; all are very filling, and I realized that they became my bread, my crunch and munch food. They replace the bread; I got the same satisfaction from them and gained more water, fiber and nutrition in my diet. I no longer needed to have bread as an appetizer or bread with a meal. Bread left my head and I just stopped eating it altogether. Sometimes I make a cabbage wedge sandwich. It's a section of red cabbage filled with avocado, my spicy humus, black olives, onions and tomatoes. That's my sandwich for the day. If you want a lot of crunch and munch, try this for a nifty lunch. Use sliced sweet potatoes as a cracker to enjoy with my Sprouted Lentil Salad, Hummus and Dip In A Whip (see recipe section.) Or put some raw hemp butter on a celery stick, it's chewy and gooey, and celery contains natural salt.

Change is not easy; if it were, everyone would do it. Be gentle with yourself as you make the transition to a healthier lifestyle. "Water seeks its own level." Treat yourself as you would a dear friend who is going through a big life change, like divorce or a death in the family, because letting go of habits, even bad ones, is a loss; you are giving it up, letting go, and giving it away. It's OK to let go and not know. Yes it's hard, but it's worth the effort because you are worth the effort. So, buy yourself flowers or mail yourself a card offering encouragement. Treat yourself to a massage, walk in nature, manicure, pedicure, haircut or sleep in. Do it for the health of it—your health of it, you deserve it, you're worth it and you're entitled to receive it. As a rule of thumb, I tell all my clients you don't have to keep getting healthy and fit, if you stay healthy and fit. Get fit, not fat. Longevity is no accident. To live longer you have to start living well now.

Raw Bites

- *Incorporate more greens into your diet, especially bitter greens; for example kale, collard greens, cilantro, dandelions, bok choy, Swiss chard, watercress, parsley, arugula, endive and spinach. They will cleanse your system, calm you down, take away your cravings and add more vitamins, minerals and fiber to your diet, while keeping you in high vibe.*

- *Let go of bread.*

- *Start writing down foods you like and recipes you enjoy. One of the reasons we go back to habit foods is because they are easy, quick to get, safe, comforting and appealing. We know what we like. When you are discovering new tastes, it's a good idea to write them down so when you have a craving, you can create a dish with a healthier substitute for that craving. That's how I came up with all my recipes in this book. I kept a notebook next to my dinner table, and while eating I would create recipes of what tasted outrageous to me. For example, goji berries, mangos, bananas, papayas, raw sweet potatoes for sugar cravings; raw black olives, sea salt and seaweed for salty and fat cravings; celery, cabbage, broccoli, and flax crackers for crunch; avocado, cacao butter, raw virgin coconut oil, olives, flax seed oil, and raw nut butters for fatty filling up; and raw cacao and cacao butter for those cacao kapow days.*

- *If you can't spell it, don't eat it.*
- *Name it, claim it and dump it. Pick your choice of food and get on with it.*
- *To get the knowledge to go even higher, food is best eaten without the fire.*
- *Keep the wisdom; lose the weight.*
- *The mind can recover from brain damage caused by processed food and chemicals, but the sooner you stop eating them, the better your brain's ability to repair itself.*
- *Do the diligence. Your life and health depend upon it.*
- *We are all living in the most powerful time the world has ever seen. Everything is at our fingertips. Reach out, take it, be it and have it.*
- *Get raw, get rich and enrich others.*
- *Believe you will have great health and you will.*
- *Stick to it and it will stick to you, and you will stick out in the world and the world will be stuck on you.*

Chapter 18

Think Outside the Box and Give Up the Boxes

*"There are people who put their dreams in a little box
and say, 'Yes, I've got dreams, of course I've got dreams.'
Then they put the box away and bring it out once in
awhile to look in it, and yep, they're still there."*
—Erma Bombeck

Our lives are filled with boxes—microwave ovens, computers, cell phones and PDAs—we drive to work in a box on wheels, and work in a lidless box called a cubicle, unless we are lucky enough to have a box with a view. We eat breakfast, lunch and dinner out of a box, and when we get home from work, we plop ourselves down on the sofa, and stare at the TV—the mother of all boxes—before going to bed. We have literally boxed ourselves in, creating compartments for everything, including ourselves. Instead of nurturing our dreams, we surf the net, flip on the television and tune into other people's dreams and lives, while mindlessly shoveling snacks into our mouths—straight from the box. Mindless television watching (especially reality TV) is a way to avoid our own issues, while we judge, and entertain ourselves with other people's issues. Instead of looking at our own issues, we overlook them.

"We love television because television brings us
a world in which television does not exist"
—Barbara Ehrenreich

The most pervasive, and invasive, box is one that 99% of us have voluntarily placed smack dab in the middle of our living rooms, and even bathrooms. Quite a few of us have more than one, and have even invited it into our bedrooms. According to the AC Nielsen Company, Americans watch an average of four hours of television every single day. That translates to 28 hours a week, and a mind-numbing two solid months per year. Another sad fact is that roughly two thirds of us plop down in front of the television to eat dinner (unconscious eating), and children spend infinitely more time in front of the television than they do talking to their parents. In fact, most kids would rather watch TV than talk to Mom and Dad. That's a pretty scary thought; especially when you consider what we are watching.

My family dinner when I was young consisted of me, my parents, the dog and the TV—all to take the attention off of our being and communicating with each other. There was no intimacy (in-to-me-see). We just discussed sports, dogs and politics and not what was going on with us as a family. No wonder there was such distance in our relationship and connection with one another.

Today, the average American kid will have witnessed 8,000 television "murders" by the time he or she will have finished elementary school. The local news dedicates more than half of its broadcast to the coverage of crime, disaster and war, feeding us a steady diet of fear. When it comes to commercials, the average child sees 20,000 thirty-second spots every year and the ones they see the most are for fast food. With all that sitting around while being bombarded with images of processed, preserved, fat filled food, should we be surprised that kids are getting fatter and feeling less valuable as their self worth plummets? And the adults aren't doing so well either—1/3 of America is overweight. The American Journal of Public Health Safety conducted a study and found that, "an adult who watches three hours of TV a day is far more likely to be obese than an adult who watches less than one hour." Excessive television watching leads to inactivity and inactivity is one of the leading causes of obesity. There is some good news however; the best way to reduce inactivity is simple: turn off the TV and get active. And, if you *must* watch TV, buy some leg weights or a stationary bicycle, or do sit-ups or yoga while you get your fix. Even better, listen to the TV; turn it on while cleaning, doing the laundry, preparing a meal, etc. You can also watch an inspiring DVD such as *The Secret*, or listen to CD's such as Dr. Wayne Dyer's *Inspiration Your Ultimate Calling* and *A Course In Miracles*. Better yet, get fit by popping in an exercise DVD. For best results, I suggest not eating and watching the TV at the same time. Do one thing at a time. When you eat, just eat.

> *"Television knows no night. It is perpetual day. TV embodies our fear of the dark, of night, of the other side of things."*
> —Jean Baudrillard

Not only does excessive TV watching lead to health problems and increased exposure to violence, it steals our time. The four hours spent in front of the tube, tuning out the world, could be spent with your family, your partner, enjoying intimacy, sex, writing, sleeping, creating goals and hobbies for yourself, or assisting someone else rather than watching life pass you by.

"Creation is a better means of self-expression than possession. It's through creating not possessing that life is revealed."
—Vida D Scudder

Watching the box keeps us boxed in and inhibits our joyful participation in life. I hear people say that they don't have time to sit down to a nice meal lovingly prepared with their own hands, yet they have plenty of time to veg out in front of the flickering light of the TV set or waste time unwisely on the computer. I promise you that truly vegging out and preparing a raw, vegan meal will not take you anywhere near four hours, and will leave you feeling energized and excited, instead of deadened and desensitized. Worst of all, when watching TV late at night or searching the Internet for games and nothingness, all the fear-based obsessive thoughts that race through our minds after TV, and before our sleep end up invading our dreams. That is what we take to bed with us in our subconscious, and that is what we create. Create good thoughts and positive visualizations before going to sleep, and your sleep and the next day will be good as well.

Merrillism #35: "Lack of Expression Equals Depression."

Look, I'm not advocating throwing your television set(s) out the window; I'm just asking you to be a little more conscious about how much of it you are feeding your brain. Are you consuming a steady diet of violent crime, and eating celebrity gossip for dessert? How much TV are you really watching? Do you find it enjoyable and engaging? Or do you use TV to tune out, turn off the world, to not feel lonely, and not feel or silence the quiet voice inside you that is telling you there is more to life than the four walls that surround you? If your own voice is too quiet to hear then let me be the booming voice you can't ignore. Ask yourself these questions and answer them honestly.

Are you giving yourself a license to waste time? If you are currently devoting more time to watching other people act out imaginary lives than you are spending living yours, it might be time to make a shift. Turn it off! Instead of watching "reality" shows, give help to others. Is your life as rich as it could be? Can you go just one day without tuning in? How about a week or a month? I encourage you to try. Just one day. Let the raw lifestyle, these tools and suggestions start you on a healing, enlightening journey.

Sidebar to the Rawbar

Twenty-one things you can do to relax, engage and create (besides watching TV):

1. Enjoy the sunset.
2. Take your dog (or your spouse, child or self) for a walk in nature.
3. Paint or draw a picture.
4. Write anything—a poem, a book, a love letter, a thank-you note, or just journal.
5. Take a bubble bath (alone or with a lover).
6. Read a book.
7. Volunteer, donate or tithe your time, your talents, or your money.
8. Play board games.
9. Talk to your kids.
10. Do a little dance.
11. Make a little love.
12. Teach yourself to play guitar, piano, flute, drums or saxophone.
13. Go skating: roller, inline or ice.
14. Prepare a meal for people you love (that includes *you*).
15. Knit a scarf or sweater for you or a friend.

16. Play in the snow, the sand, the leaves, the ocean, or sit in the jacuzzi.
17. Give or get a massage or reflexology.
18 Hold hands in front of the fire.
19. Listen to music
20. Just breathe and meditate.
21. Eat a mango with your hands, naked, and get it all over you. Have fun, it's divaliciously delicious.

> *"The greatest danger in modern technology isn't that machines will begin to think like people, but that people will begin to think like machines."*
> —Author Unknown

Then of course there is the glowing box in your office, on your dining room table, in your bedroom, on your lap, in your purse or clipped to your belt. Most of us have a least one computer in our lives, and some of you have several. Before you fly into a panic, I'll tell you right up front that I'm not going to tell you to ditch your computer. Without one, most of us would be unable to work, generate income or shop, not to mention keep in touch with business associates, friends and family around the world. Thanks, in large part, to Steve Jobs, Bill Gates and a few other visionaries, personal computers are an integral part of most people's daily lives. In fact, it is entirely possible to live a wholly virtual life. Telecommuting makes it possible to work at home, and you can buy anything you could ever possibly want or need without ever leaving the house. From furniture to clothes, DVDs and books to groceries and raw products—nothing is out of reach. You can be entertained, go to school, chat with friends, and meet your mate, without ever stepping outside. Talk about living inside the box!

There is no doubt that the computer is a wonderful tool. It shrinks the world and makes it possible to reach millions of people, all across the globe, with a few keystrokes. A computer made it possible for me to write this book, find an agent/publisher and get it into your hands. As wonderful and liberating as the computer is in some respects, our reliance on it for absolutely *everything* can be incredibly isolating. Eyestrain and carpal tunnel are nothing compared to the hazards of living a virtual life. Even though I wrote my book in longhand and spoke into a tape recorder and edited it over the telephone, my thumbs were killing me. I don't like sitting, and being confined inside for long periods of time, I get claustrophobic, antsy and irritable. Sitting for long hours does not make me feel alive and in high vibe. I like to be moving and grooving!

I am all for using computers, just don't let your computer use you. Nothing can replace human contact. Don't let your computer isolate you from others in the world. You can't look someone in the eye, and hold his or her hand online. You can't read someone's body language or be with someone else's being, online. The computer is a valuable tool, but it is not a substitute for loving, sharing, communicating, expanding, touching, inspiring, connecting, relating, building intimacy, and reaching out. So, when you leave the office tonight, leave your computer behind too. You may be surprised at what you've been missing—people, connection and intimacy. Be open to spontaneity and "what ifs." Don't take work to bed with you or on vacation. Let this book be your roadmap to divinity. Start small but think big.

> "When you cook it should be an act of love. To put a
> frozen bag in the microwave for your child is an act of hate."
> —Raymond Blanc

As a raw fooder, I obviously don't own a microwave oven or even a stove for that matter. I haven't had or used a stove in 18 years. But, to tell you the truth, I probably wouldn't own a microwave even if I still cooked my food. You may not realize it, but that little box inside your kitchen is quite possibly a big health hazard. Over 90% of American households own microwave ovens. The FDA says that they are safe for use but acknowledge that more research is needed to determine how microwaves affect the human body. The fact is, many scientific questions about exposure to low levels of microwaves have not been answered satisfactorily, yet we continue to use them—simply trusting that they are safe. Instant food isn't always instant energy, unless it's a fresh picked fruit or vegetable. God gave us hands to pick and brains to plant, so do it.

Merrillism #36: "If Your Food Is not Organic and Raw It's a Waste of Your Chewing."

I'm not a scientist, nor am I an expert on microwave ovens but I do remember that food heated in them never tasted quite as good as homemade food cooked in the oven or on the stove. It just wasn't the same. (Although, I have to admit that food cooked any which way doesn't taste right to me now that my diet has evolved.) When I was growing up my mother never owned or used a microwave, and I have never owned one. There have been numerous studies on the effects of microwave heating, and at the very least, this type of cooking can significantly deplete food of its nutrients, water, oxygen and natural flavor, even more so than other, conventional methods of heating. Not to mention the chemicals that may enter the food in the process.

I did a little digging and came across German and Russian studies on the ill effects of microwave cooking on the human body. In fact, there are numerous scientific reports which state microwaves not only distort the molecular structure of the foods, and destroy most of the nutrients, but over time, the radiation causes many problems with the immune system. Do your own research and decide for yourself. The websites www.HealingDaily.com and www.Mercola.com have very comprehensive articles citing various studies. After reading these articles, I can tell you that if I had a microwave, it would have found itself at the recycling center faster than you can heat up a TV dinner. I'm not telling you what to do, I'm just asking you to consider the possibility that microwave "cooking" may not be the most healthful way to prepare your food. It's up to you to decide for yourself. Speed is not the answer to great health. Do less in more time. The slower you go, the faster you go and know and grow.

Living inside all of these boxes keeps us from living a raw life—a meaningful, rich life. An exciting, painless, joy filled, exhilarating, peaceful existence is out there awaiting you now. The most confining box of all is the one we have created in our own minds. We become prisoners of our own thoughts, and are too afraid to step outside of what is comfortable. We stay inside our self-created box because it is familiar and safe. Like all human beings, we fear what we do not know, what we have not yet uncovered and discovered. Part of my personal success, and the reason I live a happy, fulfilled, complete, raw life is that I am willing to look, reach and teach. I consistently step outside my comfort zone, take good orderly direction, try new things, create new experiences, learn, stretch, grow and do what I don't yet know is possible. I do what I am afraid of. Don't misunderstand, I still get nervous and scared, and sometimes "what if" and doubt myself to death; but then I go out and *do it anyway*. It's an invigorating way to go through life. I hate to be afraid of anything. I feel when I am afraid of something I must do and conquer it. The process of writing this book was part of my going through the fear and willingness to step outside the box, and my comfort zone. I knew I had something to say, a story to tell, knowledge to share, inspiration and motivation to contribute to the world, but I did not know I had the means to express it. *Until I did.* Until I wrote it and shared my message.

I encourage you to step outside of *your* box. Reach beyond what you know, seize the moment, say yes to life and yourself, and look for opportunities to share, to grow, to participate, to create, and to shine. Look for opportunities to go through your fears and tears, and find your blind spots. Give up the "I wish" and say, "I am." The only way out is through it. Luck is the name losers give to failure. I love my life today, and I love that I have created what I want in my life. I want you to experience the joy of living a raw life that you love too.

Raw Bites

- **Live outside the box.** *Get rid of at least one box in your life today. Spend a day without television; turn off your computer or your cell phone. Give away the microwave. Go through your cupboard and eliminate everything that comes in a box. Let your mind run free. The raw food diet helps one maintain grace in the face of adversity.*

- *When there is a food obsession, it's all about the food but it's not about the food. Food is a symptom, a marker for a deeper problem. When we get right with ourselves, our food usually gets right. When we get right with our food, our lives get right. Look within to begin.*

- *Eat for need, not for greed.*

- *Let go of your inner critic and have more compassion for yourself.*

- *My body keeps going and my health is a reflection of that choice.*

- *Stagnation is constipation and procrastination.*

- *Raw food hits the spot, and it doesn't have to be hot.*

Chapter 19

Harvest the Fruit

"Behold, I have given you every herb yielding seed,
which is on the surface of all the earth, and every tree,
which bears fruit yielding seed. It will be your food."
—Genesis 1:29

Fruit is often called nature's candy and, as a reformed sugarholic, I can tell you that fruit is indeed a sweet treat. It's also a beauty food, natural cleanser and detoxifier. Fruit is *real* fast food. It can be eaten as a meal, a snack or dessert; or if you prefer, you can drink your fruit as a juice or blend your favorites together and create your own smoothie. According to the USDA, adults should consume at least two to four servings (a serving is one cup) of fruit every day. I say, that sounds like a great start. As part of my *Raw on the Roll Success System*, I recommend you do that amount or more if you are exercising everyday. Only consume fruit that is fresh, ripe, whole, raw and organic to ensure you receive the maximum benefit. Most fruit is not picked ripe. So, select your fruit carefully. By selecting ripe, organic fruit you'll be more effective by being more selective. With a little practice, you will actually get really good at selecting the ripest, sweetest fruits, and most flavorful vegetables by using only your eyes, smell and sense of touch. I am a great fruit and veggie picker. I intuitively know which ones are the most tasty. Strangers stop me in markets and ask me to pick fruits and veggies for them. I'm happy to help them and meet great people.

Merrillism #37: "Eat Fruit, and Stay Cute."

Water is an essential part of life and most of us don't get enough of it, or we do the opposite and try to drown ourselves in H_2O; but the truth is, you don't need to flood your system with water in order to cleanse it. You do need to drink water of course, but if you also eat foods with high water content, you won't need to drink quite as much of it. Fruit is about 80% water, and rich in nutrition. Since the human body is made up of approximately 50% water for women, to 60% water for men, doesn't it make good sense to nourish it with a food that is 80% water and contains natural sugar for energy? Let's face it, not only does fruit give us energy, its sweetness makes us sweet and happy, it makes us smile. Eat fruit, and be energized and happy. Have a great treat, eat fruit as a sweet.

Please always select organic, it's found to be more nutritious than ordinary produce and helps lengthen people's lives. There are more antioxidants in organic food, cutting the risk of cancer and heart disease. To me, an organic apple has way more flavor than a non-organic apple.

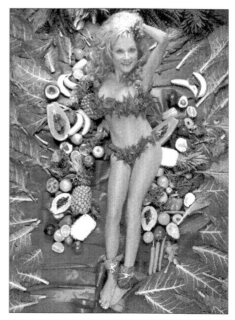

One of the main benefits you receive from eating water-filled foods is increased energy. The reason is simple. Everything you eat must be broken down and digested

I say: Eat fruit, and stay cute!

into essential elements so that the nutrition can be absorbed, and the waste eliminated. The process of digestion takes two things—time and energy. For instance, a steak can take up to ten hours to digest, which means that a T-bone eaten at lunch time, will not be fully digested until you are ready for bed or even the next day. A fruit salad only takes a half hour or so to digest, which means that its energy producing nutrition is dispersed to your body quickly and efficiently, because it has less waste and toxins to eliminate allowing energy to go right to you. If your body isn't busy digesting food, it will have more energy for other things—like thinking, dancing, skating, gardening, creating, and writing. I know that the more vegetables and fruit I consume, the quicker, clearer and brighter my thinking becomes. I feel more creative, and have more energy to spend on living my life and doing what I love with those I love. Have you ever watched someone, or even yourself, sweating after eating a high animal content or cooked meal? You don't sweat when you eat mangos, tomatoes or strawberries. That's because digesting fruit takes very little energy. The reason you feel tired, toxic and lazy when you consume a diet of cooked, overly-processed, fatty, salty foods is because of the time and energy required to digest those foods, and the toxins in those foods. As a result, your brain and body is drained of energy. You literally numb out, as if you were taking a drug. What a waste of time and chewing! You receive nothing from this type of food—no energy, inspiration, motivation or innovation. Eating watery foods, which take less time to digest, gives your body stamina, strength, cleanliness, beauty, and water which all vibrates the life force. You want to get up and get rolling, instead of sit around, resting and digesting.

There are a multitude of health benefits that come with putting down the fork and picking up the plant. For example, eating a diet rich in fruits and vegetables may reduce your risk for stroke and other cardiovascular diseases, reduce your risk for Type 2 diabetes and protect against certain cancers like mouth, stomach and colorectal cancer. Most fruits are naturally low in fat, sodium and calories, and none contain cholesterol. Fruits provide important nutrients like potassium, dietary fiber, vitamin C and A, and folate (folic acid). Potassium is important in maintaining healthy blood pressure. Fiber helps reduce blood cholesterol levels, may lower your risk of heart disease, and is essential for proper bowel function. In addition, fiber rich foods fill you up without adding unnecessary calories, which aids in weight loss and maintaining weight. Vitamin C repairs all body tissues, helps cuts and wounds heal, and keeps teeth and gums healthy. It also is the beauty vitamin. Vitamin C keeps us looking young. Folate helps the body form red blood cells, and reduces the risk of neural tube defects, such as spina bifida and anencephaly during fetal development.

Merrillism #38: "Raw Fruits and Vegetables Are the Best Snack to Give You That Rawsome, Awesome Energy to Bounce Back."

The best way to consume fruit is raw, skin and all, either alone or 30 minutes before a meal. You can eat it whole, cut up, or pressed into juice or smoothie. It's important to consume fresh squeezed juice so that you retain all the nutrients and fibers of the whole fruit. You can use a Vita-Mix® blender or juicer to create sweet, satisfying juicy drinks. Juicing is an easy way to get your daily fruit in one shot—it's portable, and gives you a quick energy boost anytime, anywhere. It is vitally important to consume fresh juice you squeeze yourself because juice found in cans, glass bottles or cartons may have been pasteurized or flash pasteurized. Pasteurization heats or cooks food to kill germs, but it also changes the enzymes found in fruits and vegetables, and diminishes their nutritional value. Watch out for "flash pasteurized," it means it has been heated quickly, but it's not raw, and it's still pasteurized. When I eat fruit, I like to let my mouth be the first to cut Mother Nature's food, so I usually eat it whole, eliminating machines, tools, utensils and gadgets, except for my delicious Mango and Persimmon Smoothie (see recipe section.) Eating fruit this way naturally eliminates preservatives in your food. Eliminate preservatives, toxins and chemicals in your food, and you will preserve your body.

As I have said again and again, the key to long term success is to start slowly. Be the turtle, not the hare. Remember, going slower gets you there faster. If you are not used to eating much (or any) fruit, your body may start to detoxify if you suddenly start eating five servings. So, take it easy. Eat one more fruit today than you ate yesterday. Do that for a week and then eat two more, until eventually you are eating three to four or more fruits every day, or less, see what works best for you. Please remember, tomatoes, olives, cucumbers, avocados and young organic Thai coconuts are fruits as well, they are just lower on the glycemic index. If you want to jump start your system, and can tolerate some of the discomfort that comes with your body's natural cleansing process, then by all means go for it. You can use fruit to accelerate the detoxification process by eating two to three or more servings per day and not eating anything except fruit until noon each day. Acid fruits like grapefruit and lemons, oranges or any citrus fruit, provide the strongest detoxifying effect. Try drinking a morning juice mix of oranges, tangerines, grapefruit and a little lemon and ginger, followed by a mid morning melon or mango smoothie with spirulina to get your blood pumping and your body glowing. Fast or slow, the most important thing is to start. Begin adding fruit to your diet today and you will feel better, have more get up and go, look younger and have more vitality. Have fruit before or after your workout instead of pasta and baked potatoes. You'll put more pep in your step and add a zip in your trip. Your skin will glow, your body will flow and you will know you are on the rawkin' raw road of happy bliss. I always tell my students, give up eating for gratification, validation and recreation. Eat for need not for greed. When you eat light and eat right, your star will shine bright. Remember these little snippets when in doubt about what to eat or what not to eat.

Raw Bites

- *Try one of my favorite fruit smoothie recipes.*
- *If you must eat at night, especially late, instead of milk and cookies, have a fruit snack. It's not heavy on your body and digests quickly. I love a persimmon, mango or papaya smoothie. Add some blueberries, banana, or apples and a little spirulina and it really hits the spot. (All these fruits help me sleep and give me peace and contentment).*
- *Instead of fast food, eat fast fruit. It's quick, easy, portable and delicious. It's truly Mother Nature's fast food. God gave us hands to pick and brains to plant. Plant a fruit tree in your backyard. Save money and get your fruit fast and organic whenever you want.*
- *Eat seasonally. I don't crave apples in the summertime. How could I when there are peaches, plums, apricots, mangoes, papayas, pineapples, nectarines, and watermelon to enjoy?*
- *Goji berries are one of my favorite treats because they contain 18 kinds of amino acids, including all 8 essential amino acids, 21 trace minerals, vitamins B1, B2, B6 and vitamin E, and they are a source of protein. To top it off, they're the number one source of carotenoids and they're known to stimulate the production of human growth hormone (HGH), which is associated with youth and longevity. (These are my favorites for snacks, toppings, trail mixes and great for traveling too.) You can also soak them in water to rehydrate them and drink the juice from the berries and then eat the berries.*

- *The key to happiness is to eat the rainbow. All those colors will keep you colorful and beautiful, inside and out.*
- *Trade your processed energy bars for fruit. Fruit will give you a quick burst of energy naturally without the high fats and sugars. Fruit is fresh; You never know how long those bars have been sitting on the shelf!*
- *Do not eat fruit and vegetables together at the same meal. Except for pineapple, papaya and avocado.*
- *Create your own Avocado Bravado dip.*
- *Eat great, exercise great, energy great.*
- *Raw foods let the good times roll.*
- *Employ Mother Nature in your home and backyard. She is the best chef in the world.*
- *The time is now. It couldn't be more ripe to eat more organic fruits and shoots (live sprouts). See the impossible become the possible for yourself with health and fitness.*

Chapter 20

Emulation: The Next Step in Creative Visualization

"What you visualize, vocalize and physicalize, you materialize. Speak it, think it, and ink it!"
—Debbie Merrill

"If you don't create change, change will create you."
—Author Unknown

Creative visualization is a transformative tool that can reshape your life, from the inside out. Your imagination acts as a preview of your life's coming attractions (Einstein), and by envisioning your life as you wish it to be—healthy, brilliant, powerfully free and bright—you will have taken the first step in making your inner vision a reality. Practicing conscious, creative visualization on a daily basis will help you become the prolific, happy, athletic, extraordinary person you were meant to be. By living a vibrant, beautiful, loving and unstoppable life, the true you emerges. Actually, you already perform visualization every day whether you are conscious of it or not. Waking dreams, or daydreams, are really just visualizations that start with a kernel of thought and expand—like a movie unfolding inside the mind. Creative visualization is the process of directing those daydreams by consciously imagining what we desire, be it an object (like a house, car, money, acting role or lover). It can be a state of being (perfect health), your perfect body shape, or a situation (such as a career change, vacation to Fiji, a new relationship or writing a book or screenplay). That's why I had you create a treasure map.

Creative visualization works on two levels: on the one hand, the scenario you imagine is impressed upon the subconscious mind, creating an unfulfilled need that your brain will continuously try to satisfy until you achieve your goal. In other words, what we believe, perceive, and conceive, we can achieve. What you visualize, vocalize and physicalize, you can manifest in your life. Your mind will look for ways to make your dream come true, and you will take actions that bring you closer to achieving it—that's the "law of attraction." The other level is a bit more abstract and may require a leap of faith. The principal is that our thoughts are the blueprints for our actions, and our emotions are the energy source that powers the thoughts into action. Speaking it into being, declaring it, announcing it and manifesting it so it can be sent back to you. By focusing on all our thoughts, feelings and words, the combined energy that goes out into the Universe will attract the object or situation that we desire. The Universe responds to our every need. We must be ready to receive it as well. Receiving is key here. In other words, ask and you shall receive! Please make sure you are not sabotaging, blocking or denying the receiving of your requests and declarations. I find that when I am in fear, I find a way to sabotage it all, i.e. get rid of it, push it away, deny it, injure myself, or block myself from receiving it. Our thoughts, especially when intensely focused, possess extraordinary power and can change the energy fields that surround us, thereby causing them to shift and manifest change in the physical world. Think of it as an advanced course in, "Fake It 'Til You Make It." The truth is, you are not faking it, you are *being* it and drawing it to you. Wow, how powerful we all are!

Creative visualization is magical but it is not magic. You don't visualize living in a mansion in Beverly Hills, and a mansion just appears out of thin air—or perhaps it may. It's more about windows of opportunities that open and allow you to make your own dreams come true—through the people, places and things that you synchronistically connect with and then act upon. You may be offered a new job that will give you the income required to increase your standard of living, or you may see an ad for a housemate in the neighborhood you have always dreamed of living in. It's about being open to the possibilities life offers you, and acting upon the opportunities when they arise with 100% of your intention and ability. When I was a little girl, I pictured myself skating in the sunshine, long blonde hair blowing back behind me, feeling like a flying angel, jumping and spinning in the sky like I was Peter Pan. I love that feeling of flying high. For years, I used to dream of flying, skating, and jumping four to five revolutions in the air. When I skate I feel like I'm flying, like a bird. Today, that is my reality. I skate on the bike path several times a week into the sunset with the ocean as my mascot, the mountains as my master, and the sun and the moon as my guiding lights. I didn't manifest that dream immediately, but in time, I was finally ready to accept that my dream could be a reality. It happened in spite of myself. I rediscovered my high school quote, "Let your dreams become your reality" while writing this book and it blew me away. How synchronistic! My path was certainly not straight and narrow, but as twisted as it was, it was always *my* road and it got me to where I am today. I am the founder of Skate Great School of Skating on lovely Santa Monica Beach, California teaching the world to skate safe, fun, and easy with the wind in their hair and mine. I want to help you discover your path so that you too can experience the joy of being on the right road—*your* road. The road you choose and desire, not someone else's wants and desires for you. Follow your heart and do what you love, trust your instincts and act now. Be fabulous, do extraordinary things, and have magnificence in your life. Make up your mind to be, do and have this now. Get on your road of happy bliss. Better yet, get on the rawkin' raw road of happy bliss.

The How of It

"Don't ask why, ask how. Why-ing is dying."

Now that you understand the *why* of creative visualization, it's time to explore the *how*. Since you are already familiar with positive affirmations and treasure mapping, taking the next step should be relatively easy. **The first step is to define your goal.** What is it, exactly, that you want to manifest? Again, you can't get what you don't know you want! Do you want something material, like a new car or a larger home, or do you desire a change in career or to fall in love, more cash flow, or do you want a fit body, a healthy mind and a happy spirit? Check in with yourself to make sure that what you say you want is what you truly desire, and that it is harmonious with the Universe. If you become stuck and fearful, ask your higher spirit to be released of the fear. So be careful of what you ask for, because you *may* get it. It is important to have integrity with yourself and others as you manifest your dreams.

Next, find a quiet place to sit or lie down, where you have some privacy and can relax. Take deep, rhythmic breaths, and relax your entire body, head to toe. Relax your mind and breathe. If you have trouble with this step, I suggest you pick up a book on meditation so you can learn some relaxation techniques. **Now, visualize the object or situation that you desire.** I used to practice this creative visualization technique with landing my skating jumps and going through my samba dance routine effortlessly, eloquently and gracefully! This creative visualization meditation is taught to Olympic athletes today and it works. It helps them achieve tremendous success and win gold medals. Once you have the vision, hold it in your mind and see it through by adding detail, clarity, color, names, sound, energy, power, time, and let it flow. Really imagine yourself doing the thing or using the object, and let the vision expand. Imagine how you would feel and behave if it were already your reality. See yourself closing the deal, walking down the aisle, getting the standing ovation. Engage all of your senses—what do you smell, taste, touch, hear and see? What is your emotional state? Really let go, and feel the feelings as you "act out" your vision. Think of it as a daydream that you control—you are writing, rewriting, recording, rehearsing, sharing it and filming the preview of your life's coming attraction. Let it be the Academy Award winning movie for your Oscar winning performance.

Practice this at least once or twice a day for about ten minutes at a time until your dreams manifest. (Preferably in the morning upon awakening and before going to bed at night.) You are powerful and you don't know it yet. That's the real truth; it's not a mystery after all. Keep your mind and spirit open so that you recognize the opportunities when they arrive. Think about your goal during the day, and when negative thoughts surrounding your goal pop in to your mind, reframe them as positive statements. Remind yourself of who you are—a powerful, extraordinary, fearless, loving person capable of it all. For now, you may want to keep your goals private but when you are comfortable, you may find it valuable to share them with others. Therefore you are declaring it out loud for all to hear, and you are also staying committed to it by letting others hear your dreams and desires. When two or more are gathered, the higher spirit will work through. Get support and acknowledgment.

It goes a long way towards building self-esteem, courage and motivation. When sharing your dreams and goals, it is important to choose wisely. Make sure you confide in someone you trust, and who will support you in your endeavors. Practice makes progress, and improves momentum. If you are eating a good 40-60% raw food diet during this process, it will definitely put some pep in your step and a zip in your trip, and keep your lights on and connected. It will help transform you from physicality to originality to spirituality, while living in reality, much quicker. If you are in love and joy, you will attract love and joy. Have an attitude of gratitude. Don't be hateful, be grateful, and keep your desires on fire.

Emulation, Declaration, Creation

Merrillism #39: "Take What You Like and Leave The Rest if It's not for Your Best."

Only you have the power to envision and create the life that you desire, but you don't have to do it alone. It is your journey, but we all need a jump-start, some inspiration and a support system. You can begin by hanging out with winners. While you are trying to find your own road to better health, make it your business to find out what healthy people are doing and do the same. I discovered early on that one of the best ways to improve my own life was to seek out people who already had what I wanted. Like many people, I learned by example by observing and trusting others. So, in order to succeed, I sought out leaders to follow until I was ready to lead myself. When I was a young skater, just starting out, Peggy Fleming was my idol. She had everything I wanted as a competitive figure skater, so I imitated her. I found out what she did to get where she was, and I did that. I practiced as hard as she did, I trained my body in the same way she did, and I emulated her style. I copied her skating moves, dressed like her, wore my hair like her, trained in the same skates, and even skated to some of her same music. You could say I discovered my inner Peggy Fleming. When Dorothy Hamill started coming up, I emulated her as well, skating and training alongside her. I even trained with her same coaches. My mom and her mom became friends. We even belonged to the same skating club in Rye, New York. I acted "as if" I was already a champion skater, and that helped propel me forward in the sport. Later on, when I turned my attention to teaching and health education, I found successful teachers, raw foodists and other gurus and mentors to coach and inspire me. Marianne Williamson was a huge inspiration to me: I read her books, listened to her tapes and lectures on *A Course In Miracles*, and I emulated her actions as well; I even completed the "Course" workbook and Teacher's Manual in her workshops, which led me to become my own teacher, author, speaker and lecturer. Four women whom I strongly admire and want to be like are Marianne Williamson, Madonna, Mother Theresa and Oprah Winfrey. I feel there is a bit of the best of all of them in me. I see myself mushrooming into this wonderful, inspirational leader. I acted my way into this role, and so can you.

Merrillism #40: "Don't Take Advice From Anyone Who Does not Have What You Want."

Life comes without instructions, so find a guru or a mentor in life—find someone you admire, someone to look up to, someone who has gone before you, and who has what you want. Work with them, listen to what they have to say, read their books, listen to audio books and go to seminars—then take what works for you and discard the rest. Please don't only listen to speeches, listen for solutions. We don't need more rhetoric, we need more reality. When you are seeking out your heroes and teachers, it is important to look for *your* people. Never listen to anyone who does not have what you want. When I seek out a teacher, healer or leader, I'm not interested in how much they know; I'm interested in how much they care. Great teachers not only show their brilliance, strength and power, they bring that out in others. They show you how to tap into your inner resources, and become the best person you can be. They empower you to empower yourself. That is true greatness. I want to learn from greatness, be around greatness and be greatness. How about you? As I said before, luck is the name losers give to failure. Practice saying, "And, so it is," and then, it *will be*, because you say so. Be extraordinary!

I said it, I meant it, and now I represent it, and you can represent it too, in your life and in the lives of those around you. Be a natural born healer and heal your life now, and the life of others you love and care about. Be rawliciously fabulous.

Your Crazy Makers

"Everybody around us really believed in us and motivated us and all the people that didn't, we dropped them. You've got to know you're a beautiful person inside and out and you shouldn't let anyone tear that away."
—Venus Williams

Get away from other people's negative thinking. It's like being behind enemy lines. Please don't let the negative thoughts of others run around rent-free in your head either. On the other side of emulation, we owe it to ourselves to get rid of the toxic people in our lives. We owe it to ourselves to hang out with people who help us shine and be powerful; in return, we help them do the same for themselves. It is the key to physical and spiritual balance. This step is not always easy, but it is necessary. Some of the crazy makers and energy vampires have been in our lives for a long time. They may be family members, friends or business associates and very often, we don't even know they are bad for us. As you become healthier yourself, you will begin to discover who the toxic people are in your life. I can walk into a room and immediately know who the negative person is, and I also know where the light is. It has become second nature for me and, as you heal, you will find it easier to differentiate between the two, become sensitive to both energies and as you grow spiritually, your instincts become sharper and you are able to identify and eliminate the crazy makers in your life.

For now, be alert to those well-meaning friends who always have a "yeah, but" when you talk about your goals, dreams and accomplishments. In an attempt to be helpful, they will give you a million reasons why something won't work in order to "protect" you from impending disappointment, and stop you from succeeding because they are not doing their own dreams. Misery loves company. If you succeed, what will happen to them and their complaining conversations with you? People make the best company when they are doing what they love. There are folks out there for whom gossip is a team sport and who rarely have anything nice or positive to share about friends, family members, colleagues or society. The Negative Nancys tend to stick together, so let them. And then there are the saboteurs who take you out for cheeseburgers right after you tell them you are a raw vegan. You also want to be alert to the victims and the martyrs; they are just as dangerous as the saboteurs. You know the type—your aunt, cousin, brother, college friend, coworker or business partner who always seems to whine, complain and have problems. It's always "Poor me" and "Why me?" They are walking victims. Nothing ever seems to go their way, and they constantly complain about their plight but never take any steps to change it, or take responsibility for it. They ask for advice but never listen and never change. They "but" you on everything. It's all a cry for love and attention. It's like a tape recording playing the same old sad song on an endless loop. I call these people energy suckers, crazy makers, energy vampires, songbirds (they sing the same old sad songs, time and time again) but if you keep them in your life—the real sucker is you. When I let go of the vampires and the crazy makers, my life took off, and I stopped sucking on LifeSavers®, candy, lollipops, gum and ice cream cones. So I didn't abandon them, mind you, I was willing to help, to be of service, but only if they were willing to let go of their victim status and do something about their issues. Whining is far from winning. Some did let go but most stayed stuck in the mud of their own martyrdom. The truth is, most people simply aren't willing to get off it, change, give up what's not working for them or let it go. Change only comes when one is willing. Willingness comes when one is willing to act move and do. They are too comfortable in the role of "martyr for the cause," self-delusions, defiance and defending their addictions and themselves. Well, I'm here to tell you that the most important cause you can fight for is your own. Only then will you be strong enough to reach out and help others. **When a man thinketh, so he is.** Surround yourself with loving, powerful, bright, healthy, creative, spiritual people, friends and family. Surround yourself with what you want to be, and let go of the toxic waste and toxic people in your life and diet. Now get going, today.

Raw Bites

- *Now go and do the best you can just for today.*
- *While you're judging yourself by your thoughts, the world is judging you by your actions.*
- *Get out, get going and get out of the complaining of the company of others.*

- *You can't go from A to Z. You have to go from A to B to C to D and so on.*
- *Learn to say "No." "No" is a complete sentence.*
- *Learn to say "Goodbye."*
- *Be willing to eliminate people, places and things that don't serve you.*
- *Your only problem is you forgot who you are and why you came here (from* A Course In Miracles*).*

Chapter 21

Three Steps Forward, Ten Steps Backwards

"The greatest glory in living lies not in never falling, but in rising every time we fall."
—Marianne Williamson

Delay is not denial, and there is no such thing as failure—only slow successes. Be a survivor in life. Survivors always win. When you survive one thing, you survive everything. There are going to be moments, hours, days, maybe even weeks, when you feel like you are going in reverse. You take three small, arduous steps forward only to run backwards ten. You can be zipping along just fine—eating foods you know are good for you, moving your body, living creatively and then POW! You fall off the wagon. Perhaps a particularly stressful day at work, a fight with your spouse, a rejection or lack of funds prompts you to indulge in fried onion rings for lunch, or to skip the gym and veg out in front of the TV while eating ice cream straight from the carton. It happens. Sometimes you fall down and get right back up, other times you fall and decide to hang out on the floor for a while. While you're down there, start asking and praying for help. I pray and take time to exercise every day. That is one of the things that work for me when I am down. Find out what's eating you so you don't eat at it. For every unshed pound there is an unexpressed emotion or tear. The less you carry around, the longer you are around. So, it's okay to stay down for a while, as long as you get back up. It doesn't have to be immediate. You may stay down for a day or two or three. The important thing is that you get up. It's okay to slip and fall, just don't take up permanent residence down there. Remember, prayer is medicine, and the spirit is your food for the soul.

The truth is, any time you endeavor to do something new, you will experience difficulties. It's inevitable. Although it doesn't seem like it at the time, those setbacks and challenges are there to prepare you for success. I suggest that instead of thinking of roadblocks, rejections and breakdowns as failures and reasons to quit, you recognize them for what they truly are: stepping-stones to huge breakthroughs, openings and new constructions; destruction equals construction. It's like taking off the eye make-up. You know, the "I" make-up. The stuff we make up to cover up what's up. (Usually the truth) That's what "I" make-up is for. Take it off and more will be revealed to you. Give up the self-delusion and illusion of perfection and you will shine through just like new, I promise you. Always do the right thing!

> *"Age wrinkles the body. Quitting wrinkles the soul."*
> —Douglas MacArthur

When the answers come from something other than you, you will believe there is something greater in you. When I was learning a new move in figure skating, trying to master a double axel for the first time, or learning a new jump, I fell down a lot. I spent more time on my behind than in the air. It's just the way it was. I accepted it, and I learned a valuable lesson. Right at the point when it seemed that I would never get it, that my body would not, could not, perform and I wanted to quit, take off my skates and give up—it would happen. I'd get up one more time and execute the perfect jump. It was as if I had wings on my feet, and I was suddenly able to perform that which previously seemed impossible—perfectly. Eventually I realized that this happened every single time. My biggest breakthroughs in skating were always preceded by breakdowns and fall downs. Every time I reached a plateau, a point where it seemed like my skill just stopped, like it was impossible, and I told myself I couldn't do it, try as I might, make it to the next level, I'd backslide. My performance would suffer for a while and then, because I persevered, a miracle would happen. I think it was the release of the rage and frustration, giving up and surrendering that allowed me to relax into it and be able to allow it to happen. Then it came to me, effortlessly and easily. Skating is a metaphor for me about how to handle stress, emotions and challenges in my life. I understand now, not to build challenges up, *catastrophize* them and make snowballs into avalanches, or to hold on tight, quit and then be resentful it didn't happen the way I planned it. Quite the contrary, it's about letting it happen, going with the flow, letting go of the attachment to how it should look. For me it's about showing up and being in the joy, fun, ease and greatness of the experience, staying committed and accepting the results.

This is a hard lesson to learn. Training as a figure skater, I learned it the hard way: hard knocks on the head, hips and knees. But, if there's no pain there's no gain. Pain is a motivator. I have a lot to show for these lessons today—knee surgery, uneven hips, broken wrist, a stress fracture in my leg and a sensitive neck. However, there are still thousands of more miles for me to roll on these wheels. I'm not done yet. I'm on a mission with a new rendition: *To skate and educate the world back to health and fitness,* back to *The Raw Truth To The Fountain of Youth.* What I can do on wheels, I can do in heels. My biggest successes always follow my biggest setbacks—in skating, my health, my career, relationships, spirituality, finances, family, everything. The saying, "It's always darkest before the dawn" is a great truth. Three days of darkness equals a ray of light. Our bodies, minds and spirits need time, space and darkness to prepare for the next level so, whether we like it or not, we fall back a bit before leaping forward. It's part of the process, of giving time, time. However good or bad a situation is, it'll change.

So, please, ***don't quit before the miracle.*** That has been the lesson of my life and, if you only remember one thing from this book, let it be that. It is the reason I say, "Always quit from a point of achievement rather than failure," knowing you have accomplished your goal. Once you do something to completion, you may make another decision. You may say, "Hey I came, I saw, I conquered and it's not for me. I'm moving on." That is success. That is quitting from a point of achievement. For instance, when a basketball player takes a shot, he completes it and moves on to the next shot. He doesn't stand there and dwell on the last shot. He keeps running to the next basket. We must do the same; complete it and move on. NEXT! Life is like a basketball game. We can't dwell on the past, we must keep on going, learn from our mistakes, and see what's missing in our greatness, not what's wrong in our greatness. Envy, greed, resentment, anger and self-righteousness are a waste of time, as you already have all you need.

Merrillism #41: "Practice, Persistence and Patience Equals Permanence."

So, while you are traveling down the road to health, keep rolling, no matter what. Celebrate when you are moving forward, and love yourself when you fall back. Don't have judgment around your mistakes, or where you are at any given time. You're going to slip, you're going to fall back, and you're going to eat junk food—just get back up on the road. Think of yourself like the punching bag at the fair that keeps popping back up every time you hit it. It's resistant and resilient. Be resilient. Please don't judge what you do as good or bad. Please don't interpret your mistakes as something wrong with you. Don't take no for an answer. Be unstoppable. You are a human being, not a human doing. If you don't make mistakes, you don't know and grow. See where you've gone wrong, correct your mistakes, then do it differently, do it better, do it over, do it again. It's no big deal. See the imperfections in it and learn the lesson instead. Laugh at yourself. Tell on yourself. It's exciting, inviting and fun. Wear life loosely. Lighten up. The lighter you are on yourself, the lighter you are on others, and the lighter your body will become. The harder you are on yourself, the heavier your heart, and your body, will become. Love yourself back to health; don't beat yourself back to health. Please don't pick up the bad in the world and others, pick up the good in you and others. And if you feel compelled to hit yourself over the head, use a feather, rather than a hammer. Let go of "shoulda, coulda, woulda," and treat yourself with patience, love, compassion and tolerance. Take the almighty pause before you judge. Compliment and acknowledge yourself and others instead. Remember you are too blessed to be stressed.

Raw Bites

- *You may not like what I have to say, but you will relate to me in a very special way.*
- *You cannot heal what you cannot feel and deal with. Learn to feel, it's okay.*
- *It's okay for you to have a fit body, a healthy mind, and a happy spirit.*
- *As you become weak in the ego, you become stronger in organic intelligence.*

- *Understand yourself and you will have great health.*
- *Challenges make us stronger. Just like lifting weights, they strengthen our bones and make them stronger. The more we challenge ourselves, the stronger we get in all areas. So challenge yourself with the raw food diet and you will get stronger. Weight lifting is my solution to osteoporosis, not drugs. I am living proof of this. I have been lifting weights for the past eight years and my bone density has improved and become stable without drugs. My doctor says to me, "Whatever you're doing, keep doing it. It's working." I keep doing weight bearing exercises everyday and I hope you will too. I keep challenging my bones, and they keep getting stronger. It's safe, fun, simple, easy and free, and it works for me.*
- *Be a trailblazer, not a dream gazer.*
- *Do one thing that you think you cannot. Keep doing it until you know that you can. There is no greater feeling in the world for me, as accomplishing something I never thought I could do. Esteemable acts give you self-esteem.*
- *You are already a winner, now be a winner at dinner.*
- *Forgive everyone for everything.*

Chapter 22

Get In the God

"Nature is the one place where miracles not only happen,
but they happen all the time."
—Thomas Wolfe

The closer to Nature you are the better you will feel with your food as well. The closer food is kept in an unheated, untreated state the more nutritionally complete it typically is and the more perfect, whole and complete you are. Eating raw for that awesome awe.

One of the best things I have ever done for myself, in addition to choosing a raw, vegan lifestyle, was to move to Southern California and create a business that allows me to spend the majority of my time outdoors in nature. I often joke that the overhead in my business is high—the sun and the sky. My office is the beach. I spend 80% of my day in GOD, what I call the "<u>G</u>ood <u>O</u>ut <u>D</u>oors." If I could sleep outside, I would. I am fortunate in that my profession as a health educator and skating instructor allows me to revel in nature on a daily basis. I am able to walk in the sand, dip my feet in the ocean, and feel the sun and wind on my face every single day. I find that being outdoors in nature centers me, and even in skates, my feet are firmly planted on the ground because I am connected to nature. I frequently go on solitary sunset skates and sun gaze; it's a rolling meditation for me: I look at the sun and say affirmations to

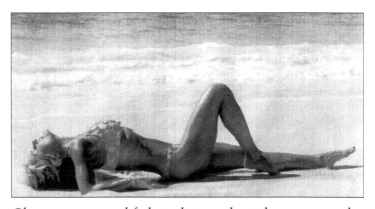

Close your eyes and feel, go deep, smile at the sun, remember to breath, delight in your senses, give in to pleasure. Prayer is asking, meditation is listening. I am the one I have been waiting for. Nature is the place I go for both.

the vast, open, abundant mountains, sky and ocean, with no music or chatter, just me and nature. I call it *sunblading*. I stare at the sun as it dips lower in the ocean and let its nourishing rays wash over and fulfill me. I leave on a high—mentally, physically, spiritually and creatively. I am so full of the life force after one of my sunblading meditation skates that I cannot eat for hours. The majesty of nature fills me to overflowing, and I am completely satisfied by the experience. I am given the gift of nourishment, creation and inspiration when I roll away. I'm dreaming while I'm awake.

Part of my *Raw on the Roll* lifestyle is connecting oneself to nature. In other words, we not only need to eat greens, we need to be around greens—walking, playing and living in nature. Nature is both magical and healing, and by getting in the good outdoors, it is possible to clear your mind, feed your body, soothe your spirit, calm your nerves, and inspire your creative juices. Get creatively juiced in nature and get your green juice in the juice bar before or after. Nature makes the best flavors and colors, and with her brilliance, boring and bland is nearly impossible both with food and outdoor activity.

*"Look deep, deep into nature, and then
you will understand everything better."*
—Albert Einstein

Our brains face constant, daily stimulation; we are bombarded with information from all directions. We receive an almost continuous stream of input from computers, the radio, television, newspapers, our spouses, kids, bosses, clients, agents, chores, and friends. We turn up the radio to drown out the sound of traffic as we fight morning gridlock, talking on our cell phones and checking our PDA's for urgent emails at every light. And that's before we even get to the office! Once there, we continue to zoom down the information super highway, taking in, sorting, filing, and discarding information like flesh and blood computers—whirling around under the glare of fluorescent lights while keyboards click, phones ring, and coworkers chatter in the background. And we wonder why we feel rushed, stressed, anxious, irritable, and overwhelmed. Now, more than ever, it is vitally important to stop the noise, step outside, get into nature and just breathe. If you are lucky enough to live or work near the mountains, the beach, a lake, a forest or even a grassy park, then take a few minutes each day to stop, breathe and connect with nature. Take off your shoes and walk in the sand or grass. It's wonderfully grounding and, with each step you take, the fog and noise in your head will gradually be released. I make all my major decisions after exercise and lunch. I am relaxed, focused, stronger, clearer, more intuitive, and empowered because I connected to my higher self through nature. You only have one ride through this life, make the most of it and enjoy the ride.

*"There is no medicine better than prayer
and no doctor better than our Creator."*
—Paul Nison, *Health According To The Scriptures*

Being in nature is good for the body as well as the brain. The sun is the best source for vitamin D, which helps the body absorb calcium and phosphorus, and promotes bone density to stave off osteoporosis. You really only need 10 minutes on your limbs during the summer, 15-20 minutes in the spring and fall, and 30 minutes in the winter (depending on the climate you live in) to receive enough vitamin D each day. Of course you should avoid peak hours (10AM to 2PM) and wear a hat if the UV index is higher than 3 or

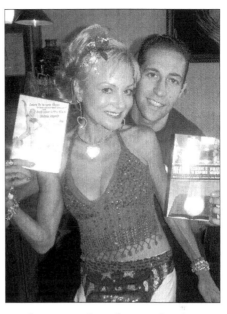

Paul Nison, the "durian king," was the first person to introduce me to the amazing durian fruit. Paul has found his kingdom in the raw food movement and he is superb at it.

you plan on staying in the sun for longer than a few minutes. If you live in a temperate climate, you can exercise outdoors, and increase your joy by "playing out" in the fresh air. Mother Earth is the best play out partner and her services are free! I rarely step foot inside a gym—except to swim and lift weights a few times a week and take a dance class. I find the sun and fresh air invigorating and energizing. That's why I moved to California. The entire state is my gym. Nature is my workout arena. In it, I can expand, play big, and think big; it's vast and abundant, and it's free for life and the only requirement is being human! Everyone can step outside while stepping outside the box that you keep yourself rigidly in as well. Live, love, laugh, life is a gift, unwrap it outdoors.

Sidebar to the Rawbar

- Finding and connecting with your spirit when in nature at the same time equals well-being.
- Expressing creatively and sensually while in nature equals well-being.
- Working in nature equals well-being.
- Quality is as important as quantity.
- Getting time in the sun, you will have won.

> *"Keep close to Nature's heart...and break clear away, once in awhile, and climb a mountain or spend a week in the woods. Wash your spirit clean."*
> —John Muir

I believe the human spirit needs to commune with nature they same way the body needs water or oxygen. Nowhere is God, our higher power, higher spirit or good orderly direction more prevalent or powerful than in nature. Spending time connected to the earth, walking in nature—exercising in nature—whether in a forest, on a beach or simply in your own backyard—revitalizes your soul. There is no better place to express and find relief from your grief, anger or spiritual sickness than outdoors. There are times when I scream at the ocean, and let the sea spray soothe my tears and free my spirit. I find that nature allows for the purest expression of spirit and, when mine needs bolstering, she is always there. I also go outdoors to get oxygen, the breath of life itself. I give thanks for the wonderful, restorative power of Mother Earth who feeds my mind, body and spirit every single day. Mother Nature, the ocean, sun, moon and mountains for me is God also. It's where I connect with the God within me. I even dedicated this book to her. If it wasn't for Mother Nature I would not have found or be given the opportunity to relish and embellish in raw, ripe, delicious, whole, untouched organic foods.

I have personally experienced the wonder of Mother Nature's restorative powers. After my mother's death, I went to Bora Bora, Tahiti to grieve, and wrote a farewell letter to her, which I promptly mailed to the waters of the beautiful, blue South Pacific. While walking back to my bungalow, the skies parted and turned bright red, orange, purple and blue. The beauty of

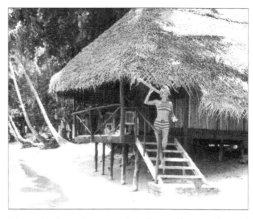

I'm a Tahiti Sweetie. It's here that I released my grief and anger after my mother's death. I found my Parawdise to revel, rejuvenate, release, regroup and relax in nature, and I indulged in some of the sweetest pineapples, mangoes and coconuts in the world.

that moment moved me. It literally opened me up and I cried, raged, conversed, apologized and pleaded for forgiveness and relief from the pain of her loss. I told the sky what I wanted to tell my mother and the spirits. And then the rain came, like divine intervention, and washed my pain away. I felt forgiven, released, healed and loved—by mom and God—thanks to Mother Nature. That moment in time helped me through the grieving process. I even have a picture hanging in my living room of the beach, the tree and the water where the healing occurred on that day, it was a stunning pristine setting I'll never forget or regret.

Raw Bites

- *Spend some time in the GOD (Good Out Doors)—thinking, creating, living, moving and breathing in nature. Take off your shoes and walk barefoot on the earth—let sand or mud slip through your toes, pad across soft grass and really feel the earth under your feet, get grounded. Even if you live in a cold climate,* you can put on a jacket and get outside for ten minutes a day in the crisp, cold air to walk in the snow, glide on ice, make snow angels or just breathe in and out. Mother Nature can be your agent for change, your companion, your miracle healer and your spiritual advisor—if you let her.

- There is a difference between slipping back and living back in the problems of your health. When you spend time in nature, you spend time living in health and the solution, not the problems.

- Enjoy the sun; do not be fearful by sunburn. Be invigorated by the sun's burn.

- When you pause in Mother Nature, you will be the cause with Mother Nature.

- Variety is the spice of life—incorporating a variety of nature's outdoor activities, and nature's raw foods provides a tantalizing range of colors, textures and seasonality to your plate, life and activities.

- Sit in silence in nature for at least ten minutes a day.

- Happiness is not contingent upon outside circumstances.

Section 3

Entrée: *Creating*

Chapter 23

Silence

"Let us be silent, that we may hear the whispers of the gods."
—Ralph Waldo Emerson

In the movie *The Hunt For Red October*, Sean Connery plays the rogue captain of a Russian submarine that is capable of operating in complete silence, allowing it to move through the water undetected. Connery's character decides to test the submarine's capabilities and launch a stealth attack on the enemy, and as he embarks on the mission, he utters a line of dialogue that, when I heard it for the first time, knew it had far greater significance than its literal meaning. To paraphrase, he says, *the world will tremble at the sound of our silence.* I was immediately struck by the truth of that line because it speaks volumes about the inherent power of silence. There is great strength in silence and even as its power is revered, it is also feared. So much so, in fact, that many of us go to great lengths to avoid it. Rather than sit quietly with our own thoughts, we turn on the television, listen to talk radio, talk on the phone, crank up our mp3 players, turn on the computer, eat, talk on the phone or go shopping in order to fill the void with someone else's thoughts or block out our own.

When is the last time you sat still for ten minutes and listened to nothing more than the beating of your own heart? How often do you go for a walk or a run without listening to music?

I used to drown out the silence too, but now I take prayer walks or spend time sun gazing on skates without music; the silence allows me to talk to the ocean and the gods and myself. I use the silence to repeat my affirmations aloud; sometimes I even sing them. Silence is frightening because we are afraid of what we might discover or hear. So what are you fearful of? Fear is False Evidence Appearing Real. When you worry and hurry through your day, bogged down by noise, food, distractions, denial and excess activity, your day is like an unopened gift thrown away, without ever being unwrapped and enjoyed. Life is not a race. Don't waste your precious energy on gossip, energy vampires, issues of the past, negative thoughts or things you cannot control. Instead, invest your energy in the positive, present moment. Take it slower and quieter. Hear the music before the song is over. Uncover and discover the recovering artist, spirit and human being that resides within you. He or she is there; don't be afraid to find what you have always wanted and have been always looking for. It's there. Just get quiet and go within to begin—and win. Do you ever take a drive without talking on the phone, turning on the radio or listening to a book on tape? Why is it that most of us feel the need to distract ourselves from ourselves? Because we are afraid of what we will see or hear or we run from our negative, fearful, obsessive thoughts.

We'd rather listen to anything but the noise inside our own heads. I believe that by constantly turning our attention outward, obsessively filling the silence, we are missing out on our rich inner lives. For it is in the silence that we discover who we really are. It is where true creativity is born, and where we connect with our spirit and find peace. It is where we hear the inspiration, aspiration and imagination to create and build. Two-thirds of our ideas and thoughts come from the silent times. The still, small voice is heard during those times. Two-thirds of God is "Go." Peace is not a season.

It doesn't come and go—it is a way of life. It's every day. Peace and health go hand in hand, each feeding the other, so that every aspect of life is imbued with a sense of ease—including diet, fitness, spirituality, creativity, family, relationships and work. But how do we find peace in a world that is buzzing with activity, where stress, anxiety and noise seem to be a part of every day? How do we go from desperation to inspiration?

The road to peace starts with silence. Silence is where true creativity and inspiration are born, where we can finally recreate ourselves as healthy, spiritual, creative beings. It is the silence that allows us to access that higher part of ourselves, the part that knows how to heal. I believe that a daily dose of silence is essential to all human beings and that by practicing quietude, we learn the meaning of gratitude. One way to get in touch with silence is to practice meditation. I realize that the idea of meditating, consciously practicing quiet relaxation, may be daunting for some of you. It is for me, too. But meditation is like clearing the clutter from your mind and letting the new energy flow, glow and go. And I believe that once you get into the habit, you will wonder how you ever lived without it. The practice of meditation needn't be intimidating. You don't have to chant, sit cross-legged or imagine yourself on a sun-drenched hilltop. There is no single, *right* way to practice meditation. It can be as simple as sitting quietly for five to ten minutes and breathing, clearing your mind and focusing on nothing more than your own breath and the beating of your heart. Or it can be on an island in Tahiti with a balmy breeze blowing in your face, the sweet smell of pineapples in the air and the sun on your body, warming it up, filling it with energy, light and vitality. It can be a moving meditation that I find so easy—skating, walking, biking, swimming, and meditating quietly in nature while saying affirmations and prayers are all forms of meditation for me.

"Meditate, Create, and Skate for the Health of It"

"There is no need to go to India or anywhere else to find peace.
You will find that deep place of silence right in your room,
your garden or even your bathtub."
—Elisabeth Kubler-Ross

To get started, find a quiet place where you can spend five to ten undisturbed minutes. Sit or lie down in a comfortable position, close your eyes, and just breathe in and out. Try to focus on nothing more than your own breathing. Empty your mind, if you can, and let the silence wash over you. You may find yourself feeling emotions like deep sadness, anger or even joy. You may find yourself moved to tears and have no idea why. Sometimes our emotions are so repressed and frozen by noise, distractions and denial that given the slightest space and silence, they emerge and overwhelm us. That's okay. Go with it. Your soul has been searching for a way to speak to you and by offering it silence, you have given it a means of expression. You may find the practice difficult and frustrating at first—your mind racing with thoughts, going through "to do" lists and rehashing the events of the day. That's okay too. Acknowledge the chatter that doesn't matter and then, *let it go.* Return to the silence. You may also find a solution to a troubling problem suddenly pops into your mind and is crystal clear. Or you may gain the courage to take a difficult action. Just let whatever comes, come and then let it go. It's all good. There is not a right way to experience silence. Once you become comfortable with the practice of meditation, tapping into the still, silent voice within, you can practice it anywhere, any time. What I like to do and works for me is to mediate while sun gazing on the beach, skating and biking into the sunset, also while eating my raw meals and visualizing all the good things I want to experience the next moment. Meditation for me is also visualizing things working out in divine right order in the way I want them to. Reciting my daily affirmations to the ocean, sky, moon or mountains is also a form of meditation for me. As is doing yoga silently outdoors or in my home. It's just me, my breath and nature, and then I invite in my higher spirit. I invite you to discover the power of silence for yourself. Meditate, don't medicate.

Raw Bites

- *Look for opportunities to experience silence throughout your regular daily routine: while preparing a meal, writing, taking a bubble bath, commuting to work, exercising, going for a walk, eating dinner—all can be done in silence. I call it active meditation. Try eating dinner without talking, or listening to something and thinking about negative things. Look at eating as a form of meditation. Eating is a spiritual time to put love in your body, mind and spirit. Eating in silence allows for proper digestion and assimilation of your food. It is a good time to replenish your spirit. What we put in, we give out. Loving thoughts and loving foods give out love. Negative thoughts and CRAP food put out negativity and a negative persona. Feed your spirit, relax and quiet your mind. A quiet mind is an open mind. Where there is an open mind there will always be a frontier.*

- *Spend five minutes in the morning sitting quietly, thinking about how you would like to experience your day. Visualize, vocalize and physicalize it, all through meditation. Create a purpose for the day when you wake up. Say, "my purpose is to _____ today."*

- *Play monk for a day. Spend one whole day without television, radio, music, or talking on the phone. See if you can get your family to play along. If you can refrain from talking all day too, that would be sensational and such a peaceful, restful experience for your body, mind and spirit. The word vacation means to vacate. Meditation vacates the mind.*

- *Practice silent communication with your partner. Non-verbal communication is a powerful way to connect with the person you love. Instead of whispering sweet nothings in your partner's ear, practice being a sweet something. As they say, actions speak louder than words.*

- *Silence also stands for not having the last word. You don't have to win every argument, so agree to disagree. In fact, not saying anything in response to a request or a gossip conversation is very beneficial. Zip the lip. Silence gives us time to think and ponder, to reason things out, to evaluate and digest them, and to make up our minds before we decide. I use silence in my three businesses a lot. I call it "the silent pause." I say, "I'll get back to you," or "I need to run it by my dream team (me and my higher spirit in silence)." I say this to give myself time for silent thought and meditation. I need to pray on it and wait for the decision to make me.*

- *Silence is not always tactful, and it is tactfulness that is golden, not silence.*

- *If I do not leave, I will come to believe.*

- *A candle loses nothing of its light by lighting another candle. Meditation is like lighting another candle of information, hope and guidance for oneself.*

- *When you pause in Mother Nature, you will be the cause with Mother Nature.*

- *Go into meditation and see that the pain will push until the vision pulls.*

- *Meditation will help you come to believe you can do it. Then the "how to do it" will appear.*

- *We are spiritual beings having a human experience, not human beings having a spiritual experience.*
- *Let us find the miracle-go-round by not uttering a sound.*
- *Empty space is the best place. Empty your mind through meditation.*
- *Through meditation your mind will transcend limitations. Know that you can create limitless possibilities with your health and well-being.*
- *To get what you have never had, you must do what you have never done.*
- *Let the body show up and the mind will catch up.*
- *Denial is not a good style, meditate and go within and gain a mile of a smile.*

Chapter 24

Picasso

"The secret of life is in art."
—Oscar Wilde

rt must be integrated into every aspect of life, including our education system. I also think that art, in conjunction with today's technology, can help us achieve great health. Feeding your soul a healthy diet of creative expression is as important as feeding your body nutritious foods; without both types of nourishment, we will atrophy and die. I believe that the best chefs are artists, and great art is as fulfilling as wonderful food.

Figure skating was my art, my first love, my everything—for a while. Eventually my art expanded to include acting, singing, dancing, writing, producing, lecturing, and health educating. What elevates figure skating to art is the ability to infuse athleticism with grace and beauty. Part of my challenge with figure skating was that I had the body of an athlete and the soul of an artist, and it was sometimes difficult to reconcile the two within myself. There is an element of figure skating that has nothing to do with technique, with turning two-and-a-half times in the air and landing backwards on one foot. It is a certain something that cannot be quantified. The judges try to quantify that which is unquantifiable, but **art** cannot be measured out in points, it just is. It defies measurement. You know it when you see it. It seems easy, effortless and natural.

I believe that art is, can, and should be part of everything we do. I also believe that everyone is an artist. That doesn't mean that everyone can make a living from his or her art or even that everyone is a great artist, it simply means that every one of us possesses the soul of an artist. Art is a means of expression that is as varied as our experience. What we think of as traditional art forms—painting, sculpture, poetry, song, dance and theatre—are only the tip of the iceberg. Of course what we think of as art has expanded; there is installation art, video, film and mixed media. People use materials such as glass, yarns, rocks and even garbage and reshape it into works of fine art. You may not think it's art, but somebody does. The definition of what constitutes art is always changing. There is no real definitive answer to the question, "What is art?" The answer is different for each of us, depending on our experience, education and outlook. Art is God and God is Art. Art has the power to heal, enrich and empower, inspire and motivate—not only the person who sees or experiences it, but the artist who creates it. And today, that artist is you.

> *"Love the art in yourself, not yourself in the art."*
> —Konstantin Stanislavsky

That's right. **You are an artist.** You might not know it yet but you are about to find out. The truth is, anyone can paint a picture, form a sculpture, write a poem, choreograph a dance, sing a song or perform a soliloquy. Not everyone will see their painting hanging in the Louvre or perform at the Met, but everyone (including you) has the innate ability to create a work of art. To prove it, I want you to create your very own work of art right now. It can be as simple or elaborate as you want to make it. So, put down this book and pick up a pencil, pen, crayon, paintbrush or magic marker. Try your hand at watercolor or oil painting, make a sculpture out of molding clay, Play-Doh® or even flour and water. Draw a picture, paint your heart, or a flower or the beach. Use your body, your imagination and your spirit to express your creativity. It doesn't have to be right. It doesn't even have to be good. As long as you are freely expressing what you are feeling, it's art.

"Imagination is more important than knowledge.
For knowledge is limited, whereas imagination enhances the entire
world, stimulating progress, giving birth to evolution."
—Albert Einstein

Remember, you are the artist, so whatever you do is right for *you*. You don't need to take a class, read a book or have any idea of what you are doing. All you need to create art is to be a human being. Let yourself go, have fun with it, and most importantly, don't judge or critique your creation. When you don't judge it, nothing occurs, and there is peace and acceptance around it. The best way to kill a creative idea is to take it to a meeting. So don't, this one is just for you. Once you are finished, if you feel like it, display your art somewhere you can see it every day. Frame it with a colorful, beautiful frame, and then hang it up where you can enjoy and revel in it every day. Or, if you prefer, place it in your treasure chest, notebook or on your treasure map to remind yourself of the artist that lives inside of you. If you prefer, let someone else see it, read it, give it away, sell it, teach it, perform it, copyright it, share it or do whatever you want with it.

"I don't want life to imitate art. I want life to be art."
—Ernst Fischer

Now that you have completed your art project you are probably thinking, "Well that was fun, but what does it have to do with raw food and health?" The answer is, *everything*. All great works of art, and even the not so great ones, begin with an open heart and the desire to nourish and enrich the lives of those who see and experience it—even if the only person who sees it is the person who created it. Close your mouth, open your heart and get to your art. If it enriches you, it is enough. Food is the same as art. When you prepare a meal with love, it elevates it to an art form—one that is just as valuable as a Picasso or a Rembrandt. I wanted you to experience creating your own work of art to prove that you could, yes, but also to open your eyes and heart to the infinite possibilities of what art *can* be. You will have vibrant energy and more enjoyment in your life through creativity. Your newfound freedom and full self-expression will bring you long-lasting health, and a sense of aliveness. I always say, "Lack of creative expression equals depression."

Art is an expression of emotion. As I have said before, food prepared with love is the most nourishing and fulfilling kind, and I hope that you will approach *un*cooking with an open heart and the desire to feed your soul, as well as your body. If you do those two things, you cannot fail. Perhaps one day you will even be a master raw chef, designing and preparing culinary masterpieces of your own. I have included a couple dozen of my personal recipes in this book, made by my own process of trial and error, so you don't have to start from scratch. While I have not attended culinary school, I have become a skilled raw chef with the imagination, recreation and inspiration for raw foods. I want you to feel free to add to, change and alter any recipe you endeavor to prepare. Think of the recipes as a guide, a place from which to start, and then expand them to suit your own tastes and satisfy your own inner artist/master chef. There are two kinds of failures: those who think and never do and those who do, but never think. Go to raw restaurants and seek inspiration from the presentations of other raw chefs. Ask them to explain what's in the dish and go home and recreate one like it or tweak it to create a fancier or simpler version that is all your own. I learned how to be a vegetarian, and a raw vegan by imitating and recreating the dishes I ordered out in vegetarian restaurants. I always add a little extra of this and more or less of that because the Italian in me loves to mix everything together and I love flavor, nutrition and tradition. For example, I usually add garlic, olive oil, cinnamon, dill, lemon, cayenne pepper, ginger, raw stevia powder, raw buckwheat kernels or some other dash of flavor to whatever recipe I am making to add a little bit of zest and to spice it up a bit. That's how I became a creative raw chef. The more you experiment, the more you will learn what you like, and you will begin to discover a whole raw universe you never knew existed. It is important to play, branch out, try new things—not only in the kitchen, but in all areas of your life. If you are not failing, you are not taking enough risks. Eating is a metaphor for how you live your life. How you prepare your food is how you prepare your life. I encourage you to live, connect, relate, generate, create, exercise, work, give, receive and *uncook* with passion, love and a sense of play. This could be the most important step you take in your life. Transitioning to a more raw, vegetarian, vegan diet can be fun, fulfilling and flavorful. It can also be frightening. Please let go of the fears that appear, they are the termites that devour any foundation of health we try to build. If you do little things well, you'll do big things even better.

Raw Bites

- *Pretend that you are a master raw chef and create a dish out of your own imagination. Feed it to your lover, friend or child. Don't tell them it's raw or vegan, just watch them enjoy it. Bring love and conversation to the meal and you will both be fed and nourished enormously with what I call the feeling of going from raw to awe. From raw to richness. Create a raw sculpture made of fruits and vegetables, design a plate full of raw wonders using all the colors of the rainbow, "paint" a face with blueberry eyes, flax seed freckles and a bean sprout goatee. You are only limited by your knowledge, not your imagination. Above all, have fun. I made a red, white and blue raw roller skate cake for my show out of coconut, blueberries, strawberries and cacao for the wheels, and it was delicious. On Thanksgiving, my artistic dish is a raw turkey. I make it out of sprouted nuts, seeds and veggies, and shape it into a big turkey. Become a Picasso or a Michelangelo and skip the Leaning Tower of Pisa and make a raw pizza.*

- *It's okay to play with your food. Get your kids involved—they love to play with food! When you are finished, take a picture of your masterpiece to remind yourself that food is art and art is love and God. Place the picture on your treasure map and on those days when everything seems lost, know that the future is just a moment away. Sit down and eat your divine design.*
- *Start where you are. Where you are is exactly where you are supposed to begin.*
- *Put love in your food. "Love cures. It cures those who give it and cures those who receive it." (Dr. Karl Menninger)*
- *Change any negative thoughts you have about health, creativity and food, and you will change your world. Move a muscle, change a thought. Change your thoughts, change your world.*
- *Success is when preparation meets opportunity.*
- *You will achieve more if you don't mind who gets the credit. Let others help you and give you knowledge. You don't have to do this alone. Ask for help and be willing to receive it.*
- *Now is the time to eat to look and feel great forever.*
- *Everything is impermanent. Fear comes from attachment to permanence. Nothing lasts forever, so there is nothing to hold on to.*

Chapter 25

Have a Green Party

Merrillism #42: "Eat Green and Stay Keen, Clean, Lean and Serene."

Green is a magical color—it is the color of money, the center of the rainbow, the symbol of the environment and, as everyone knows, a green light means go! The key to recovering my own health was by adding more green in my diet. When I was a vegetarian, I was still eating a lot of sugar, also in the form of carrots, beets, wheat, fruit, and starches like cooked rice, sweet potatoes, pasta, and rice cakes, which all turn into sugar, along with processed and cooked foods, and I ate very little in the way of green, leafy vegetables. As I made the transition from a vegetarian to a vegan diet, I began eating more greens—green leaves, celery, zucchini, parsley, kale, collard greens, dandelion, cilantro, broccoli and sprouts as opposed to carrots, beets, butternut and kabocha squash, peas, corn, turnips and rutabagas—all of which are sweet, starchy and higher on the glycemic index chart. At one point I ate so many orange, sweet vegetables (to get my sugar fix) that the palms of my hands, the bottoms of my feet and my face turned orange. Once I added more green, leafy vegetables to my diet, my body became more alkaline, and my blood sugar leveled out. I had fewer sugar cravings and ate less sugary, starchy vegetables, and my tendencies towards hypoglycemia disappeared. I was so grateful that I needed to snack less, and sustained more energy without eating more food more frequently. However, those sweet, orange vege-

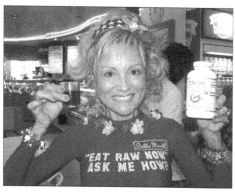

"I eat green to stay clean, keen, lean and serene."

tables did serve an important purpose by helping me overcome my craving for bad sugar, because they replaced it. You could say sweet veggies were the lesser of two evils. I ate them for the first 18 years of my vegetarian/vegan lifestyle, until I discovered the miraculous miracle of eating green. Then I let go, went green and got keen, lean and serene. For 28 years, I've been drinking two ounces of wheatgrass juice a day, every single day. I also eliminated processed, refined and cooked foods from my diet. That's when I really started to detoxify my body of all the funguses, Candida, and toxins that had built up over the years. Inflammation left my system along with pain, and my digestive problems disappeared as well. I began to believe in the miracle of eating green because my energy was better, my skin cleared up, I lost weight and I experienced a renewed sense of vitality, clarity, energy, strength and peace. And because my blood sugar was normalizing, I felt calmer. I also lost my sweet cravings and started craving bitter foods—kale, collard greens, dandelion, parsley, celery and cilantro. Hail to the kale! I learned that greens are the key to healing, brilliance, eliminating addictions, and disease-free living and abundant health and vitality.

Merrillism #43: "Don't Get Nutty on Nuts or Fruity on Fruit, Have a Green Party and Invite Yourself To It."

Even though cashews, Brazil nuts, pistachios, almonds, and hazelnuts contain large amounts of fiber, protein, antioxidants, Vitamin B, phosphorous, copper, magnesium, folates, calcium, Omega 3's and selenium we still need to eat green to be keen and clean. Green vegetables are an important source of many nutrients the body needs to function at an optimum level. Greens, like all vegetables, are an excellent source of dietary fiber, which is important for proper bowel function, and for reducing constipation and diverticulosis. Fiber also helps reduce and manage blood cholesterol levels, which may lower the risk of heart disease. Beet greens, spinach and kale are all good sources of calcium and potassium, which is helpful in maintaining fluid and electrolyte balance in the body, and is thought to promote healthy blood pressure and strong bones. Leafy green vegetables contain folate, which helps the body make red blood cells, reduces the risk of neural tube defects, spina bifida and anencephaly during fetal development and, according to some studies, may protect against cognitive loss in older adults.

Lacinato kale and regular kale are both rich in vitamin A and calcium, which promotes healthy eyes and skin, and helps protect the body from infection. Avocado is an excellent source of vitamin E and protein, as well as a healthy fat, which prevents the oxidation of fats and vitamin A, and is believed to help in the prevention of prostate and breast cancer. Green veggies like broccoli, spinach and zucchini contain vitamin C, which is essential for healthy bones, teeth, gums, and blood vessels. Vitamin C also aids in iron and calcium absorption and wound healing, and contributes to brain function. It's also the beauty vitamin. It keeps us young. Greens are healing foods and people who eat more of them are less likely to experience some chronic diseases including stroke, type 2 diabetes and certain cancers, such as colorectal, mouth and stomach cancer. Since vegetables, including greens, are lower in calories and naturally cholesterol free, eating more of them helps reduce caloric intake. Also, bitter green foods help take away cravings for "bad" foods. I used to crave cookies and crackers and cakes, now I crave parsley, cilantro, celery, kale and collard greens. I have acquired a taste for bitter foods and you may discover, as you begin to heal, that your taste buds will actually change and that you prefer the taste of greens to sweets. You begin to crave that bitter bite that makes you feel all right! I believe that one cannot heal completely until they develop a taste for bitter greens.

Greens also slow down sugar entering the blood system, so when you eat a lot of sweet foods, it's good to eat greens as well. They'll slow down the spike in sugar levels in your system. Also, when you eat a steak or a meal heavy in carbohydrates, eat a big salad with plenty of greens. The enzymes and chlorophyll in the greens will help digest the meat and sugar. Greens contain tons of chlorophyll. In fact, the greener the leaf, the more chlorophyll and oxygen that leaf contains. Yes, you can also get it from the packaged green powders, but there's nothing like eating or juicing the real deal and getting the enzymes, oxygen, water and nutrients so fresh and alive. I always choose the fresh leaves first, but when I'm traveling and can't get my greens, I substitute green powders. My breakfast for many years was three dates and three almonds rolled inside kale or collard greens and it provided everything I needed—the sugar, the fat and the chlorophyll in a delicious combination. I was right in my center zone. Not too high, not too low, just right. Try this combo with any fruit or nut. I love it and I recommend it. It keeps you at an even keel to start the day.

Tips to Help you Increase the Green

Eat it, juice it, chop it, slice it, blend it, drink it. Let go of the stinking thinking about greens. It's not what you're drinking, it's what you're thinking. They are delicioso!

- **Be a local.** Buy fresh, seasonal, locally grown, organic vegetables—preferably at your local farmers market or organic produce store, or grow your own. Create a garden. Locally grown, seasonal vegetables cost less, and are likely to be at their peak of flavor. You get them right away instead of having to pay someone to fly them to you, which means you're not contributing to carbon monoxide fumes or paying for transportation costs. Organic vegetables tend to cost a bit more, but are the best (and my only) choice. I don't choose to eat pesticides, fumicides, fungicides, and herbicides and then feel like suicide. The increased nutritional value and taste are well worth the extra pennies. Organic foods are my health insurance premiums.

- **Take the easy way out.** You can buy bags of pre-washed, organic salad greens, organic radishes, grape or cherry tomatoes and pre-sliced zucchini for a fast, easy salad. You can also buy prepackaged celery sticks, broccoli florets and snow peas. Keep cut up broccoli, celery, red bell peppers, zucchini, okra, asparagus spears and sprouts (i.e. broccoli, clover, sunflower and alfalfa) in the fridge—perfect for dipping in my yummy Dip In A Whip found in the recipe section.

- **Presentation is everything.** Use vegetables to decorate individual plates or serving platters and then eat your art! When I go to a party, I eat the kale and parsley they use to decorate the plate (after it's been washed.) There is always an exorbitant amount of it because no one wants it. They all go for the cooked, sweet, fatty food.

- **Have a green salad with dinner every night.** Try using turnip greens, arugula, Swiss chard, bok choy or endive for a change of pace, dress it with your favorite oil or my special Spritty Spirulina Dressing or Japanese Salad Dressing in the recipe section.
- **If you are still eating meat and cooked foods,** shred zucchini, basil, cilantro, spinach, celery, cucumbers, parsley and kale into casseroles, quick breads, muffins, pasta sauce and lasagna.
- **Instead** of steak and potatoes, have steak and a salad, or eat a spinach salad (skip the bacon). Have a salad with your chicken, instead of rice. Try my Raw Hummus or Sprouted Lentil Salad (in the recipe section) instead of the steak and chicken. It's just as filling, nutritious and delicious, and it's raw vegan. Totally rawsome.
- **Order a veggie pizza** with toppings like spinach, red peppers, and broccoli, or better yet, make your own. Try my raw Pizza Pizazz recipe and you'll forget that Dominos delivers.
- **Keep it interesting.** Try these greens from *A to Z*. There's the creative you and the chef in you; now that's a dynamic duo.

Arugula

Asparagus

Baby Greens

Basil

Beet Greens

Bok Choy

Boston Lettuce

Broccoli & Broccoli Rabe

Brussels Sprouts

Celery

Chicory

Chives

Cilantro

Collard Greens

Dandelion Greens

Dark Green Leafy Lettuce

Escarole

Endive

Fennel

Kale

Kohlrabi

Lettuce: Romaine, Red Leaf, Green Leaf

Mesclun

Mint

Mustard Greens

Parsley

Spinach

Swiss Chard, Red and Green

Turnip Greens

Watercress

Zucchini

These suggestions are guides to progress, not perfection. There is no need for excellence, speed, brilliance and perfection your first time around. There is more to life and health than making it go faster. I always say that when I pray for patience, God gives me long lines and traffic jams. Be patient with your progress. Practice makes progress. Have fun with the green, lean machine that you are becoming. Keep trying and enjoy it.

Wheatgrass

*Wheatgrass juice is an inexpensive way
to chase health and catch it.*

I believe it has magical, cleansing properties and is one of the most perfect, raw, live foods you can get. For that reason, it is often called "solar powered food" or "sunshine in a cup." Because it is made of 70% chlorophyll (the substance that gives plants their color), wheatgrass is the greenest of all the greens. Like its name suggests, wheatgrass is made from the young wheat plant and is packed with vitamins (A, C, E, K, B-complex and B-17), minerals (including calcium, phosphorus, iron, magnesium and potassium), as well as 17 amino acids (the building blocks of protein). In fact, wheatgrass is so nutrient dense, it is said that one ounce of wheatgrass is nutritionally equivalent to two pounds of fresh produce. Wheatgrass juice is a remarkable body cleanser, body re-builder and toxin neutralizer, and many people believe it can cure cancer. I don't know for sure if that is true, but there have been numerous examples to support the claim that wheatgrass juice has the ability to heal chronic disorders including anemia, high blood pressure, arthritis and is often used therapeutically (along with traditional treatments) in the treatment of some cancers and AIDS. Wheatgrass juice draws toxins out of the body, purifies the liver, improves blood sugar problems, and washes drug deposits from the body. Many of the healing properties attributed to wheatgrass juice come from its exceptionally high concentration of chlorophyll, which is often called the "blood of plants" and is similar in molecular structure to human blood. Chlorophyll has been shown to inhibit the growth of bacteria, build red blood cells, normalize high blood pressure, and stimulate healthy tissue cell growth. Its cleansing properties are well known; it is an effective cleanser for the digestive tracts and has been shown to reduce and eliminate body and breath odors. For me, wheatgrass also takes away my sugar cravings, and is very alkalizing. It energizes me as well as calms me down. It keeps me in my zone. I love it. Sometimes when the market is out, I will rotate on E3Live or my lean, keen, green machine cocktail and get my raw on the roll, out of control boost. Remember to chew it. After chewing it, roll it around in your mouth so your gums and teeth and throat absorb it, and then swallow it slowly. I try and drink wheatgrass juice on an empty stomach or two hours after eating. Then I wait one to two hours to eat or drink anything. That is the ideal way I enjoy doing it. But, it doesn't always work out that way for me with my rawsome awesome, busy lifestyle. So, I take my own advice—I do it the best way I can do it until I can do it the way I want to do it—but I do it.

There is no doubt that wheatgrass juice is wonderful for your insides but it is quite beneficial to your outsides as well. It can be used as a skin cleanser and astringent, a treatment for allergies or blocked sinuses (by placing several drops in each nostril), a circulation stimulant and skin softener (add several ounces to bath or rub directly on skin), and it helps cuts and bruises heal quickly. You can even gargle with it to help with a sore throat. It's also been used for enemas, colonics and hemorrhoids. I believe it's a cure for everything and anything. When my ribs were broken for a time in the ice shows, I would apply the pulp to my ribs and I healed much faster. Who would have thought that a little grass on my rib would help speed up the healing? I thought grass was only used for people to smoke and mow or dogs to eat before or after they vomited to settle their stomachs. Actually what it does is alkalize an acidic system. An entire world of possibilities opened up to me through wheatgrass.

Wheatgrass juice is best consumed fresh, right after juicing. You can find it at most juice bars; if you have trouble locating one in your area, ask your local health food store to carry it or for a recommendation. You can also grow wheatgrass yourself at home and make your own juice; all you need is a wheatgrass juicer, and a little bit of a green thumb. I drink two ounces every day, but you can drink more for therapeutic purposes. If you are eating loads of fresh fruit and veggies already, two ounces should be plenty. If you are a newcomer to this, a little green juice with a green apple in it or a little bit of water can be used as a chaser. But I suggest you avoid fruit juice, smoothies, coffee or tea. It's really best consumed alone and on its own with no assistance. Try to set a goal for that. I can't say enough about the wonders of wheatgrass, and if you try it for two weeks, I think you'll fall in love with the way it makes you feel. You'll find that, if you drink it regularly, you will avoid colds, flu's, sinus problems, viruses, allergies, cravings, sicknesses, etc.

I'll say it again, when anyone acquires a taste for bitter green foods, true healing begins in the body. Greens are the key to great health, which is why I always tell people to have a green party and invite yourself to it. Oh, I love my sweet fruits, orange and yellow squashes, carrots, mangoes, persimmons and figs, (they are some of my favorites), and I love nuts and grains. However, I think we tend to forget about the green and we need to revel in it—because green is the queen and it's where the magic is. If we eat green, think green and live green, we will experience great health, wealth and happiness. The grass really is greener on the other side! If you're on the go, cereal grass juice powders or fresh cereal grass juices are great to drink. They are so nutrient dense and are some of the best superfoods on the planet. They provide us with all the life-giving nutrients we need to build lean healthy bodies. Please don't deprive yourself of these superfoods as well!

Raw Bites

- *Make today a green day. Incorporate green leaves and vegetables into every meal.*
- *Start your day off right. Down a two-ounce shot of wheatgrass instead of coffee.*

- *Try my Green Keen Lean Machine Cocktail (in the recipe section). I drink it for great health!*
- *Try my Green Blended Rawsome Awesome Soup (in the recipe section).*
- *Have some celery with raw almond butter or hemp seed butter (See the Resources section for recommendations.)*
- *Cultured veggies are loaded with probiotics, which are good for digestion and reestablishing your inner ecosystem. They increase longevity, control cravings, and are alkaline and very cleansing. They are great for the colon, adding good flora and bacteria to the digestive tract. Eat raw, cultured vegetables when you are constipated. They also greatly enhance the digestion of protein. I eat a little after every meal, even a fruit meal, to act as a digestive enzyme for myself.*
- *When you realize you've made a mistake, take immediate steps to correct it.*
- *Peace begins on your plate.*
- *Don't believe all you hear, spend all you have, or sleep all you want. Take what you like and save the rest for when you are ready.*
- *One is ready when one is willing. Pray for willingness.*
- *Act as if you already have it.*
- *It's easier to stay green than to get green.*

Chapter 26

Success is a Habit

"Motivation is what gets you started.
Habit is what keeps you going."
—Jim Rohn

T he dictionary's definition of a *habit* is, "A recurrent, often unconscious pattern of behavior that is acquired through frequent repetition." The first step in changing an unhealthy habit is to bring it into consciousness. Part of the reason so-called bad or negative habits are powerful is because they are hidden in our subconscious minds, causing us to act, without knowing why. He who conquers his mind, masters his mind. By bringing that habit into the light, you can work on it, transform it and replace it with a new healthy habit that moves you closer to the good. Since habits, good or bad, are part of the human condition, why not decide to make good health your habit? Like I said before, eating junk food is just a bad habit; habit hunger and bad habits can be broken. Eating nutritious foods and exercising are habits, just like brushing your teeth is a habit. You don't have to think about brushing your teeth every morning, you just do it, and if for some reason you don't, you are likely to experience feelings of discomfort. Not to mention bad breath! That is why it's so diffi-cult to break harmful habits, even though you *know* they are bad for you and even though you *want* to change, you are so used to doing the thing, whatever it is—overeating fatty foods, thinking negative self defeating thoughts, not exercising, complaining or eating late at night while watching TV. Not doing the bad habit causes you extreme anxiety and discomfort. You are so used to that bad feeling it's hard to imagine anything better or believe there is another way, so you get stuck there. You continue to do the same thing expecting different results. This is the definition of insanity. You say, "just this time it will be different," and it's usually the same or worse. Nothing changes till something changes.

It is our daily experiences (our habits) that help us achieve our goals, so it is important to create your day so that it brings you closer to your goals. In other words, you need to plan. I always say, *not* planning is planning to fail. And there is always room for improvement. It's the biggest room in the house and we all need to spend a lot more time there, myself included. I found the best way to develop good habits and give myself the best chance for success is to plan for it. For me that means I plan my meals, my wardrobe, activities, phone calls, errands, exercise, and downtime the night before. My days are busy; I wake up and hit the ground rolling, so in order to ensure I eat the way I want to eat, I prepare my meals at night. I put everything I need, and only what I need, in my lunch bag and glass jars, and I'm good to go. I call my car Café Honda so I don't have to be at the mercy of fast food drive-thrus, vending machines or hunger. The important part is that I take what I need, and no more. If I have more, I'll eat more. I may be stressed out or tired or whatever, so I'll eat just because it's there and rationalize the eating. What I'm saying is, don't tease or appease by tempting yourself unnecessarily. Another great tip is to cut up your fruits and veggies as soon as you get home from the market. Wash them, cut them, and have them ready to go. That way, when you have a snack attack, you have something good to grab, instead of a bag of chips, bars or cookies. I also separate other items like nuts, dried fruits and crackers into individual portions.

I get small snack bags and put a handful of nuts or cacao nibs, or goji berries in there and then I can just grab my snack bags and go because I know that if I take the whole bag, I'll keep going and eat all of that too. I call it emotional and anxiety eating—it's not real hunger. Also, when I'm stressed or tired or going through a hard time, I don't keep certain trigger foods in the house or buy them. If you have to keep them, put them in the trunk of your car and believe me, you won't want to go out to get them in the middle of the night, so you'll be safe. Another way to plan ahead is when you are preparing meals for yourself or your family, make extra so that you have healthy leftovers on hand for lunches or another dinner during the week. Even refrigerated raw meals are good for at least one more day. That way you won't get stuck, and feel like you need to grab fast food or a microwave meal.

Planning is vital with exercise too, especially now that you are trying to create a new habit. So, schedule it into your day, everyday. Don't leave it to chance and hope you will find some time to squeeze it in. You won't. Schedule it like you would any other important business meeting, lunch date or conference call. Think of it as an appointment with your most valuable client, *you.* And if something comes up and you have to cancel, make sure you reschedule or take something else off your plate and substitute it for exercise. It's the most important appointment of the day for you. You wouldn't leave an important client hanging, so show yourself the same respect. Please don't rip yourself off, or let yourself down. Many people find it's easiest to exercise first thing in the morning because you get up, you don't think about it, you just do it and it's done. The rest of your day goes great, and you feel energized, organized, motivated and inspired. It's unlikely that something will come up at six or seven in the morning to take you off course. Others prefer to go during lunch or take a class after work. Find out what works for you, and then do it.

As I have said, growth is messy. It's uncomfortable. It's going to take time for you to transition. Studies have shown that it takes 21 days to establish a new habit. I suggest you start today. Pick one habit you want to add, one bad habit to change or eliminate and just begin. Don't make it an option, make it a priority and do it every day. This is key. Habits are habits because we repeat them. The trick to 21 days is that if you skip a day, you start over. That doesn't mean you have failed, it just means that you haven't made it a habit—*yet.*

Raw Bites

- *Pick one old habit to change or one new habit to create. And make it happen. Start today.*
- *Plan all your meals and snacks ahead of time for tomorrow.*
- *This book is The Raw Truth To Fountain of Youth.*
- *Our problem is not that we have lack of power, it's lack of a problem that is our power.*
- *It's easier to stay in shape than to get in shape.*

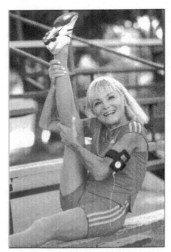

I stretch every day to keep the aches, pains, and doctors away. It gives me energy mobility and agility.

Chapter 27

Over the Hump Lesson #3:

Put the Weights in Your
Cookie Jar, Not Cookies

"You take your life in your own hands, and what happens?
A terrible thing: no one to blame."
—Erica Jong

Take responsibility for your own ability to transform your health (responsibility means that you respond to your own ability). As you continue to grow in your health, you will find that there will always be obstacles to overcome, plateaus to conquer and mountains to climb. There will also be new discoveries to make, fresh solutions to find, and new answers to old questions. That is the nature of life. Let today be the first day of the rest of your life, not the tomorrow you worried about yesterday. I am always in process and have learned, over time, to be comfortable with that. TIME equals Things I Must Earn. Transitioning and transformation is my status quo. I have lived the raw lifestyle for many years, yet I continue to discover new things to enrich my journey. Raw foods have opened up a whole new world of exotic tastes I never knew existed. I'm a nice Italian girl from Yonkers, New York. What did I know about exotic fruits like durian, sapotes and goji berries? Heck, I used to think a 'mango' was a type of dance, a rambutan was a hammock, mamay was a Spanish mother, durian was a book and sapote was the Spanish pronunciation of shoes (zapatos). Today, I am happier eating jicama, persimmons, dried mulberries, goji berries, raw cashews, cultured veggies, spirulina and maca than I ever was drinking champagne and drowning my sorrows in ice cream. Before I moved to California, I had never heard of any of these foods. I used to eat canned peaches and cottage cheese, half a cantaloupe with Melba toast, and thought I was eating naturally and healthy. Carrot cake, popcorn, and creamed corn, I reasoned, were vegetables and complex carbohydrates. Now, I eat kale, collard greens, sprouts, sprouted lentils, okra and blue-green algae, chlorella and crystal blue manna. There is a whole world of amazing flavor out there if you look for it. I don't miss all the processed junk foods I used to eat because I don't eat them anymore. I replaced them with foods I love that are also good for my body and taste better, fill me up quicker, give me more energy and are full of vitamins, nutrients, minerals, water, oxygen and enzymes—the beauty foods my body requires and desires to be beautiful. Beautiful = Be-You-To-Be-Full.

> *"Replace, Recreate, Rejoice!"*
> *"Enjoy your achievements as well as your plans."*
> —Max Ehrmann

One of the keys to success in transitioning your diet is finding replacement foods. For example, try trading cooked peanut butter, which goes rancid, for other nut butters, such as raw, organic almond, hemp, coconut, pecan or cashew butter. Or, try replacing your favorite creamy chocolate desserts with my *Chocolate Coconut Ganache.* You can use sapotes and bananas to make the best banana cream pie your mother *never* made. Learn how to make raw ice cream—it's so tasty and satisfying, you will never know it's not the real thing. Find what you love and recreate it as a raw dish. If you love pumpkin pie, go out and buy a pumpkin, put it in the blender, add some cinnamon and raw honey or stevia, some vanilla, nutmeg, pumpkin pie spice, and coconut butter. Add a little bit of ginger and blend it up to make pumpkin pie pudding. And if you want to dehydrate some crust, you can make it out of almonds, pecans or your favorite nuts. This is real pumpkin pie with no sugar, no dairy and no cooking required. Take a little time to find foods you love to replace foods you crave, and put some love, energy and thought into the preparation of it. One of my favorite Italian dressings is parsley, olive oil, sun dried tomatoes, garlic, basil, rosemary and sea salt; I dunk broccoli in this fabulous dressing. I also drizzle it on crackers, in salads or with zucchini pasta. It helps with that Italian pasta cravings and reminds me of my Mamma Mia's Sunday dinners. Your health will blossom and your body will reflect it in your shape, your weight and your newfound love for it. Greed and gluttony are still two of the seven deadly sins. I don't care if it's raw or cooked food, eating less is still living more. Be fortuitous, not gluttonous. Be a MIRAWCLE, and become a RAWRIOR now!

The Final Transition

As you become more committed to eating raw, organic, whole foods with maximum nutritional impact, your body will become more sensitive. In other words, you will feel the negative effects when indulging in unhealthy food much more intensely. It's like when a high performance automobile that is used to getting high octane fuel starts to lurch and clunk when it's switched to cheap gas; your body will react when you switch to lower grade food—it's like putting sugar in your gas tank. Your body adapts to cleaner, more nutritious, fulfilling, efficient fuel, so when you feed it junk, the system gets clogged and malfunctions. By going raw, the body will transform from an old junker to a sexy sports car.

That's what my body was doing during my Brazil trip—transforming. When I was in the rain forest, I gave up cooked foods because I was afraid of getting sick, from eating cooked food in a foreign country, so I spent 30 days eating nuts and fruits and vegetables, and some fresh raw acai (a Brazilian antioxidant berry and juice). I gave up tofu, which is cooked, and replaced it with spirulina to get my protein—I was cleaning out my system, getting healthy and I felt amazing. After my trip, I landed in Miami for a week; I wanted to indulge myself so I gave in to my old cravings for cooked carbs, processed foods and my addiction to tofu and soy. Tofu was the last house on the block for me and the hardest to give up. I didn't realize I was allergic to soy, and I ate a lot of it. I wanted tofu and rice cakes so badly, so I said to myself, "You know what, I want it, I deserve it and I'm gonna eat it." So I did. And a funny thing happened. It didn't taste good to me. It tasted stale, starchy, old, dead and dry; which is what all cooked, packaged, processed food that's been on the shelf tastes like. It didn't taste alive. It didn't have that fresh taste I was used to; it didn't give me that "life." Cooked food doesn't have the water and oxygen whole ripe, raw fruits and veggies have. My body had adapted to eating fruits, vegetables and watery food in Brazil. After I indulged in all my old favorites, all I wanted to do was go to sleep, which was odd because I never wanted to sleep when I was in Miami. I always wanted to swim, dance, sun, shop and party. But I felt repressed, depressed, drained and lethargic. When I returned home to L.A. from Miami, I stopped craving food and started craving life. I believe I experienced divine intervention in Brazil, because that's when my diet and my health really took off. I didn't know I could eat like that but out of my commitment and persistence and willingness, I found out I could. I gave up tofu and cooked foods, and I never looked back. Tofu is "nofu" for me today. If I eat it I feel Tired, Old, Fat and Ugly. Today, my body is my barometer for how I feel and what I should do. So let your body be your barometer; it will tell you what to eat if you listen, really listen.

It will happen naturally, without your even having to think about it. You'll see that when you have been eating healthfully for a week or so, and you go back and eat something unhealthy, you won't feel as good. So you'll naturally stay away from things that make you feel bad. It's like aversion therapy. You'll eat something and, if you don't feel energized, you'll know it wasn't in your best interest and you won't eat it again. Remember, if after you eat you don't feel like dancing or walking around the block, then what you ate did not work for you. Eventually, the cravings will disappear, the habits will disappear, the depression, as well as the fat and the fear, and you will feel better, stronger and more in control of your life. When you are doing something about your issues, the issues usually get better because you are in action. Stay in action or detour into destruction. Inaction threatens any bit of success for health you may have.

Remember, the key to getting over the hump is to get over the hump. Keep going. Take a step and then take another step, and then another. Find someone to step with you. Remember, you can always take the elevator going down, but you have to take the steps going up. Look at how far you have come and look at where you are going. Keep the end in sight! Rawllelujah! Continue to explore, learn and grow and keep peeling the onion, as *you are almost there*. Then when *there* becomes *here*, you will keep going and going and growing and glowing!

Food Obsession
by Debbie Merrill

It's not what I'm eating, It's what's eating me
Thinking only about dinner, and it's just 5 past 3
I see it's to avoid my feelings and responsibilities
To give back to the world all my talents and abilities
It feels like such a burden and hard work to put out
The alternative, to stay with thoughts and obsessions,
which only scream and shout

If only I could eat what I want when I want it
I guess I really could but my jeans would not fit
Uncover, discover, take risk and the actions
Or be stuck on the couch, disabled and in traction

Food obsession will guilt and shame me to stillness
It's cunning and baffling because it's an illness
I must die the death of self in order to get well
Seeking only money, fame and prestige is the reason I fell

Trusting God as my source, an infallible friend
Will carry me through all the way to the end
I worry about nothing to avoid everything, relying solely on me
If I have to find a God, I don't have a God, that's the problem I see

The answer to stay grateful, committed, in the present, do God's will
Like when you are hiking you trudge up the hill
It works, it's simple, an easy remedy
It need not be tough for all of us to see

Just listen for guidance and put ego on the shelf
What you'll gain by losing is the love of yourself
Food is not love!

Raw Bites

- *Eat a raw, vegan, or vegetarian diet for 30 days and see how you feel.*

- *Make a new recipe to replace your sweet cravings.* My Splendid Spectacular Persimmon Smoothie *is orgasmic and can be made into a pudding or ice cream.*

- *Take a field trip to an exotic foods market, natural foods or farmer's market. Buy three organic fruits and veggies you've never had before and give your taste buds a treat.*

- *By eating more raw fruits and vegetables, you will gradually experience strength, serenity, spirituality and creativity.*

- *You are lovable, loving and loved.*

- *You are a unique, precious creation.*

- *Educate and celebrate yourself, and know that you never graduate.*

- *Let today be the first day of the rest of your life—not the tomorrow you worried about yesterday.*

- *"A spoon does not know the taste of soup, nor a learned fool the taste of wisdom." (Welsh Proverb) I say educate, create and end the debate.*

- *Become a MI<u>RAW</u>CLE and a <u>RAW</u>RIOR now!*

- *Get back on the roll if you slip and fall. See it as an interruption, not a failure.*

Chapter 28

Debbie Merrill's Skate Great USA School of Skating

"Live with intention. Walk to the edge. Listen hard.
Practice wellness. Play with abandon. Laugh.
Choose with no regret. Appreciate your friends. Continue to learn.
Do what you love. Live as if this is all there is."
—Mary Anne Radmacher

O ne of the best reasons to get healthy, and stay healthy, is so that we can pursue our dreams, follow our bliss, achieve our goals, be a mira̲wcle, and live our lives fully. If food is how we nourish our bodies, then finding and doing our right work is how we nourish our souls. Sometimes, if we are lucky and we are committed, we can make a living doing what we love. For me, that is an absolute necessity. I used to do all kinds of odd jobs—I have worked as a temp, handed out flyers for a nail salon on the streets of NYC, picked oranges in Ojai carrying a 50 pound sack on my front and back, I've laid asphalt in driveways, worked as a movie extra for $40 working a 16-hour day, waited tables, and taught yoga, skating and dance—all so I could make enough money to pursue my dreams. Until one day I decided to stop waiting for someone to give me a break, and decided to give myself one instead. I stopped waiting for someone to produce me and I produced my own opportunities: I opened my own skating school, created a "Learn to In-Line Skate" DVD, produced and starred in my own public TV show and wrote this book as well as starred in TV and commercials (which are my real dreams). Waiting is nothing more than idle movement for me. Wishing, hoping, and not doing, being and creating. So I decided to take a stand, find my power, and put my talent out in the world for all to see. I began taking risks. He who doesn't risk, doesn't live. You see, by sharing myself with the world in the form of service and love, I'm not only letting the world know who I am, I am contributing, serving, being vulnerable, real, open and powerful. When I do that, I can make a difference in the lives of others, as well as my own, through whatever work I choose for the day. And believe me, I wear many hats each day. I am a producer, an author, a lecturer, a teacher, health educator, skater/skating instructor, performer, actress, singer, dancer, coach, fitness trainer, friend, student, family member and child of the Universe. I do more in one day than most people do in a week. And I do it with joy, contentment, and energy. I get the job done because, as I often say, completion is perfection.

Skating and dancing are my most enduring loves. I spent the first half of my life on the ice and, after landing in Venice Beach, I fulfilled my dream of bringing the artistry of figure skating out of the ice rink and onto the beach—from the blades to the wheels. I created it and called it Figure-Blading. The very next year I was inspired to open California's first and longest running inline skate school and named it, "Skate Great USA School of Skating." I believe skating is childlike; it works on posture, carriage and confidence. It makes you look, act and feel younger and besides, it's fun! The basic premise of my instruction is that every person possesses the potential for increased athletic ability, happiness, health and success, and my primary goal is to empower each student with

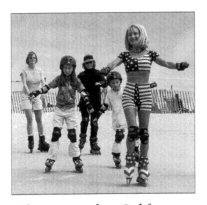

When I moved to California, it wasn't long before I realized that this was the only place I wanted to be, so I started the first and longest running skating school in Southern California—Skate Great USA School of Skating. The sky is my overhead and the beach is my office.

a sense of connection to his or her potential. A great teacher shares her knowledge, strength and experience, and is also able to show students how to tap into their own unique talents. My goal with everyone I teach and come in contact with in my life is to acknowledge and appreciate their gifts and help him or her discover their own. This was a talent I had hidden away from myself, along with many more I uncovered and discovered. Whether it is my raw food educating, skating, writing, singing, dancing or performing, I say bring it out and bling it on!

I believe that the best way to expand as an artist and as a person is to share your talent with as many people as possible. I love performing and I find teaching to be gratifying in the most amazing ways. It's a way of turning on the steam and building esteem, multiplying your gift—by giving others the opportunity to shine. It's a joy to watch a new skater go from wobbling along self-consciously to flying down the boardwalk with wings on their feet. Teaching expanded my world. My students really taught and inspired me to be a brilliant and prolific coach. And every student was heaven sent to me at the perfect time, and in the perfect order. I believe that when the student is ready, the teacher appears. It also works in reverse: when the teacher is ready, the student appears (from *A Course In Miracles*). So for over 20 years, I have been the student disguised as the teacher. What a great way to learn, earn and get the sun's healing burn at the beach. Thank you, Universe! I believe that when you live your dream fully, when you follow your heart, your dreams grow even greater; forces greater than you are at work to assist you in the process. A favorite quote of mine is, "What lies behind us and what lies before us are tiny matters compared to what lies within us" (Ralph Waldo Emerson). When I opened my school, I simply wanted to share my gift and my dream with others. I didn't realize then that I would receive so much in return. I went on to produce my own public television show, *The Debbie Merrill Show: Raw Foods On The Roll—Getting America Healthy*, which was shown in eleven cities throughout the United States. Raw on the Roll! Then I produced a successful DVD, *"Learn to In-Line Skate: To Look and Feel Great at Any Age,"* and have become a health educator, lecturer and author, empowering people with the gift of raw foods. I believe eating raw foods opens the gates of heaven to enter the fountain of youth. This book is a manifestation of my private one-on-one consultations, tips, tricks, notes, quotes, skills, drills, secrets,

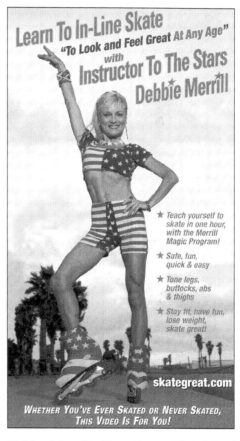

Debbie Merrill's Skate Great USA School of Skating, Learn to In-line Skate to Look and Feel Great At Any Age *DVD, available now at Skategreat.com*

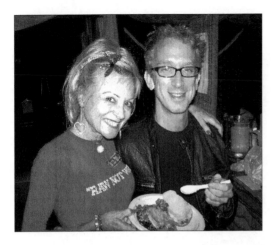

Andy Dick is a fellow raw vegan enthusiast and was a special guest on my TV show. I love being around his humorous, electric energy as I meet him spreading the raw message around town.

Gabriel Cousens, M.D. is one of my favorite raw food mentors, healers and educators. I love all his books, insightful wisdom, love and events, especially his Tree of Life Rejuvenation Center in Patagonia, Arizona.

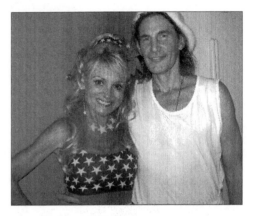

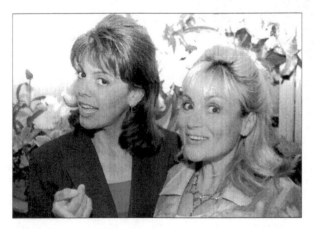

I'm so glad I met Jane Velez-Mitchell; I thank and applaud her for motivating me to be a pioneer in my pledge to go veg and for finishing this book.

suggestions, concepts, formulas and recipes, which allows me to reach more people and share not only my experiences, but also the wonder world of raw, live food. I have truly become a Raw Veggie Vegan Diva and I am living my dream with energy, vitality, success, enthusiasm, lust and excitement for life. I share these accomplishments, not to toot my own horn, but to illustrate the power of living raw, truthfully, walking the walk and talking the talk and really "going for it in life," by being committed and not attached to the outcome, but just the fun of the race. I'm enjoying the being and doing it all. Be convinced that everything is All-Right-Now. When you do that, anything can happen.

Merrillism #44: "If You Spend Your Health Chasing Wealth, You'll Spend Your Wealth Chasing Health."

So, I've talked about my goals and dreams, I encourage you to find your own. Find your own "skate school" creation. I recognize that not everyone wants, or needs, to make their work their play—I understand that. But I also think everyone needs to have *something* to do that makes their heart sing. It doesn't have to be work, it can be a hobby, an avocation, or just something fun and inspiring that you enjoy. Remember to have fun. The more fun you have, the more your health and life works. Life is limiting, fun is not. Fun is limitless, and so is health. For example, one the many things I do for fun is take a dance class with a great instructor and friend of mine, Jeff Costa of Cardio Striptease®. In his classes, 20 to 30 women are all together laughing and dancing around in lingerie, skirts, shirts, tights and panties, bumping and grinding, doing the "shake it 'til you break it." Shaking it to celebrate and rejoice in our bodies and souls, expressing our sensuality, sexuality and creativity while doing cardio sensual dancing. This is an example of real exercise and real fun. It works the mid-section and lower areas where downward gravity takes hold. When I take this class, I feel alive and fulfilled afterwards, because I fully express my true self in all ways: cardiovascularly, creatively, sensually, aerobically and powerfully. This is how I choose which exercise I do and which sport I participate in. These are the kind of dance classes I teach as well, combining all of the above. It has to include all those ingredients or I don't do it. And the more fun it is, the longer you do it, so you wind up burning more calories if you need to. You lose track of time and it doesn't even feel like a workout, it's a playout. How great is that? In the class, we're all releasing our "inner strippers" and it's fantastic, silly, freeing, fun, energizing and enlivening. It's also excellent exercise, but that's just a bonus. I invite you to let out your inner stripper, skater, writer, rock star, comedian, teacher, painter, or dreamer. What would you do if money and time were not a factor? Find a way to do it. Start where you are, and then expand.

Raw Bites

- *Start a dream journal. As I have said, writing is one of the best ways to get in touch with your inner being. Spend a few minutes each day dreaming about what you want, what you want your future to look like, who you want to be in it. I make a list of five things that I want, five things I'm grateful for and five things I'm learning every day. That way I am at least in touch with what I want, and I start writing what I want, instead of what I don't want. Then I see it, feel it, think it, thank it and manifest it into being. It's possible to think great thoughts, eat healthy live food, have fabulous creative expression and a wonderful life. That is what you will have in your life when you do this, instead of when you don't. What a great life to live! That is true wealth. I write things right. As Julia Cameron says in The Artist's Way, "Write to drain the brain daily." Don't go to bed with it all in your head.*

- *Dabble. If you have an idea about what you may want to do or be, try it out. The more you risk, the safer you are, the more you succeed.*

- *Find a mentor. Find someone who does what you want to do and pick his or her brain. Find out how your mentor achieved his or her goals and follow the path they have laid out. 1) Meet them for lunch or tea and take their good, orderly directions. 2) Call them every day or several times a week to check in and declare your creative actions and successes. 3) Celebrate your accomplishments. 4) See your failures as slow successes, and as God's protection, redirection and guidance.*

- *What you are visualizing, you are materializing.*

- *If you are in love and joy, you will attract love and joy in all areas of your life.*

- *Once you make one small advancement in your health and creative expression, you have the rest of your life to reap the rewards.*

- *The number of vegetarians, vegans and raw fooders is rising everyday.*

- *The ocean is always in motion. Flow in, flow out, "and move flowly like the ocean."*

- *"Try not to become a person of success, but a person of value." (Albert Einstein)*

- *Courage is fear that has been converted into dignity, integrity and power.*

- *"Anyone bored these days is not paying attention." (Bill Copeland)*

- *My concerns don't keep me from living my dreams, they keep me from enjoying them.*

Chapter 29

Feel the Wow
with Cacao Ka-Pow!

*"All you need is love. But a little chocolate now
and then doesn't hurt."*
—Charles M. Schulz

I believe the only way to live life is passionately, completely and deeply—that is the way to become happy and content. You might get hurt, but nothing hurts so much that a little cacao (raw chocolate) won't fix. What if I told you that you could be a healthy, raw, organic, vegan, and could lose weight, look great, feel fantastic, and have a clear and sharp mind—without giving up chocolate? I know that for many of you, giving up chocolate is as inconceivable as giving up air, so the fact that chocolate is actually good for you should come as a pleasant surprise. You know I ended my love affair with sugar and junk food to embrace the raw lifestyle many years ago. Giving up processed foods, refined sugar, alcohol, caffeine, illicit and prescription drugs, and tobacco wasn't easy, but thankfully it didn't mean I had to give up pleasure, and neither do you. If you are a secret chocoholic, it's time to come out of the closet and embrace your love of the dark, delicious treat in its natural state. Cacao beans taste like dark chocolate because that is precisely what they are. All chocolate comes from cacao beans, and cacao nibs are the seeds of the cacao fruit, so essentially cacao is raw, organic, unprocessed chocolate. It is my secret weapon to open the heart, sharpen the mind, lift the spirit, increase the abundance and bliss, and put you in a good mood. That's why they call it the good mood food. Cacao promotes that blissful, loving feeling, which is why lovers give gifts of chocolate to express their love for one another on Valentine's Day.

Sidebar to the Rawbar

Raw cacao…

- Is great for weight control. It diminishes appetite and assists in weight loss.
- Helps to open the heart and improve brain function.
- Contains 20 times the antioxidant levels of red wine and 30 times the amount of antioxidants in green tea.
- Contains theobromine, magnesium (the mineral most lacking in the S.A.D diet) PEA and anandamide (the bliss chemical associated with feeling great).

Now you can give up alcohol and caffeine for something utterly delectable and nutritious. I feel delicious, and my friends call me Delicious Debbie, thanks to raw cacao. Cacao is one of my 10 Superfoods. It contributes to good physical and mental health because cacao promotes brain focus, alertness and functioning. Cacao is thought to be the best source of magnesium, which is effective in lowering blood pressure, regulating heartbeat, balancing brain chemistry and building strong bones. This is particularly significant when you consider the fact that 80% of Americans are magnesium deficient, which is a leading cause of heart problems. Additionally, cacao is ultra rich in antioxidants. Antioxidants promote cardiovascular health, protect and help repair damage caused by free radicals, and may reduce the risk of certain cancers. Antioxidants, sometimes called the beauty minerals, are also found in cacao and are important in building strong hair, nails, bones and teeth, promoting healthy skin and detoxifying the liver.

"And Charlie, don't forget about what happened to the man who suddenly got everything he ever wanted. He lived happily ever after."
—Roald Dahl, Charlie and the Chocolate Factory

One reason people eat chocolate when they want to "feel good" and why many women crave chocolate before or during menstruation, is because cacao contains substances known to promote feelings of well-being and combat mild depression. Among these are anandamide, also known as the "bliss chemical," because the brain releases it when we are feeling great. It promotes relaxation and helps prolong our feeling of well-being. Phenylethylamine is a substance created in the brain when we are in love, which is why eating chocolate naturally lifts our mood, increases alertness and acts as a mild antidepressant. Cacao raises serotonin levels in the brain, which contributes to the antidepressant effect, and also stimulates endorphins, the "feel good" chemical that the brain releases after vigorous exercise. Cacao does contain small amounts of caffeine and theobromine, but I believe the benefits obtained by eating a small amount of it far outweighs the potential harmful effects of consuming it. Besides, if the only little caffeine you consume comes from cacao, you are much better off than if you drink coffee, tea, caffeinated "energy" drinks, soda, alcohol, take stimulants or prescription drugs.

Merrillism #45: "Go Raw Now; I Am Teaching You How to Find the Wow While Eating Your Cacao."

With all the minerals, antioxidants and beneficial chemical properties contained in cacao, it's no wonder it is often called, "the food of the gods." We are used to thinking of chocolate as a guilty treat, something so yummy that we eat it, even though we know it is bad for us. Recent studies have shown that chocolate, at least in its natural state, has gotten a bad rap. What makes good chocolate "bad," is the processing, refining and the addition of white sugar, dairy products and other chemical additives and the overeating of it. Overeating any food is not good, whether it's cacao, nuts, mangoes or french fries. I believe in moderation not deprivation, even in the raw food diet. Eat less and live more, and never be too shy to ask for a doggie bag. You are what you eat, think, assimilate, eliminate and absorb. Raw cacao beans and nibs contain no sugar and between 12% and 50% fat, depending on the variety. Given its fat content, it is important to consume cacao in moderation. Since I have a very small frame, being a figure skater, four to six beans or two tablespoons at a sitting is enough for me. Depending on your height, weight and fitness goals, a little more or less may work for you. The important point, however, is to eat cacao as Mother Nature intended, raw, unprocessed and unrefined.

I always have cacao nibs or beans (the seeds of the cacao bean with the outer shell removed) on hand. They're delicious eaten straight, or you can add agave nectar, honey or berries such as goji berries to add sweetness. Cacao nibs are a yummy addition to smoothies, raw ice cream and add a burst of flavor to trail mix. Try my Raw on the Roll High-Energy Trail Mix with raw goji berries, raw mulberries, Brazil nuts, cashews, almonds and raw cacao nibs—or create your own crunch and munch. I also put them in my Mocha Choca Toca Maca Chino Tea to add a chocolate flavor and crunch. Sometimes I freeze them and add them like frozen chocolate chips on fruit salads, and in my Coconut Spirulina Spread. You can also add them to my Heaven's Coconut Butter Spread and to

Debbie's Spritty Spirulina Spread. Mmmmmm. It's divaliciously delicious! Get creative with your food and you will get creative with your life. See my recipes in the back for more delicious ways to add my favorite superfoods into your *Raw on the Roll* lifestyle. I tell all my clients and friends, "When eating raw organic there's no need to panic."

Raw Bites

- *Trade your chocolate candy, cooked nutrition bars and gourmet chocolates for raw, organic cacao beans and nibs. You can be a chocoholic everyday if you do it the raw way! Look in your local health food stores, there are raw chocolate bars that are just as good as the cooked ones, and much better for you.*

- *Instead of saying "no" to chocolate, make a sweet treat that your kids will love to eat. Make my Raw CoComoco Corn Chewies today and enjoy. You won't miss those other cooked crispy treats, brownies or chocolate chip cookies, I promise!*

- *When I eat and sell my cacao to the masses, I dine with the classes. Cacao is rawliciously, eviliciously delicious. Dine like a delicious diva now.*

- *I don't eat cacao at night but some of my Raw on the Roll Dream Team say it helps them sleep better. Try it and see how it works for you. Sometimes cacao helps me with elimination. It improves my peristalsis action. So plunge the prunes and try cacao for that Ka-Pow on the toilet.*

- *Say NO to cooked chocolate, desserts and bars, and find the Next Opportunity, which is raw cacao.*

- *Be the best, enjoy the best and forget the rest.*

- *A few beans a day and you're on your way.*

- *Eat cacao and make one person happy each day, even if it's you.*

- *Eat cacao and have a life with raw food, tradition and nutrition.*

- *David Wolfe, one of my mentors in the raw movement, always says, "Today is the best day ever." Especially after eating his rawsome, awesome cacao. (See resource section.)*

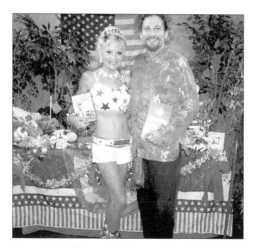

David Wolfe with his exuberant energy and knowledge of exquisite food and super nutrition inspired me to go 100% raw vegan 17 years ago and I've never looked back.

Chapter 30

Drink Your Solids and Chew Your Liquids

"Wisely, and slow. They stumble that run fast."
—William Shakespeare

We live in a fast world. We do everything fast and then complain because, somehow, top speed is still not fast enough. In our rush to hurry up and get there already, we are missing out on the journey and forgetting the old adage, "Speed kills." There is much more to life than making it go faster. We are racing through and we are missing out. Nowhere is it more apparent than at the dining room table—or more likely, the kitchen counter, in front of the TV, or at our desks. Eating a meal has evolved into nothing more than a chore we race through as quickly as possible so we can check it off our ever expanding "to do" list. Even at meal times, we have become human doings instead of human beings. We do everything except enjoy our food. How can we enjoy it when we gobble it down standing over the sink or shovel in mouthfuls of food while driving, walking, reading or talking on the phone, barely stopping to chew, as we sit in front of the computer screen, answering email, surfing the web and returning phone calls between bites—multitasking ourselves to death? Drinking our meals, eating bars and shakes to replace meals, and wondering why we don't feel or look our best. I try and put my fork down and breathe between bites. I chew slowly and close my eyes when I eat alone, and try not to talk, read, watch TV or write, (I said I try). I just eat, savor, relish and cherish my meal so that it truly fills me, feeds me and nourishes my mind, body and spirit with its divine life force. Quiet eating is a form of meditation for me. When I eat this way, I digest my food well and I feel satiated, relaxed and content and I don't feel like I need a second helping because I enjoy my food the first time around. When I

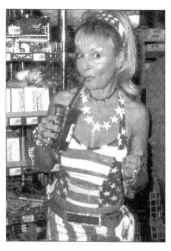

I learned to chew my liquids and drink my solids to improve digestion and get my alkaline greens in.

eat my meals rushing, racing, driving, talking on the phone or in a hurry, I don't feel like I have eaten, like somehow it didn't count, so I get to do it again. I used to think that if no one saw me eat, or if I didn't sit down to a "real" meal, or if I just nibbled as I prepared a meal, it didn't count. So therefore, I got another "real meal." That type of deluded thinking and behavior always equates to overeating, weight gain, lethargy, feelings of guilt, remorse and foggy thinking. When I make the time and take the time to eat my treat, I'm ready to handle any feat on my own two feet!

> *"You can find your way across this country using*
> *burger joints the way a navigator uses stars."*
> —Charles Kuralt

There is an international organization known as Slow Food that was founded in Italy almost 20 years ago, shortly after McDonald's opened in Rome's Piazza di Sapgna. The organization abhors fast food and encourages people to slow down and enjoy their food again by reconnecting with culture and tradition. To that I say, "Bravo!" Fast food is antithetical to everything Italians stand for. Italy is a country that loves good food, good wine, good conversation, art, history, music and one another. Dinner with friends takes the whole night and the preparation and enjoyment of food is an integral part of everyday life. There is so much passion in preparation and demonstration. Meals are meant to be eaten, enjoyed and, most importantly, shared with family and friends. Sadly, enjoying life and spending time with loved ones around the dinner table has fallen by the wayside in today's society because we "just don't have the time." As a result, we eat more food faster, and enjoy life and family less, creating less passion and time for one another. We have become a number, an email address, a code or a social security number. We somehow have lost our names and existence with one another.

We are killing ourselves with fast food. Children are dying on basketball courts, ice-skating rinks and football fields at very young ages because of our national obsession with and addiction to drive-thrus and fast food. The high cholesterol, fat and sugar contained in these foods is causing problems like diabetes, high blood pressure, high cholesterol, obesity and heart disease in children and adults, just to name a few. One out of every three children will develop diabetes in their lifetime. 15% of children and adolescents ages 6 to 19 are considered overweight and obese and an additional 15% are at risk of becoming overweight. Even worse, is the fact that more than 10% of children between the ages of 2 and 5 are overweight. They are overweight before can they even walk or run. The added pounds that contribute to certain health conditions and diseases in adults contribute to the same problems in children. Physicians are reporting an increase in serious health problems such as hypertension, ADD, cancer and strokes. What we eat today could have a significant impact on the future of our health in this world. I believe it is the broken link to the chain in our health. You still are what you eat! Children need to spend more time exercising and eating foods that allow them to *want* to do exercise. They need to be educated and inspired regarding the benefits of eating healthy, live food. If you are a parent, be a role model for your child. Don't keep junk food at home or on the counter. Exercise as a family outdoors, spend time together, and serve fruit for dessert. Have healthy snacks readily available. Studies show that kids are much more likely to pick up a banana or grapes than a candy bar if it's available and visible. Keep fruit on the counter. Avoid eating fast food for dinner. If you must dine out, find a healthy, affordable place where you can all eat together and order healthy salads and foods. Please refrain from fried, fatty, salty, sweet foods. These types of foods cause overeating and addiction to these foods and establishments. Families that eat together stay together. Remember, this is your valuable, precious family time. If you don't take the time and make the time, you will never find the time. Time will pass you by and so will your loved ones.

Merrillism #46: "If You Don't Taste it, You Waste it", Eat Organic, it Tastes Better.

Non-organic and processed food is a waste of chewing time. I'd rather use my mouth to sing, and speak pearls of wisdom and eat real raw food. Eating on fast forward is unhealthy on many levels. By slowing down, even just a little, and by taking time to breathe, you'll enjoy your food more, stress less, taste more and experience better health. Part of the reason many of us eat too much is simply because of the speed with which we eat. It takes 20 minutes for our brains to receive the "full" signal from our stomachs, and by eating too quickly we bypass the "off" switch and end up eating past the point of satisfaction. The simple act of eating slowly means we will eat less food and therefore, lose or maintain weight with ease. Raw, organic foods are nutrient dense, so you need to eat less quantity to receive nourishment and fulfillment. Some studies suggest that eating every meal slowly, to the point of satisfaction, could result in losing as much as 20 pounds in one year. Another benefit of slowing down is pure pleasure. Since you are not gulping your food down, thinking only of your next bite, you can really focus on what you are eating—your current bite, rather than the next. How much more enjoyment could you get out of your meal if you savored every single bite? It's like living in the present moment, not the future. Embellish, relish and cherish the flavors, textures, tastes, colors, shapes, smells and feelings of the food. Find passion in your eating. Now that's Italian!

You are in control of how, where and how much you eat, not just what you eat. If you're eating meat and processed food, how much are you eating? Where are you getting it, and where are you eating it? What's your frame of mind while eating? This is something very important to look at for your good health. Eating slowly is better for digestion. This is especially important when eating raw foods, which are more difficult for some people to digest. Digestion starts in the eyes, the tongue and the mouth, so chewing your food more thoroughly and for a longer time means your stomach won't have to do all the work, and you will have fewer digestive problems. It makes sense when you think of how much harder your stomach has to work to break down chunks of barely chewed food as opposed to small, finely ground pieces, fruits and blended foods. It's the reason baby food is mushy—they don't have teeth to start the process so, in order to digest it (and so they don't choke), the food needs to arrive in their stomachs liquefied and blended. So, pretend that you are as delicate as a baby and chew your food completely and you will taste more, digest better, enjoy more and eat less. If you do have digestive problems, you may find it helpful to blend your meals in a blender for a few days (this is called a blended fast). Also, eating cultured veggies helps. Or, if you really need it, try taking raw digestive enzymes. Finally, eating slowly and mindfully will decrease your stress and give you the opportunity to answer some unanswered questions, and help you resolve problems and come up with solutions, inspirations, and imaginative ideas. Part of our "go, go, go" mentality is due to the pressure we feel to complete everything we want or need to accomplish in the space of one day, prompting us to try and do everything faster. One way we can lessen the stress is to force ourselves to slow down while we are eating and enjoy the process. Look at eating a meal as a pleasurable break from the rat race and hustle and bustle of life. Think of mealtimes as active meditations and you will not only enjoy your meal more, you will enjoy your life and your body more. You will enjoy your own company and in turn the company of others. People make good company when they are healthy and doing what they love.

Merrillism #47: "Eat Slowly, Think Quickly."

Drink Your Solids…

When you eat, do nothing else. Always sit down to eat and, even if you are eating alone, resist the urge to watch television, read, work, email, surf the web, talk, make phone calls or write. Just eat. Pray before you eat, then ask that it be enough and give thanks for the gracious gift that you are about to receive. **Start eating with your eyes first**. Take the time to appreciate what your hands or someone else's have prepared with love and intention. Admire the care, colors, shapes and artistry of the chef, friend or loved one who created the meal you are about to enjoy. See it, smell it, touch it, love it, and eat it. Mangiare! **Put down your fork between bites,** and chew, masticate and enjoy each bite completely. Experience the texture of each morsel on your tongue and let the different flavors mix, meld and burst inside your mouth in many different phases. Enjoy the salty, sweet, bitter, sour and spicy tastes on your tongue. Deepak Chopra says it's good to experience all five flavors at one meal for satiation and contentment. I practice this and it works. I don't crave more. I'm satisfied and content. Don't swallow until you have thoroughly chewed each bite, breathe between bites, and don't pick up your fork for the next bite until you are finished with the one you are currently eating. Please don't drink anything while you're eating. Wait at least an hour or two after you have eaten to drink anything. This is so you do not dilute your digestive juices that are working so hard to help digest your food. Try drinking a glass of water at least half an hour before meals instead so that you are not dehydrated and feeling thirsty during the meal. This is a great tip, you will also feel less bloated and full when done eating. All meals have a beginning, middle and end so savor each moment. Know when the end is near and get ready to walk away when you are still a little hungry, not stuffed. Try not to have one of those "I'm so bloated I can't eat for three days" kind of meals.

"Chew Your Liquids…"

Drinking fresh squeezed, organic fruit juice is a wonderful way to increase your raw food and water intake. I recommend drinking fresh, squeezed fruit juice in the morning for cleansing, and vegetable juice in the afternoon and evening for healing, strengthening and building. Of course you always want to drink fresh squeezed, organic juice rather than the kind that comes from a bottle or can, which is usually pasteurized or flash pasteurized (heated with ultraviolet light—in other words, cooked) and therefore devoid of healthy enzymes. Making your own juice is also better for your taste buds, your pocketbook and saves you travel time. When you drink it fresh, you are receiving the maximum nutrition available instantly, and because fresh unstrained juice contains some pulp and fiber, you can almost literally chew your juice. Try it. I do it on my public TV show and get a big laugh because I swish it around to get it in my gums, tongue, cheeks and throat, while making funny noises and faces. This way, it easily gets absorbed into my bloodstream. Make a chewing motion as you drink and you will really squeeze the maximum amount of flavor out of every sip. You may feel kind of silly at first, but chewing your liquids is an effective way to slow down and savor the flavor longer so you'll feel more satisfied with less. Also, a 16 oz. glass of orange juice is a lot of sugar. Please do the math. Do you know how many oranges it takes to make 16 oz. of juice? Pay attention to your body. You may only need 4 oz., or try dividing the 16 oz. throughout the day. Fructose is still a form of sugar. Raw juice has no fiber but it is still a valuable source of vitamins, minerals and phytonutrients. A four-ounce serving of 100% raw juice satisfies a fruit serving. Let the flavors of all your foods and juices burst in your mouth. Let the taste last in your mouth and on your tongue so you can relish in the taste and experience, and have a wonderful rawsome experience.

Merrillism #48: "Water Is Like Prayer, We Need It Every Day."

Many times, we mistake thirst for hunger. We think we need to eat, but we are actually dehydrated. So, next time you feel what you perceive as hunger, drink a glass of water and wait 20 minutes. If you are still hungry, then eat something. I drink about one to two quarts a day because drinking water is one of the best things you can do for your body. If you aren't a water lover now, become one. The following H_2O facts will probably amaze and startle you:

1. One glass of water shuts down midnight hunger pangs for almost 100% of the dieters studied in a university study.
2. Dehydration is the number one source of daytime fatigue.
3. Preliminary research indicates that 8-10 glasses of water a

day could significantly ease back and joint pain for up to 80% of sufferers.

4. A mere 2% drop in body water can trigger fuzzy short-term memory, trouble with basic math and difficulty focusing on the computer screen or intricate work.

5. Drinking five glasses of water daily decreases the risk of colon cancer by 45%, slashes the risk of breast cancer by 79%, and cuts the risk of bladder cancer by 50%.

Are you drinking the amount of water you could everyday?

Here's how you can begin:

1. Make your water come alive. Add some fresh chopped or whole sprigs of peppermint, parsley, dill, cilantro or green leaves to a glass or pitcher of water before you go to bed. When you wake up the next morning, you will have "live" water to drink because the enzymes from the parsley or greens will have infused it with energy.

2. Add flavor. A lot of people fail to drink enough water because they think it's boring. So, flavor it up by adding the juice of fresh lime, lemon or orange to it. Another delicious alternative is to make your own "spa water" by cutting up a whole cucumber and adding it to a pitcher of chilled water.

3. Add water to your favorite fresh-squeezed fruit juice and freeze it. I did this when I went to college in Miami. I'd eat frozen orange juice with lots of water in it for breakfast when I walked to school. Because it was so hot and humid, it was delicious, nutritious and hit the spot when it was hot. Kids really love this one. They think it's a frozen, sugary ice

pop. Trick them into eating healthy—I did it with my dad when he was sick and he loved it.

Raw Bites

- *Eat one slow meal, preferably one you make yourself. Take time to appreciate your handiwork. If it took you one hour to prepare, give yourself at least that time to eat and enjoy it.*

- *Lay off the fast food. Make today the day you eliminate fast food from your diet for good. Fast food takes your money fast. Fast food takes fast money. Fast food takes down your health fast as well.*

- *Drink more water. Water is like soap for your insides. Water cleanses, heals, repairs and maintains the body.*

- *Eating is a time to meditate, invigorate and rejuvenate.*

- *Masticate your food to improve digestion. Chewing your food 50 times before swallowing kick-starts the digestive process, which begins in the mouth.*

- *Eat at least one meal a day outdoors with great scenery, to bring beauty, peace and joy into your meal, mind and mannerisms.*

Section 4

Dessert: Living and Giving

Chapter 31

From Raw to Richness

"Live life fully while you're here. Experience everything.
Take care of yourself and your friends. Have fun, be crazy, be weird.
Go out and screw up! You're going to anyway, so you might as well
enjoy the process. Take the opportunity to learn from your mistakes:
find the cause of your problem and eliminate it. Don't try to be
perfect; just be an excellent example of being human."
—Anthony Robbins

I started my journey on the *road to raw* without really knowing where it would lead. I had no expectations, I just knew I wanted it and wanted to do it. I was hoping and praying it would take me in the right direction, and away from myself. I wanted to leave the girl that I was in the dust. I wanted to ditch the angry, sad, unhealthy, insecure girl who looked good on the outside, but who didn't know how to fix the inside—or even know that the inside needed to be fixed.

"Man struggles to find life outside himself,
unaware that the life he is seeking is within."
—Kalil Gibran

If living raw could get me away from *that* girl and into the girl I knew I really was, I was all for it. And you know something? It worked. I traveled all the way deep, deep down and around and around the road, far away from the mess and stress, until the road curved and I made a perfect figure eight that led me right back to myself—with one important difference. The Debbie I encounter today is the Debbie I always knew I was and wanted to be. I didn't know what I needed until I heard it, and raw food opened my ears so that I could hear it, and raw living food put wings on my feet so I could get into action and do it. I had to see it, hear it, seize the opportunity and go for it. That is what I am asking and encouraging you to do. Seize the moment and do it now! Get in gear, put on the gear, and shift gears. You are ready for the ride of your wild life. Please don't apologize for your past behavior, don't analyze it, just utilize this knowledge to make positive changes in your life now. Ask your feet to carry you on this rawkin' raw road of happy, healthy bliss. Don't live in fear, just live in the here and now, "Go For It!" Learn to be humble, instead of numb, by applying this system now. My journey has taken me from raw to the rich life I always hoped for. Living raw has transformed me in every way—it transformed my health, brought me wealth, enriched my spirit, infused my life with creativity, love, community, brilliance, vitality, spirituality and the freedom to be, loving and fully self-expressed. I finally found what it means to be fully self-expressed, and what a joyful reality it is to live in. Not needing the O.K. and approval of others to be and express myself. I didn't need the score of a perfect 10 to keep going at life again. What a relief! It's true; health is an inside job. It's my job (and I believe everyone's job) to turn the inside out and share it with the world. Go from health to health, success to success, love to love, joy to joy, prosperity to abundance, extraordinary to mastery, creativity to excellence, and from spirituality to enlightenment. I did, I am and I will continue to do so as I spread the message. Living raw gives me the truth and the word. Once you grow in health and spirituality, your words have more power to affect others.

"Life is what happens to you while you're busy making other plans."
—John Lennon

I plan and the Universe laughs. Planning and worrying are not the same action. In the past, I had a tendency to worry, worry, worry and worry some more because it made me feel like I was doing something about the problem, but the reality is all I was doing was obsessing, ruminating, stressing and creating drama and stories around everything. I thought it would fix things (especially my health) if I worried, obsessed and talked about it. Then I realized that worrying is trying to fix things that haven't happened yet, and may never happen. All worries are reruns. It's like being on a rocking horse and going nowhere. Worry is an ironic form of hope. Don't worry about it—just do it. So I decided to save the drama for the page and the stage. Remember, write things right, and write things out. Planning is action. Stay in action, or else detour into destruction. Action keeps us grounded in the present. Where our health is concerned, I believe we have to take constructive, contrary, courageous action instead of worrying about what may or may not happen. When in doubt, "quote it out" like I do to get me through. It works. Use one of the 365 quotes in this book, create your own or use this one: *"My body is thin, healthy, firm and beautiful, always and forever."*

When I first embarked upon this journey, I wanted to lose some weight, look good, feel more energetic, alive and vital, look healthy, never get sick again and have creative, joyful success in my life. I wanted to make more money, be rid of fear and negativity—that is what drew me to the raw lifestyle. Perhaps it is what attracted you as well. I didn't realize at the time how deep the raw lifestyle would take me into myself, and how far out I would then be able to go. As Shirley MacLaine says, "You have to go out on the limb, that's where the fruit is." By digging deep, I was able to explode outward and share the important lessons I have learned with the world. I love sharing the message and not the mess all over the world, in my lectures, education, videos, book, TV and radio appearances, skating and dance classes. It fills my raw spirit. I believe that the healing process is not really complete until we are able to share our experience and help heal our fellow man. I love the one-on-one with all of my students. I learned from them how to be brilliant. It's the act of sharing that completes the circle. I teach, consult, write, lecture, perform and share what I know in order to serve others, and also to reinforce it for myself. I will say it again, it's not *about* me, it's *through* me. It's not about me, it's about *we*!

> "Big heartedness is the most essential
> virtue on the spiritual journey."
> —Matthew Fox

I hope that living raw will help give you the life you so richly deserve. Extraordinary living is about more than eating healthy foods, exercising and breathing; it's about more than going to work, paying the bills, getting the kids ready for school, exercising and planning for retirement. Being healthy isn't only about the physical—true health is achieved by nurturing your spiritual and creative side—as well as by being, loving and giving all of yourself to yourself and others. Be healthy by taking risks, being fearless, unstoppable, powerful, compassionate, tolerant and vulnerable every day. Living is giving. So, as you explore this last section, don't make the mistake of saving the best for last. Enjoy the dessert of life *right now*. Don't just eat your food raw, eat your *life* raw—take big bites, little bites, mini-bites, chew well and live thoroughly in the *no limit* zone. Seek pleasure, find peace, accept help, give help and give it your all. Go for it all. Grab life by the handful and dig in.

> "I am here to live out loud."
> —Emile Zola

Raw Bites

- "It takes a long time to bring excellence to maturity." (Publilius Cyrus)

- Sometimes it's about spiritual solutions and not physical ones.

- Before you put things into words and actions, put them into images in your mind.

- I am the "I" and the Eye in my life. I see what I see, not what I want to see.

- Uncover, discover, and recover the power within you. Look within and use this book to begin.

- If a creative work of art or health is in you, it has to come out. Give up the "yeah, but" syndrome. After but, everything else is BS anyway. Have faith and trust you will because you are and you can.

- "Art enables us to find ourselves and lose ourselves at the same time." (Thomas Merton)

- Some people give and forgive, others get and forget.

- The gift of health and happiness belongs to those who unwrap it.

- "My life is my message." (Gandhi)

- How high I am, how much I see, how far I reach depends on me.

Chapter 32

Rhyming and Jhymin' are the Way I Express,

Glitter, Sequins And Rhinestones is The Way That I Dress—it's My Quirky, Creative, Wild Need to Express

"Unbeing dead isn't being alive."
—e. e. cummings

When I was a young girl, I needed to fit in almost as much as I wanted to stand out. Yes, I loved my sparkly getups and I adored being in the spotlight, but I also felt pressure to look like all the other figure skaters. I hated the fact that I had breasts and a butt when everyone else had narrow hips and flat chests, so I hid my assets and tried to diet myself into looking like a prepubescent boy, instead of the young woman I was rapidly becoming. The pressure to fit in and look like all the other ten-year-old figure skaters caused me to under eat and over exercise. I even dressed like a boy, trading my shiny getups for athletic wear, tie-dyes and overalls. I turned into a jockaholic and hid my glitter, rhinestones and feather boas in the back of my mind and closet. Of course, I eventually came out of the closet and let my inner crown-wearing queen run free. I was fortunate that I had a lot of people to help me transform from a skater jock to an ice skating, dancing diva. In my first professional skating show, I performed a version of Sonja Henie's "Lovely Hula Hands." My choreographer, Bobby Denard, having performed with Sonja Henie, choreographed the entire show so that I could replicate her performance and style. I'll never forget the two chorus boys skating over my long, silky, straight hair as I was turned upside down in a swirling spin. I was on the road for seven years with this show as the Hawaiian Princess on ice. I performed one false eyelash at a time and learned how to apply them as well. I was living La Vida Loca, "My name is Debbie, I am a show girl," and boy was I showing the world who I really was. I was learning, living and loving life in the spotlight. My professional transition from competitive skater to performer not only supported my true desire to perform, be different and stand out from the crowd, it demanded it.

Your profession may not demand that you stand center stage, but you can still be a star in your own life. One of my inspirations is Marianne Williamson, who wrote two of my favorite books, *A Return to Love* and *Illumination*. I studied with her when she was teaching the material from *A Course In Miracles*. This is one of my favorite books about love and forgiveness. I highly recommend reading it for your health. I love it so much that I framed her picture on my treasure map to serve as a constant reminder that I can shine for the world and be a leader, an educator, and a powerful, brilliant woman like her. It's about how each one of us has not only the ability, but the sacred responsibility, to shine in our own lives. She wrote a fabulous speech for Nelson Mandela's inauguration that so inspired me that I printed it out and framed it to serve as a constant reminder to be my own brightest light:

Our deepest fear is not that we are inadequate.

Our deepest fear is that we are powerful beyond measure.

It is our light, not our darkness that most frightens us.

We ask ourselves, who am I to be brilliant,
gorgeous, talented, fabulous?

Actually, who are you not to be?

You are a child of God. Your playing small does not serve the world.

There is nothing enlightened about shrinking
so that other people won't feel insecure around you.

We are all meant to shine, as children do.

We were born to make manifest the glory of God that is within us.

It's not just in some of us; it's in everyone.

And as we let our own light shine,
we unconsciously give other people permission to do the same.

As we are liberated from our own fear,
our presence automatically liberates others.

—Marianne Williamson

Merrillism #49: "Bling it On; Let Raw Foods Give You a More Creative Life."

I say bring it on. Give me the rings, bling and all the things. I'm ready for anything in my creative life. Eating raw foods gives me alertness, awareness and an awakening to all the joy life has to offer. I'm unstoppable. Being raw doesn't mean being plain or boring. It's quite the opposite. Just as I encourage you to eat all the colors of the rainbow, I encourage you to live the rainbow. Taste all the flavors of life and dress to express and impress. If wearing pink hot pants and a pink tie with silver tennis shoes makes you feel like a star, go for it—with gusto! The point is not to literally wear glitter and rhinestones (unless you want to), the point is to give yourself the freedom to glow and grow and be the star in your own show. Life is a stage, a school, a gym and we are all working out our performance and refining our act. The way you dress is just another way of telling the world who you are and announcing your presence. What you wear is not about fashion as much as it's about passion. Passion for our freedom of speech, choice, food, dress, work and spirituality.

I know a high-powered financial analyst who works from home. He spends the majority of his day on the phone, wheeling and dealing and making million dollar decisions. He could choose to go to work in his pajamas or old sweats, but instead, he gets up every morning and puts on a business suit—right down to a pressed shirt, necktie and cuff links. He says it makes him feel powerful, successful and in control. It's his uniform, like Superman's big red "S." I love to wear red, white and blue—the shinier, the better—and top it off with red, white and blue skates or skate covers and glow-in-the-dark wheels. It's my uniform and reminds me that I am a star in my own unique life shining for all the world to see, me being me, but most of all—inspiring others to set free and be.

What do you like to wear? What makes you feel like a star? I say, "Bling it on!" Shine on me and I'll shine on you, because you are a star. Everything about you shines, and if you don't know it yet, I am here to tell you that you are, (as we all are) here to inspire the world with your energy, your gifts, your talents and your being-ness. Living raw is about more than diet; it's how you live every part of your life. So give yourself permission to be extraordinary, incredible, fabulous and miraculous from something as simple as the way you dress to how you choose to live each day. Be the big "F" in your life. Be Fun, Fair, Firm, Fatherly, Friendly, Fantastic and Fabulous every day. So eat raw, live raw, wear raw and *be* raw— every day and in every way.

Sidebar to the Rawbar
Raw In Rio

When I shimmied my way into Brazilian samba dancing, I happily traded my leg warmers and skating skirts for g-strings and boas. Rio De Janeiro Carnival, here comes the new Girl from Ipanema! I displayed my dancing feet in Rio with Mangueira Samba School at the Sambalbrome and was digging the crowd of 50,000 cheering, yelling, dancing and partying revelers. I got to shake it and not break it. As I said earlier, Brazil is where I first went 100% raw 18 years ago. It's where my entire raw food life began, because I didn't want to eat chorizo, fijoda and drink Caipirinhas (Brazil's version of a margarita). I didn't want to get food poisoning, so I lived on the fruits and shoots of those gracious people and their generous tropical gifts for a month. That trip was the catalyst for me to become a 100% raw fooder. *Obrigado*, Brazil!

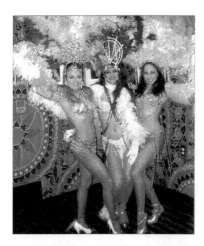

My dance troupe, Taste of Brazil Dancers, put wings on my feet. I loved performing at House of Blues in Hollywood, California for Carnival. What I do on wheels, I also do in heels.

Going Raw In Rio got me on the rawkin' raw road of happy bliss. I'm having fun having fun, living forever young, expressing the best and the rest in me.

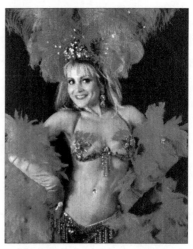

Raw Bites

- *Dress up in your favorite getup—the one that makes you feel sassy, and classy, so you'll want to strut your chassis. Wear it even if the only thing you have planned is a trip to the grocery store or to exercise class. Notice how what you wear affects how you live, feel, be, do and have fun and how people connect with you.*

- *Wear pink or red—yes, that means guys, too. Nothing says confidence like a pink or red hat, shirt, handkerchief or dress. It exudes power, sensuality, brightness, aliveness and it's alluring. It vibrates how you feel about yourself- you feel bright, alive, colorful, vibrant, present and visible. Be flashy, trashy or classy—whatever is clever for you.*

- *Be bright, bold and beautiful. When you feel like fading and resigning, step up, stand up, twirl, shout out loud, dress loud, make a statement, and bling it on.*

- *Have fun every day.*

- *Life's a drag, so dress it up.*

- *Be a leader and a winner, not a follower and a spectator. It's your birthright to shine and help others to do the same.*

- *"The mistake of art and creativity is to assume it's serious." (Lester Bangs)*

- *"Art is an experience, not the formation of a problem." (Lindsay Anderson)*

- *"Creativity is to make visible what without you might perhaps never have been seen." (Robert Bresson)*

- *"True creativity starts where language ends." (Arthur Koesther)*

- *"An original is a creation motivated by desire." (Man Ray)*

- *"To create is divine, to reproduce is human." (Man Ray)*

Chapter 33

Intimacy—
In-To-Me-See

Merrillism #50: "Uncover, Discover, Discard and Recover."

Some of the most delicious and satisfying flavors in life are tasted through our relationships—some are spicy, some are sweet, and others sour over time or leave us with a bitter aftertaste. Occasionally we encounter someone with whom we experience all the flavors at once. I, like many people, used to look to my relationships with men to provide the seasoning for my life. I craved love and attention but feared rejection, so I sought out men with whom I had relationships, but little intimacy. I would substitute sexual intimacy for emotional intimacy, because what I really feared was that I would be seen—really seen, and then be rejected. So I attracted the wrong men again and again, until one day I realized that the problem wasn't that they were the wrong guys, the problem was, I was the wrong girl. I realized that I was addicted to bad relationships just like I was addicted to junk food. Part of my personal journey was to uncover the truth of who I really was and was not, and to recover the real me, discover the person I wanted to be, and throw out the rest. For me, living raw means being truthful with myself and with others, honoring my word and commitments, being seen and, most important, honoring myself.

Intimacy is the fine art of letting another person inside, allowing yourself to be open and vulnerable and revealing yourself—all of your self— good and bad included. The most important and enduring intimate relationship you will ever have is with

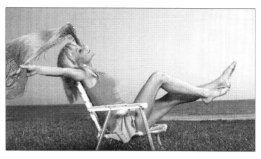

I always make time for silence and intimacy, [in-to-me-see] with myself, sun and higher spirit, at my favorite place, the ocean and nature. My Pa-raw-dise.

yourself. How can you expect to have love, empathy and trust for another human being if you don't love, trust and have empathy for yourself? As the cliché goes, *you cannot truly love another unless you love yourself first.* So, how do you do that? How do you go from berating, criticizing and judging yourself to loving, praising and caring for yourself? For me, the answer begins and ends with raw. As I began to care for and respect my body, feeding it live, raw foods, I was then able to become more loving and compassionate with my soul. And because I was more generous with my inner being, I was more generous with others. I began to care more for the body that housed it—it was a circular process. It's the reason I say you cannot separate your physical, mental and spiritual health. It's all one thing. Our minds do not operate on a different plane than our bodies; we are integrated. Therefore, in order to experience true health, we've got to be healthy on the inside as well. Part of that health means accepting and loving who we are right now and allowing others to love and accept us, to feel worthy, entitled and fulfilled. That was the hardest jump for me to land. You cannot be loved, if you don't open the door first. Let others in, let others help, love, fulfill and contribute to you.

As you begin to peel back the layers and get to the heart of who you really are, you will begin to develop an intimate relationship with yourself—you will discover what you really think, feel and care about. Intimacy requires transparency and connection and is hindered by secret keeping. You are as sick as your secrets. So, get to know yourself. Be honest. It may be difficult at times, and you may not always like what you see, but look at it anyway. Please give up self-delusion. It is suicidal intimacy. Forgive yourself and dig deeper. As I have said many times, writing is an extraordinary tool; it is through journaling that I have been able to let go and delve deep into myself, find the answers and the blind spots in my shortcomings. There is something magically freeing about moving the pen across the page and letting your feelings flow. I encourage you to write everyday. I also find meditation to be a wonderful tool for connecting to the soul. The stillness allows your true self to emerge and be seen. The Latin word for confidence is confideao, which equals faith in God, which means courage. Some people have a harder time than others developing intimacy and find therapy immensely helpful in uncovering emotions that have been locked away, frozen for too long. Whatever method you choose, I encourage you to begin the journey inward, so that you can then find the courage to venture outside of yourself and connect with others. Go within to begin and win.

Merrillism #51: "An Open Heart Is a Healthy Heart; a Closed Heart Is a Heart Attack."

Opening your heart to yourself is the first step in developing healthy intimate relationships with others. When prepared with love, relationships are truly the spice of life. And while you cannot always avoid the sour, a couple of bites of bitter are well worth the sweetness that comes from true connection with another person. Today, I wear my emotions on my sleeve. I express myself fully and completely and live with an open heart. That doesn't mean that everyone likes me, agrees with me or even gets me. But none of that matters because *I* get me; I love myself enough to accept that not everyone will. And that's okay. The good news is I don't need it to shine my light anymore. I shine because I choose to, love to, want to and it's my divine right. I'm here to glorify greatness of the spirit, regardless of who likes and approves of me. It doesn't matter anymore. I'm past that, I don't have the time for the chatter that doesn't matter. I can stand here today with my arms open, embrace life, and say here I am, Intimacy—*in-to-me-see*. Eating raw can help you get there, you only have to open your heart and be a part, get it out, and let it in.

Raw Bites

- *Take yourself on a date. Go to the park, take a walk on the beach or in the woods, have tea at an outdoor cafe, or take yourself out to dinner. Get to know yourself.*
- *Spend time with your partner. Intimacy is built on shared moments, so make time for just the two of you. Go on a date (like you used to), prepare a meal together, go for a drive, hold hands or stay up and talk.*
- *Take a chance. Ask someone you admire out on a date. Make a new friend. Risk saying, "I love you" first. Open your heart and be seen.*
- *Believe in love at first bite (and sight).*
- *Ask your higher self the hard questions in the early morning. Often the answers will come by mid-day or sunset.*
- *Ask for forgiveness, not permission.*

Chapter 34

The Ocean of Motion:
The Unlimited Abundance

Merrillism #52: "You Cannot Keep it Until You Give it Away; Give to Live; Giving Is Oxygen and the Bloodline of Life Itself."

I used to say that the ocean was my God. I said my prayers to the sea, and when I was angry or scared, I'd rage and scream at the top of my lungs while taking a prayer walk, during my skating meditation, or while I swam in the ocean. I'd go underwater and scream at the top of my voice, a high C, and then finish it off with a good cry. I'd rail at the waves as they crashed against the shore. I let the sea absorb my sorrows and celebrate my joys; it was my solace and my salvation and the place I always found peace. Afterwards, I'd feel great. I guess you could say that the ocean is my church—my peace, my spiritual sanctuary. It is the place I feel closest to God, most connected to my higher spirit and most abundant. I have since discovered that every place is a church and everyone is my ministry. When I am near the sea, I feel peaceful, grounded, connected to nature and at one with the Universe. The reason I started my skating school on the beach was because the moment I arrived, it felt like home to me. I felt safe, free, happy, fun, alive, energized, abundant, and in motion—like the ocean. Being near the sea gives me the sense that I can do and be anything. I feel that people are more open to learning new things and taking risks when they are close to the ocean because it's expansive, limitless, vast and free and reminds us that we are, too. The ocean flows in and out and reminds us to breathe. What a fantastic feeling. The same power that created the ocean is within us to learn to skate or do anything we want to do.

> *There is a wonderful mythical law of nature that the three things we crave most in life—happiness, freedom, and peace of mind—are always attained by giving them to someone else.*
> —Peyton Conway March

The ocean reminds me to keep an open mind so I will always have an open frontier and its constancy reinforces that for me on a daily basis. The ebb and flow of the tides represents the ebb and flow of life and the human experience. The ocean's natural state is movement—the tide goes out, gathering strength along the way, and comes in with a crash, depositing treasures on the shore. It doesn't hold on to what it has, because the ocean, like the universe, understands that there is an abundant supply of riches and treasures, it lets go. It all flows in and out like money; money in, money out. Love in, love out. The raw lifestyle continues to send me the riches of the Universe day in and day out. I now see that we are not the bubbles in the ocean, nor the ripples or the waves. We are the ocean. It demonstrates the truth that you cannot keep "it" until you give "it" away. You can't hold on; you must let go of the tight grip and let water flow

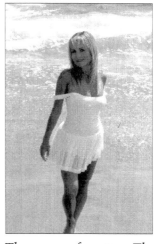

The ocean of motion. The ocean is my favorite spot on the entire planet it is my higher spirit, my sanctuary, my place of peace, meditation, contemplation, and recreation.

through your hands, let life flow through you. That goes for every-thing. "It" can be anything—love, money, success, knowledge, joy, time, ideas, and happiness—anything of value. Giving completes the circle. You cannot create happiness by holding on—you've got to give joy to others in order to receive joy in your heart. Love cannot be taken by force, it must be given freely and then, and only then, will it be returned abundantly. It works with everything in life. Judge others and you will be judged. That is why I do what I do. I know that my health is a gift that I cherish and don't take for granted. I value my health and work at it everyday. I try to be the best person that I can be, and only the best. I enjoy bringing that out in others who I meet, greet and teach. By sharing it with you, I am receiving even greater health in return.

I teach, I educate, lecture, perform and write in order to help others grow. It comes into me like a wave and I send it back out to you with a crash and a bang to wake you up. The more that comes in, the more I am able to send out again and again and again. I am just like the ocean—always in motion, giving and receiving. I am repeatedly being gifted with the potion of notion like the flow of the ocean. Then I send it right back to you. I call it my easy flow and glow to go. This is the process of life. If you are bored in life, you are not paying attention. I hope that my trials will be your triumphs. The only way that I can continue to grow is to give what I know away. Giving takes many forms—you can give money, time, energy, talent, knowledge, listening and love. All spiritual believers believe, as I do, that truth and teaching are the most precious of all gifts. For it is by giving knowledge that we are able to hold on to the truth of what we have learned and what we have discovered. You gain nothing by hoarding and being stingy with your secrets, talents and knowledge and locking away what you know. Miser and pauper mentality gives you lack of abundance in all areas of your life, along with barriers and misfortune. One of my favorite affirmations is, *I am enough, I have enough, I do enough, there is enough. Enough is a feast.* Try it yourself; it's a great confidence builder.

I didn't know I could sing until I started singing. I didn't know I had the talent to be such a prolific writer until I started writing. I didn't know I could be an accomplished skater in all three varieties—ice, inline and roller—until I began skating and teaching, I didn't know I could produce until I started producing my own public TV show, *The Debbie Merrill Show Raw on the Roll Getting America Healthy.* We discover our gifts by doing them and giving them to others. It is in the doing, sharing and teaching that we claim ownership in who we are and what we've got. Enjoy and share your achievements. Once again, your life is not about you, it's through you. Be a vehicle for enlightenment, healing, health and inspiration for others, and you'll be and have joy, fulfillment, contentment, wholeness and mastery in your life. Doing the best you can today ensures you will do the best you can tomorrow.

> *We make a living by what we get,*
> *but we make a life by what we give.*
> —Winston Churchill

The simple truth is that, as I give to you and you give to the world, the world gives to me. It's the easy flow and go of life. My health is your health and your health is mine because we are all one. As you learn and grow and become the person you want to be, as you experience life and gain confidence, strength, courage and self-esteem, it is your sacred duty to share your knowledge with others. What you give away will expand, it's the ripple effect. Go out and live your life, but more importantly, go out and *give* your life, and you will receive an abundance of health, wealth, happiness, peace and fulfillment in return. Share who you are and what you have with everyone. Give freely of what you have and accompany me on this rawkin' raw road of happy bliss.

Raw Bites

- *Give to your favorite charity or church; tithe. Pay the toll for the guy in the car behind you. Pay a compliment to the next person you see on the street. Let someone cut in front of you in line at the post office, on the freeway or grocery store. Kindness is food for the soul. It is better that we should err and give too much, than refuse to give.*

- *Give to your neighbor. Offer to go grocery shopping for the lady upstairs (buy organic of course). Walk your neighbor's dog. Make a fruit salad for the family at the end of the block. Smile at everyone you meet. Smile all day. Create a mile of a smile on your face. Talk to a stranger. Ask someone how he or she is doing. Give food to the homeless or the poor. Visit the sick and elderly.*

- *Giving to others is giving to yourself. Giving is food for the soul. It keeps us alive and vibrant and in love with life, ourselves, and others. Caring is medicine. I know, for me, one of the most fulfilling and important roles in my life was being caretaker for my beautiful and loving dad, Nano, and I learned that by helping him I helped myself be the person I knew I could be. Love never asks me how much must I do but how much I'm willing to do.*

- *Give to your loved ones. Tell your kids, spouse, boyfriend, girlfriend, mom, dad, relatives and best friend that you love them. Send a love letter to your Mom. Laugh. Write a poem for your lover and read it aloud. Teach your niece or nephew how to skate, dance, swim, or ride a bike. Acknowledge, compliment, contribute, thank and be gracious of others. They'll feel better, and so will you.*

- *Be a fountain of giving and your life will become rich as you become raw. Then you've gone from raw to richness, you've literally found the Raw Truth to the Fountain of Youth. Congratulations on your graduation.*

- *To have something is to give it room enough to grow. Fig trees and sapote trees cannot grow on top of one another or too close to one another. Neither can we humans.*

- *Weeds grow fast. Flowers take time to bloom. So do we humans.*

- *It is not a matter of growing old; it's getting old if you don't grow.*

- *It's better to be open, giving and loving than closed and wise.*

- *"Give more. You must do the things you think you cannot do." (Eleanor Roosevelt)*

- *"Within our dreams and aspirations we find opportunities." (Sue Atchley Ebaugh)*

- *"We are the flowers. We are the ebb. We are the weavers. We are the web." (Shekinah Mountainwater)*

- *Expect the best and accept what you get. Let it flow capriciously through you. All that is in motion is you.*

Nano, Loving You & Letting You Go

Dad,

You know you were the best Man I ever had
And your absence from here on, I will truly be sad

Your qualities of generosity, forgiveness and kindness, I want
    to attain
Along with your sense of humor, charisma and style, a man
    with no shame
Your Cadillac and suits were your alter ego, I see

But I knew the real Man, who never said "No" to me

Always a joker, always a smile
With your cigar and a cap, always in style

My skating, the shoe store, the chores and your wife
You juggled it all and still enjoyed life

You loved all the kids, walking the dog and the sun
When you had time you golfed and even scored a hole-in-one

You called me "Monkey" and I still don't know why?
The stuffed one I gave you in your arms watched you die

You taught me to swim, to drive and to spell
And played all those Sinatra tunes that I learned so well

Like a good dad, you always checked if I had gas in my car
And when I traveled, you slipped me a bill, no matter how far

Up at 4AM, off to the ice rink we would speed
You laced up my skates, massaged my feet and took care of my
    every need

With my Mom, your wife, you truly were her friend
She never lacked or wanted, all the way to the end

Your work in The Navy that you did for a while
You became a lieutenant and mastered it in style

Your dedication to family and your work, all for us
You never complained or quit, nor made a big fuss
Your battle with Alzheimer's, you fought it in stride

And with all your pain, you
    maintained your great pride

Dad, I love that you had
    tenacity and drive
That's why at 88, you were
    feisty and still alive

Your courage, your strength and
    your ever-so-strong will
Made me want what you had,
    even though you were ill

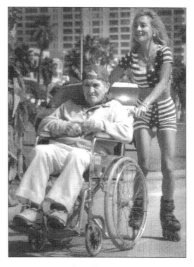

*I so enjoyed rolling with my dad
along the beach. If he only knew
about a plant-based diet back then,
he may not have suffered from
the one of many eating-related
diseases such as Alzheimer's.*

Your compassion and kind heart
    were an asset I see
And the best part of all, now I
    see them in me

As I skate around in my red,
    white and blue
I wouldn't be who I am, if it wasn't for you

Your spirit moves on as a legacy through me
As I move forward without guilt and ever so free

In my heart there's a space, for your love I still keep
As you soar with the angels in your blissful new sleep

Thank You for being my Daddy in every way
Now you're off with your new family, March 13th was
    your day
We all love you and are happy you're resting in the end

With love from "Your Monkey" and all of her friends.

Until we meet again...
Love Always and Forever,
Your Daughter,
Debbie

Chapter 35

Bless You = Be-Less-You

"Wisdom is a blessing only to those prepared to absorb it."
—Author Unknown

When Buddha was asked, "Are you a man or a god," he said, "I am aware." To me, being aware, alert, alive and accountable is true awe. Raw has empowered me to go from raw to awe, true wisdom and true enlightenment. Enlightenment means to lighten up. I began writing this book with one simple goal: *to help heal my fellow man back to health and fitness.* I believe that true health, encompassing mind, body and spirit, is all-inclusive. It's not just for me, or for elite athletes, celebrities or the very rich—health belongs to everybody. Health belongs to you. This is a "we" world, not an "I " or "me" world. It's all about community. We all need to be healthy together because the healthier we all are, the healthier this planet we all share will be. If it works for me, it works for you, I don't get it until we all get it. My responsibility and my mission is *to inspire, educate, and enroll the world back to health and fitness* through a plant-based diet, skating, dancing, creativity and spirituality. That is why I say, "As you give to the world, so the world gives back to you." We may be on our own individual journeys, taking our own roads, but in the end, we are all in this together, so let's help each other get there in good health. All for one and one for all. We are all one and we are all children of the same Universe, here to reap the gifts of the kingdom. Receive, give and enjoy!

Merrillism #53: "Don't Think Less of Yourself; Think About Your Self Less."

I find when I think about myself less, I get less depressed, accomplish more and the things I was over-thinking and worrying about get managed, get done or never happen. My concerns about myself transfer to the concerns of others. That is so contrary to the way I was raised, how I used to think and what I used to believe, but it works, so I had to shift my thinking. Try it. I highly recommend it. Focus on things outside yourself for a portion of your day and your problems, issues, concerns and worries will be resolved. Or at least not seem as important. Try not to let everything be an emergency. In my mind, if it's "urgent" it's probably not that important in the big scheme of things.

The following is a poem I wrote while transitioning to a raw food diet. It helped me, and my wish is that it will help you, too.

Transition is Safe

This transition has given me pleasure, so much knowledge
    and pain
Who knows what will happen next, only growth will there
    be to gain

Sometimes the fear paralyzes and the voices ever so real
Then I look in the mirror and tell myself, "I love You and all
    your appeal"

So I'm taking many new actions not knowing what to expect
Trusting spirit will not lose my file and label me a reject

It's important to love the excitement and admit I'm really in joy
Forgetting the negativity, knowing it's only a ploy

Believing all will get done, there's more time than I say
Slowing down is a must, so I'll be guided every day and
    all the way

It will all be a memory in just no time flat
Why not embellish this place, and rejoice where I am at!

Everything Is All-Right-Now!

If this book has helped you to transform even just one thing—if it has inspired you to eat a little healthier, move your body more, practice being kind to yourself and others, live more simply, open up to intimacy, live more truthfully, more richly, to express yourself, get outdoors, and find a spiritual connection, then I feel I have succeeded—and so have you. I believe that we are all meant to participate fully in our own lives and that each of us has a higher purpose. I came here with the desire to be a healer—to motivate, inspire and touch people, and to bring joy, purpose and belief into people's lives. I have achieved this mission by being a teacher, a health educator, a fitness trainer, leader, author and performer with a raw, organic lifestyle. As I shine, I give you permission to shine. Whatever one can perceive, conceive and believe, one can achieve. I know this to be true, because I did it. I am a living example of what is possible. I climbed out of the gutter and onto the sidewalk and reached for the stars until I became my own star. I know one thing for sure. If I can do it, you can do it too. What you visualize, vocalize, and physicalize, you can materialize in your life through affirmations, visualizations, acting "as if," dressing up and showing up, faking it until you make it, acting your way into right thinking, being at cause and unstoppable in all your actions, thinking outside the box, taking contrary action, finding your blind-spots and finding out what you don't know you don't know, you can create as dreams and goals for yourself that you never thought or imagined possible.

Think big. Think success. Think, "why not me?" The word "Think" is an acronym for Thoughtfulness Honesty Intelligence Niceness and Kindness. Why not indeed? You have discovered the Raw Truth to the Fountain of Youth, and it's your turn now. In fact, it's always been your turn, you just haven't taken it. You are worthy. Move from less than, to self-worth. Eat less and live more! Think less and be more. The less you carry around, the longer you are around. Please *stop* doing the things that are making you sick and *start* doing the things that make *you* better. There are three important words there—stop, start and you. Only you can take responsibility for your own ability with your health. Do it for the health of it—your health of it. You deserve it. It's your birthright. You don't have to live in the shadows of someone else's dreams and actions. Think less, be more, live to give.

"A painting is never finished—it simply stops in interesting places."
—Paul Gardner

I'm not stopping yet. I'm still going for the gusto while I have the raw gusto. I'm going to glide with pride, get a firm hide and stay on this ride to raw bliss, and not a trick will I miss. My hope is that you let my *Raw On The Roll Success System* work for you and allow some of this information and knowledge to stay in your mind, consciousness and heart for your entire life. Don't deny it 'til you try it and apply it, and you don't even have to buy it; it's given to you free by Mother Nature.

I thank God for raw foods and I thank raw foods for my God. Without them, I would not have moved from physicality to spirituality, to originality while living in reality; and from raw to awe and from raw to richness. You can too. Try the tricks, tips, skills, drills, notes, quotes and recipes in this book and you will be amazed at how much better you feel and look before you are even halfway through. Don't quit before the miracle. With you and your higher spirit as the majority, all else is the minority. If your higher spirit is with you, who can be against you?

Bless You. Be-Less You!

I Love You All!

Raw Bites

- *Only when you truly inhabit your body can you begin the healing journey.*
- *Economy is making the most of life.*
- *As you grow spiritually, your words have more power to affect others.*
- *He who has no fire in himself cannot warm others.*
- *Clean up your mess in all areas and be your own mess-iah.*
- *Organize your body, mind and spirit and gain access to organic intelligence.*
- *You cannot sit on the rawkin' raw road of success, or you will get run over, so get rolling now!*
- *Enjoy yourself. It's never what you think it is. Marry into that.*
- *Be a <u>RAW</u>IOR. Spread your raw bliss.*
- *Be gentle with Mother Earth.*
- *Great love and great achievement involve great risks.*
- *You are endowed with the harmonious, priceless gifts of life's force. Congratulate and celebrate your blessings by Being-Less you.*

Section 5

Final Course

Chapter 36

The Essential Raw Kitchen

*"Nothing would be more tiresome than eating and drinking if
God had not made them a pleasure as well as a necessity."*
—Voltaire

A house is not a home unless it contains food for the soul as well as for the body. I used to love cooking and I was good at it—I inherited that from my mother. I enjoyed playing around in the kitchen, making up new, exotic dishes. I used to love cooking for my dad because he ate whatever I made him. I used to burn toast, scramble eggs, make banana splits with no bananas and peanut butter and jelly sandwiches with half a jar of jam and a whole jar of peanut butter. He devoured every bite. So, I gained confidence in cooking and preparing food. Then I watched my mom, who was a fabulous Italian chef and master baker. Everything was home grown and made from scratch. Even the parsley and tomatoes came from the garden. Whenever my mother cooked a meal, neighbors and friends were clamoring at our front door to come for dinner, especially on holidays. So, I learned from the best. I loved baking too because, as you know, I loved my sweets. I'd bake cakes, cookies, Italian donuts, muffins, and shortbreads. You name it, anything sweet, I'd bake up and eat! I'm still a whiz in the kitchen, but now I eat a lot more whole, living foods, like fruits and vegetables, so I spend less time preparing my food and more time preparing my life. I have become quite adept at the art of *un*cooking and can make anything with a blender, a dehydrator, a wooden spoon and my own two hands. Of course, I have never forgotten the most important ingredient my mother used: *love.* Along with putting love into the food you eat, it is important to put love into yourself. Think loving thoughts, do loving acts for yourself and others, and you will successfully love your way back to health and fitness. Have a love affair with yourself. Write a love song or a love letter, make a love potion, write or tell a love story, be a love child or tidy up your love nest. Get into love making, get a love making massage, a colonic, or a facial. Whatever floats your boat, do it with love. Have regard for, benevolence toward and endearment for yourself. You are lovable, likeable and desirable. Let your food be the same in this game. Have faith in yourself as well. (Faith means For All I Trust in Him or Her)

Merrillism #54: "You Can Be Whatever You Believe You Can Be."

As you continue to travel down your own road to abundant health, it is important to watch what you think, about *everything.* It is all connected. What you think about food, yes, but also what you think about love, exercise, wealth, success, happiness, and relationships—everything. When I first started to pay attention to my thinking (my reasoning, rationalizations, judgments, interpretations, justifications, and excuses), I noticed that when I identified with my negative thoughts, I lost my power. By watching my thoughts, without judging, berating or hating, I held on to my power. The watcher is not the doer. I no longer fill in the blanks and create drama because most of it is just plain worrying and negativity and a beat up job on myself, or someone else. The bad things I imagine usually never happen. So, just watch your thinking when it comes to your health and see how you justify taking that extra bite or adding a little bit more chocolate sauce to your ice cream, eating more than you need, having seconds or eating late at night right before bed, or even in the middle of the night! Pay attention to the rationalizing, but don't identify with it or act on it. Have the feeling but don't act on it. You cannot hate yourself into eating right. You need to love yourself into eating right. Love yourself back to health, wealth, prosperity, abundance, fitness and peace. Remember, it's an inside job. As we know from *The Secret*, "Incurable is curable from within." If the cure works, chances are you have the problem. You probably feel undesirable, unloved and unworthy, so you eat and overeat unhealthy food to fill the hole in your soul. Share your misery, pain, and fears and get to the tears. Don't go to bed with it all in your head. Please remember, that the most important thing is to prepare your food and life with love, fun, and get ready to *rawmble*.

Seven Basic Kitchen Tools to Put More Raw in Your Drawer

1. *The Raw Truth to the Fountain of Youth Food-for-Life* plan found in this book, and super food list.
2. Vita-Mix® blender. Essential for grinding grains, making smoothies, soups, salad dressings, dips, purees, nut butters, frozen treats, desserts and puddings. You can use any blender, but nothing compares to Vita-Mix® because it has a lot of power and has different blades for multiple purposes, and it lasts forever.
3. Glass storage jars. For storing dry goods, soups, sauces, salad dressings, sprouts, nuts, dried fruit, nut butters and fruit butters, sweeteners, water and juices, gourmet raw leftovers, dehydrated crackers.
4. Always have fresh, ripe, raw, organic fruits and vegetables washed and ready to eat, juice, blend and snack on. Keep fruits

on the counter for yourself, your family and your kids. Fruits and vegetables readily available makes it easy for them to reach for a healthy snack. You can even core apples or pre-slice them so they are ready to crunch and munch. Instead of candy bars, cakes and cookies, keep a week's worth of cut-up veggies in the fridge ready to munch on—that's what I call real fast food. This helps everyone resist temptation for cooked, dead, dry, nutritionless food. The latest survey from the Department of Agriculture says that only 28% of American adults get the basic two servings of fruit a day, and only 32% eat three servings of vegetables. Ironically, even though 50% of Americans know the importance of eating fruits and vegetables, 90% do not eat their recommended daily intake! Three reasons: 1) We are culturally programmed to like salty, fatty, sweet foods—which hardly describes fruits and vegetables. 2) Fast food restaurants spend *1 billion* dollars a year on marketing. The budget for the Produce for Better Health Foundation is only $9.6 million. That's a drop in the advertising bucket when it comes to the money spent on reaching and talking to consumers. 3) Many feel that they don't know how to prepare fruits and veggies. If it doesn't come out of a box, jar, package or can, people often don't know what to do with it. I say, just eat it raw, natural style. That's why raw fruits and vegetables are great. They are safe, fast, fun and easy. Nothing to do or think about. Nothing to it, but to eat it. How much more convenient can you get than a banana? You just peel it and eat it.

5. Food Processor. Similar to a blender but with more power and versatility for making salsas, pudding, hummus, dips, spreads, nut cheeses and sauces.

6. Dehydrator. I use this instead of a stove (I don't even have a stove in my home, and haven't in ten years). Make sure

you buy one with temperature controls and use non-stick, reusable dehydrator sheets. I don't dehydrate over 110 or 114 degrees. Great for making my crackers, squash jerky and dehydrating fruit, tomatoes, veggies or whatever is clever.

7. Juicer/Wheatgrass juicer. You really need two juicers; one for citrus, fruits and veggies and one for wheatgrass. There are a couple of vegetable juicers that will work for wheatgrass too such as Green Star® and Omega®. Because I'm constantly on the go, I usually buy my wheatgrass at juice bars while I'm out. It's quicker, easier, less work, there's no cleanup and I can get on with life. I meet people while in line and have developed friendly relationships with the staff and customers and wind up educating people on the healing powers of green juice and wheatgrass. It's a rawsome experience for me every day. Actually my body craves it and looks forward to it. Have a glass of wheat for a treat.

Seven more to grow on...

These are items that are nice to have, but are not necessities

1. Spiral slicer for slicing veggies into delicate strands of "pasta."
2. Sprouting / nut milk bags
3. Sprouting jars with mesh lids
4. Water filter
5. A good knife for dicing, slicing, cutting and chopping (Or let your teeth be the first instrument to open nature's gift).
6. Wooden bowls, wooden forks, wooden spoons, wooden knives and chopsticks if you like (I often eat with my hands, they are clean and always available).
7. Fiber in the fridge. Fruits and vegetables are loaded with fiber as well. Numerous studies on fiber have shown that the risk of colon cancer is much lower among people with diets low in meat and high in fiber. Eating more fiber helps

lower cholesterol levels, which will help lower your risk for developing cardiovascular disease. More fiber in the diet also helps to stabilize blood sugar levels, important in preventing and healing from diabetes. Additionally, it helps to relieve constipation and hemorrhoids, by making it easier and quicker for waste to pass through the digestive system.

Ten Things to Eliminate:

1. All the "boxes" in your house: Microwave, toaster, toaster oven, breadbox and cookie box—or keep it and put hand weights in them instead.
2. Excessive time in front of the TV and computer.
3. All meats: beef, lamb, pork, wild game, fish, poultry.
4. Cooked foods: roasted, heated, sautéed, fried, boiled, baked, cured, smoked, flash pasteurized and pasteurized. Start reducing cooked foods a little at a time, or all at once, whatever works for you.
5. Bottles, jars, cans, boxes and bags of chemically treated, artificially flavored and colored, processed and preserved foods and supplements.
6. Toxic substances such as alcohol, prescription drugs, over the counter drugs, illegal drugs and tobacco. I do not drink alcohol; it's not an option for me. Even though plenty of experts say red wine is good for you because it has so many antioxidants, I don't drink it. Not even a sip. Cacao, green tea, goji berries and acai (a Brazilian berry) and blueberries also contain antioxidants. So I don't need to rationalize why I need to drink alcohol anymore. I haven't had alcohol or drugs in 28 years, and I intend to keep it that way. I don't need it, want it, crave it, give it or buy it. I find it to be a mood altering substance, addictive, a junk food

loaded with sugar and calories. It always leads to more. It's a set up for cravings of sugar, cigarettes, drugs and more alcohol—and more trouble. I highly suggest eliminating it from your life. It's one less thing to decide upon. Have my Persimmon Spectacular Splendid Smoothie instead. It lasts longer and does more for you. Drinking alcohol takes me out of my zone, my vibe, vibrato and frequency. "Drunkenness is temporary suicide / Drunkenness is voluntary madness." (Bertrand Russell)

7. The unhealthy white foods, including white flours, dairy products such as ice cream, milk, cheese, butter, sour cream, cream cheese and yogurt, as well as refined iodized salt, processed sugar in any form (for example, sucrose, dextrose, fructose, high-fructose corn syrup, maltodextrin), and artificial sugar substitutes [aspartame, saccharin, acesulfame potassium, sucralose, neotame, and cyclamate).

8. Caffeine and other stimulants produced from herbs or chemicals. Often found in teas, coffee, colas, "energy" pills, drinks, and bars, fiber and herbal mixes, these substances are known to alter your body's natural rest cycle, and can also be downright dangerous depending upon your heath status. Be cautious, careful and conscientious. "Natural" does not always mean "safe." Read labels and get to know your ingredients.

9. Food preparation and storage containers and tools made with toxic materials such as Teflon®, aluminum or plastic.

10. Any food that is looking old, discolored, black, shriveled, limp and past its peak of freshness. If it's not fresh and alive, toss it. Even live foods have a shelf life.

Raw Bites

- *When you create yourself for the day, ask yourself, "Is who I am and what I am, who I am being?"*
- *If the cure works, you probably have the problem.*
- *For every problem there is an opportunity. Seize the moment; learn the lesson.*
- *A fault recognized is half corrected.*
- *Life can only be understood backwards, but it must be lived forwards.*
- *The grass is greener on the other side, but it's just as hard to mow.*
- *A man wrapped up in himself makes a very small bundle.*
- *"Things turn out best for people who make the best of the way things turn out." (Art Linkletter)*
- *Raw, living foods give you the health you need to live the life you love.*

Chapter 37

Debbie's Top Ten Superfoods for Eternal Life

An extraordinary life is an expensive proposition for health

Please choose live superfoods made by companies that are all raw, all **organic**, have a pristine selection, and practice quality control and ethical production. If you can't find the following items in your local produce market, see resource section.

1. **Spirulina.** See *Have a Green Party* for benefits. Start with 2 T. a day with your morning and evening meal. I like Nutrex Hawaiian Spirulina.
2. **Wheatgrass.** See *Have a Green Party* for benefits. Start with 1 oz. a day and drink or eat on an empty stomach; try to build to 2-3 oz. a day. Affordable yet priceless.
3. **Organic, raw Maca.** A root vegetable from Peru that's dried into a powder, it's unheated, untreated and tan in color. Maca balances hormones, improves human growth hormone (HGH) levels and memory, fights depression, improves stamina, energy and strength, and is also used as an aphrodisiac. Athletes, body builders and Olympic athletes often use maca to improve endurance, strength and

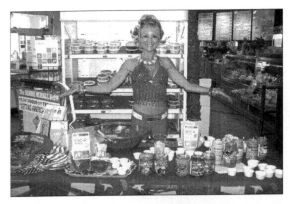

My uncooking classes, raw food demonstrations and recipes with my super foods are always a big hit with the crowd. I love educating people on the why and how of raw.

Chocolate is allowed on my food plan as long as it is raw vegan organic cacao, one of my favorite super foods. I love creating and teaching people all about my raw cacao recipes and the extraordinary wow of cacao!

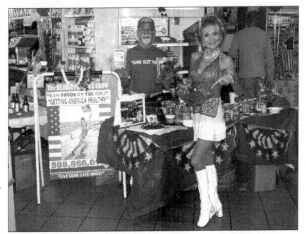

stamina. Start with 2 T. a day; one in the morning, one in the afternoon.

4. **Organic, raw Cacao.** See *Feel the Wow with Cacao Ka-Pow!* for benefits. Start with a handful of nibs, beans or powder twice a day.

5. **Organic, raw Sea Vegetables (seaweed).** Sea vegetables contain a wide range of nutrients such as calcium, vitamin A, vitamin C, magnesium, potassium, enzymes, chlorophyll, B vitamins, iron, protein and 16% more dietary fiber than oat bran. Sea vegetables act as a chelating agent and help to eliminate heavy metals in the body. The rich, dark colors add

vivid contrast and tasty flavor to any meal. There are many varieties to choose from, including Nori, wakame, sea lettuce, hijiki, Irish moss, kelp, kombu, dulse, arame, bladderwrack, and Corsican.

6. **Organic, raw Hemp Seed, Hemp Seed Powder or Hemp Seed Butter.** Hemp is one of the most nutritionally complete proteins. It contains Omega 3 and 6, and other essential fatty acids, and is high in dietary fiber. Hemp seed builds strength, and energy. Start with 2-4 T. a day in a shake or smoothie, or sprinkle on cereals and salads. You can also add to Debbie's Spritty Spirulina Spread or my Heavenly Coconut Butter Spread.

7. **Organic, raw Goji Berries.** Goji berries contain 500 times more vitamin C than oranges, as well as 18 amino acids, 8 essential acids, 21 trace minerals. They are red, ripe, raw, ravishing and ready to eat. Great for the blood and nervous system. Goji berries enhance sexual function, stimulate HGH production, relieve insomnia, improve sleep, decrease cholesterol and help you look and feel younger. Start with two handfuls a day as a snack or in my cereal, my smoothies, *Debbie's Raw on the Roll High-Energy Trail Mix* or *Quinoa Goji Crackers*. You can also toss in *Debbie's Italian Stallion Salad*.

8. **Organic, raw Coconut Butter and Coconut Oil.** Rich in vitamin E and other antioxidants, these raw coconut products are good for your skin, hair and nails, regulates the thyroid and improves hormone balance. Coconut butter is as good for your outsides as it is for your insides. You can eat it, wear it or hair it. Start with 2 T. a day. Eat it right off the spoon, put in smoothies, on crackers, salads, vegetables or use in dips and sauces. I use these fabulous superfoods in most of the recipes and meals I prepare.

9. **Organic, raw Flax Seed and Flax Seed Oil**. A great source of Omega 3, 6 and all essential fatty acids (EFAs), Flax promotes proper immune system development, is good for muscle tone and smooth skin, helps strengthen the circulatory system, and contains lignans, which provide a natural source of antioxidant and phytoestrogens. The flax seeds make for a great Flax Cracker as well. The oil is great for salads, smoothies, dips, dressings and as a hair treatment. Start with 2 T. a day in any way.

10. **Organic Live Aloe Vera Plant or organic, raw 100% Aloe Vera Juice**. Use aloe topically for burns, insect bites and abrasions, or blended with fruit smoothies. It is a powerful detoxifier and, because it soothes the intestines and colon, it can be used as a laxative. I seer off the skin of an aloe vera leaf, take a slice and eat a piece twice a day everyday. Then I rub the rest all over my face. Wrinkles away with a sliver of aloe vera a day. Then there's no urgency for plastic surgery.

Additional Bonus Foods

Raw Organic Olive Oil is very therapeutic for gall bladder and liver, helps reduce cholesterol, contains nutrients and great for hair and skin. 1-2 T. a day.

Celtic Sea Salt or Pink Himalayan Crystal Sea Salt is 80% mineral content with many different types of minerals, and there's no increase in blood pressure when using these salts. A teaspoon of salt daily is good for the adrenal glands, you can also add some form of seaweed or kelp to get your iodine. Never use table salt.

Organic, raw Bee Pollen has all the vitamins, minerals, nutrients and enzymes that we need. Also contains B12 and protein; you can actually live on this substance (An option for vegans because bees are not harmed or killed in the harvesting of bee pollen).

Organic, raw Tocotrienols. A rice bran protein, high in Vitamins E and B complex, tocotrienols act as a probiotic, contains alpha lipoic acid and fatty acids, 22 essential amino acids, and assist in liver detoxification and rejuvenation. Start with 2 T. a day; one in the morning, one at night.

Sweeteners

Stevia Powder. I always recommend it in its organic, raw, green, and unprocessed form. It is a non glycemic sweetener and great for diabetics. I use it in everything that requires sweetness. You can buy it in health food stores in bulk.

Organic, raw Agave Nectar . This is where tequila comes from and has an essential sweet flavor. It's about 10-30% on the glycemic scale and is slow in raising blood sugar, but still safe to use.

Organic, raw Yacon Syrup. The yacon is a tropical tuber plant found in a jungle-like environment (i.e. Peru, South America.) The juice is pressed out of the root to make a syrup-like substance. Low on the glycemic scale so it's good for diabetics. It doesn't raise blood sugar and doesn't metabolize as a carbohydrate. And the FOS sugars act as a pro-biotic for your colon and intestines.

Organic, raw Natural Sugars. Use fresh oranges or grapefruits, mashed bananas, pureed figs, dates, soaked berries (goji, Incan, mulberries) for their juice and natural sugars.

Organic, raw Honey. There are lots of raw honeys on the market, please make sure your selection is unheated and unstrained, preserving its healthful properties such as enzymes, antioxidants, bioflavonoids and bee pollen. Make sure it is 100% certified raw organic honey, made without pesticides, chemicals or antibiotics. Note: Traditional organic beekeeping prevents deforestation. Manuka honey harvested from flowers of the tea tree is very healing. Local honey can also be purchased from farmers markets and natural food markets as long as it is 100% certified organic and raw. Personally, I choose not to eat honey.

Local farmers and small co-ops practice sustainable farming, which supports a cleaner safer environment for everyone. Locally grown produce is often picked the day you buy it which means it can be harvested at its peak for the freshest flavor. Keep the earth green with fewer miles from the farm to your plate. Did you know that most produce travels over 1,500 miles? Local produce travels less distance and helps conserve energy! There is also less production of carbon monoxide in the air, from planes, trains and automobiles used in the transporting process. Your produce is picked and eaten fresh from Nature to you, quicker and easier.

"To the world you may be one person
but to one person you may be the world."

Chapter 38

The Raw Truth to the Fountain of Youth™ Food-for-Life Plan

"Eat Less, Live More."

"The less you carry around, the longer you are around."

"There is nothing to it but to do it."

*"This plan will help you overturn your overeating
and overturn your undereating."*

The following food plan works for me, and it can work for you too, if you do it. You may do this plan in its entirety or add it to your existing plan and slowly transition 20% to 40% to 60% to 80% to 100% raw foods. Your plan for good health should also include any type of exercise that you enjoy at least one hour a day, six days a week. Exercise releases disease 8% faster from your body. Eat less food and live longer with less disease. Please see your health professional (i.e. homeopathic, M.D. or someone with the knowledge and practice of a plant-based diet) before embarking on this plan. And remember, whenever possible, always select fresh, ripe, whole, raw, seasonal and organic foods.

Here are the rules to never lose with your health. Here's how to find the Raw Truth to Fountain of Youth: If you apply it, Mother Nature will supply it. Good Luck and Good Health.

Here are the best foods to choose from the Garden of Vegan: "Moderation, not deprivation," "Diet less, taste more."

Fruits

You should aim for 2-3 servings of fruit every day or more according to your height, weight and exercise output. The quantities listed below constitute one serving. Give these incredible fruits a try and if you already have tried them, get to know them better: quince, Asian pears, kumquats, passion fruit, cranberries, pomegranates, persimmons, papaya and guava. Fruit with seeds are fertile, original and pure, and still not genetically modified.

- apple, 1
- banana, 1
- cantaloupe, ½
- casaba melon, 2 c.
- cherimoya, 1
- cherries, ½ c.
- crenshaw melon, 2 c.
- dates, 4 fresh (medjool, bari, or whatever kind you like)
- dried fruit, 2 oz. (w/o sugar and sulfites/preservatives)
- durian 4 oz. (includes 1 serving of fat)
- figs, 2 large, fresh or 2 oz. dried figs
- goji berries, 2 oz.
- grapefruit, 1
- grapes, 1 bunch medium size
- guava, 1
- honeydew melon, 2 c.
- Incan berries, 2 oz.

- kiwis, 2
- lemons, 2
- limes, 2
- mango, 1
- mulberries, 2 oz. dried
- nectarine, 1
- orange, 1
- papaya, ¾ Mexican, organic papaya/1 Hawaiian papaya.
- peach, 1
- pear, 1
- persimmon, (hachiya or fuyu) 1 large or 2 small
- pineapple, ½ c. or 4 oz.
- plum, 1
- prunes, 4
- pomegranate, 1
- quince, 1
- rhubarb, 1 c.
- rambutan, 4-6
- sapodillas, 2 small
- sapotes, 1 large or 2 small
- tangerine, 1
- watermelon, 2 c.

And any fruit you like in moderation

Vegetables

You should aim for 5-6 servings of vegetables, including green, leafy vegetables, every day. Unless otherwise noted, one serving is 1 c. or 8oz., raw, juiced or blended is best and slightly steamed for the transition diet.

- alfalfa sprouts
- asparagus
- artichokes, Jerusalem artichokes, sunchokes

- bean sprouts/all sprouts (i.e. sunflower, mung, broccoli, clover, onion)
- beets
- bok choy
- broccoli
- bamboo shoots
- brussel sprouts
- carrots in small amounts (¼ c.)
- cabbage
- cauliflower
- celery
- Swiss chard
- cucumbers
- eggplant
- endive
- greens, all (kale, lacinato kale, collard greens, Swiss chard, dandelion, baby greens, romaine lettuce, spinach, parsley, cilantro, Irish moss, malva, arugula, watercress)
- jicama
- kohlrabi
- mushrooms
- okra
- onions
- peppers
- parsnips
- ½ c. pumpkin (i.e. kabocha, butternut, acorn, spaghetti, all squashes with seeds)
- ½ c. raw hearts of palm
- rutabagas
- ½ c. peas
- sauerkraut—raw, salt-free is the best

- corn, 1 whole on the cob or 1 c. raw corn kernels cut off the cob
- string beans
- tomatoes
- turnips
- ½ c. water chestnuts, raw
- zucchini, yellow, green
- seaweed (arame, dulse, hijiki, nori, wakame (see Super Foods)
- ½ c. tomato sauce raw (see my *Titillating Tomato Sauce Supreme* recipes)
- ¼ c. sun dried tomatoes
- 1 large or small vegetable juice, preferably all green (may add green apple or small amount of carrots or beets for beginning juicers)
- ½ c. oil free salsa (see my *Titillating Tomato Sauce Supreme* - ketchup variation)
- ½ raw, organic sweet potato or yam (no white potatoes)

Proteins

You should aim for 2-3 servings of protein every day. The quantities listed below constitute one serving and usually 2 oz. of protein. Please soak and sprout all nuts before eating when possible. You may dehydrate the nuts and seeds at 115 degrees after soaking and sprouting for a crunchier nut.

- 2 T. chia seeds (includes 2 servings of fat and 2 oz. of protein)
- ½ c. almond milk or other nut milks (includes 2 servings of fat and 2 oz. of protein)
- 2 T. almond or any nut butter (includes 2 servings of fat and 2 oz. of protein)

- 2 T. flax seeds or flax seed powder (includes 2 servings of fat and 2 oz. of protein)
- 2 T. hemp seeds or 2 T. hemp seed powder (includes 2 servings of fat and 2 oz. of protein)
- 2 T. pine nuts (includes 2 servings of fat and 2 oz. of protein)
- 2 T. pumpkin seeds (includes 2 servings of fat and 2 oz. of protein)
- 2 T. sesame seeds (includes 2 servings of fat and 2 oz. of protein)
- 2 T. sunflower seeds (includes 2 servings of fat and 2 oz. of protein)
- 2 T. tahini (includes 2 servings of fat and 2 oz. of protein)
- 4 oz. seitan—this is for the transitioning stage but this is not a raw food
- 12 cashews (includes 2 serving of fat and 2 oz. of protein)
- 12 macadamia nuts (includes 2 serving of fat and 2 oz. of protein)
- 12 whole pecans (includes 2 serving of fat and 2 oz. of protein)
- 12 almonds (includes 2 serving of fat and 2 oz. of protein)
- 8 Brazil nuts (includes 2 serving of fat and 2 oz. of protein)
- 8 oz. raw hummus (includes 2 servings of fat if contains oil and tahini and 4 oz. of protein)
- 4 oz. tempeh—this is for the transitioning stage as this is not a raw food, (includes 2 servings of fat and 4 oz. of protein)
- 8 oz. raw soy hummus (includes 2 servings of fat if contains oil and tahini, and 4oz. of protein)
- 8 oz. or 1 cup sprouted legumes (equals 4 oz. of protein)
- 8 oz. tofu—this is for the transitioning stage as this is not a

raw food,(includes 2 servings of fat and 4 oz. of protein)

- 8 oz. mock salmon pate (includes 2 servings of fat and 4 oz. of protein)
- 4 oz. sprouted nut cheese (includes 2 servings of fat and 2 oz. of protein)

Fats

You should aim for 3-6 servings of fat every day based on your height, weight and exercise output. Less fat is better. Fat is not where it's at. The quantities listed below constitute one serving of fat.

- ¼ slice of avocado
- 2 medium flax crackers
- 2 oz. dehydrated cracker with seeds and nuts
- ¼ slice coconut meat from organic young coconut
- 1 T. coconut oil, coconut butter or shredded coconut
- 2 T. tocotrienols equals 1 fat
- 2 T. salad dressing (containing no sugar. Honey, stevia, agave or yacon are okay) Try and make your own, it's best. You know what's in it, and it's made with love and joy.
- 6 whole olives
- ⅛ c. olive tapanade
- ¼ raw power bar—(Jake's Unbaked, Raw Revolution®, Lydia's Organics®, Ancient Sun®, or any raw bars on the market that you enjoy)
- 6 of any type of nut (if peanuts, then only raw and preferably soaked. Raw jungle peanuts are best)

- 1 tsp. oil (Udo's Oil, Total EPA's, flax, borage, hemp, olive, canola, sesame, grape seed, Brazil nut, walnut, macadamia nut and almond) no peanut, heated or treated oils
- 1 T. raw cacao nibs
- 1 T. raw cacao beans
- 1 T. raw cacao butter
- 1 T. raw cacao powder
- 1 T. raw nut butters—pecan, almond, black sesame, hemp and cashew
- 1 T. seeds— sesame, pumpkin, sunflower, hemp, chia

Grains

You should aim for 1-2 servings of sprouted or steamed whole grains every day or one to three days a week. If you suspect you might be allergic to wheat or gluten, limit your consumption of these foods. The quantities listed below constitute one serving.

- 1 slice of sprouted, raw bread
- 4 raw dehydrated grain crackers equals 1 grain and 2 fats if seeds and nuts are included
- ½ c. raw, soaked and sprouted millet, buckwheat, amaranth, kamut, teft, wild rice and quinoa equals 1 grain. Steaming is okay for transition diet only. (Steaming is not raw.)

Free Foods

Free foods. Use the concept of moderation—less is more. The quantities listed below constitute one serving.

- 2- 4 sheets of raw nori
- ¼ c. raw mustard and ketchup
  (See my *Titillating Tomato Sauce Supreme* recipe - ketchup variation.)

- 1-4 T. Bragg® raw apple cider vinegar per day
- 2 T. raw miso
- 2-4 T. spirulina, chlorella, Blue Manna, crystal blue-green algae, or your favorite green powder formula
- herbal teas and sun teas
- plenty of water
- 2 oz. wheat grass juice or 2 oz. e-3-live every day on empty stomach or 2 hours after a meal.
- Fresh herbs and spices including Celtic sea salt and pink Himalayan crystal sea salt, kelp or Bragg® Liquid Aminos if desired, 1- 4 T. a day
- High quality Kombucha Tea 2-4 oz. a day, dilute with water.

Additional Suggestions

What you don't eat is as important as what you do eat. The following are a few suggestions for great health. Try and set this as a goal if you can. Remember, progress not perfection. This is what I do, and if you want what I have, you can follow me. If not, take what you like and leave the rest for when you're ready!

- Drink fresh squeezed vegetable juice daily, preferably all green (may add carrots, beets and/or green apples in small amounts). Try and reach the goal of all green juice, remembering green is clean and gets you lean.
- Take digestive enzymes if needed at each meal. If eating meat and heavy starches take more.
- Take a multi-vitamin daily, if needed and as recommended (raw, whole food vitamins are preferred).
- Take acidophilus daily or eat fermented foods, cultured veggies, raw sauerkraut, Kombucha Tea, and coconut kefir all are great as they contain probiotics.
- No caffeine or diet carbonated soda, juices, energy drinks.
- No pasteurized or flash pasteurized fruit or vegetable juices

- No gum or candy (not even sugarless candy)
- No fried foods
- No cough drops (unless recommended by a health professional)
- No tobacco products
- No prescription or illegal drugs
- No alcohol (that includes wine and beer!)
- No preservatives, processed foods, additives, chemicals, pesticides, fumicides, fungicides, herbicides, insecticides. They all equal suicide.
- No animal products if possible. Remember, peel the onion and allow yourself to transition.
- No "bad" white foods—dairy, white flour, sugar. Use soy only while transitioning, and only if it's non-GMO.
- No cooked breads, there is danger ahead
- No cooked food. Remember, peel the onion and make progress, not perfection. Take baby steps towards your goal.
- YES—Engage in any exercise, for one hour, 6-7 days per week

Raw Bites

- *Your life is your choice. Take a stand with your choice and live it to the fullest now.*
- *Remember, people are dying because they are sick of living.*
- *It works if you let it, if you want it, if you're willing and you work it. So work it now.*
- *Sing for your supper and sing to your food and you will have energy, vitality, longevity and beauty. You will go from Raw to Awe to Richness. You will lose weight and feel great!*

- *Follow the suggested guidelines from this food plan and select your protein, fat, grain, fruit and vegetable amounts daily and then work it and enjoy it. Have fun with it.*

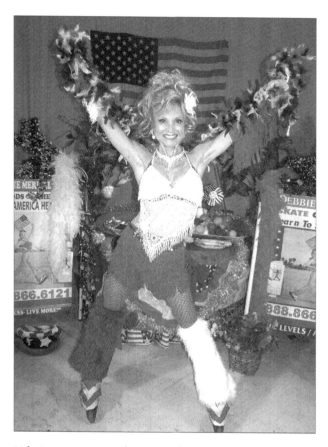

V for Victory, it's time for me to celebrate! I made it this far—18 years 100% raw vegan. I'm now America's RAW VEGAN DIVA with the FEVA so catch it! The Fountain of Youth is inside me now.

Section 6

Recipes

Chapter 39

Rawsome Recipes

If your food is a drag and you're not, dress it up with a few of my favorite rawsome awesome recipes. They're fun, easy and fashionable.

Cooked, processed, preserved food was my addiction, but it wasn't my first. My first addiction was fear. I find that most addicts are fanatics who have a way of taking a good thing and going overboard. Their philosophy is, "if a little bit of something is good, more must be better." Addicts are even capable, at least in their own minds, of turning bad into good, but the addict's tendency toward excess inevitably means that *use* will eventually turn into *abuse*. The recovering addict's mission is the search for moderation.

I have found that the *Raw Truth To The Fountain Of Youth* lifestyle gives me the balance and moderation I need. It certainly eliminates a lot of my food choices that are unhealthy for me to begin with. I replaced my old motto of: "If some is good, more must be better," with a new, healthier mantra: "When in doubt, leave it out" or "Moderation, not deprivation." I found that once I made these small, simple advances toward my health on a daily basis, I began receiving the benefits and reaping the rewards on a daily basis as well. I eat to look and feel great, not to fill my emotional holes. Food is not the center of my life anymore, life is. Three meals a day with life in-between.

It is time to start eating fruits and vegetables as if your life depended on it. Organic fruits and veggies are the only real health foods found in the supermarket, and even a little dirt won't hurt because it contains minerals. In fact, I rarely wash my fruits and veggies because, since I only buy organic, locally grown, seasonal vegetables and fruit, I trust nature and my body to do the cleaning. I usually let my teeth open Mother Nature's food, rather than an appliance, knife or another person. You don't have to be a raw food vegan or vegetarian to eat more fruits and vegetables. Everyone can benefit from doing this. Mother Nature is the best chef in the Universe and I suggest you hire her to work in your kitchen full time.

Please follow my gentle suggestions. I have traveled this road for 28 years, and my experience has paved the way for you so that you don't slip and fall as you follow your own road. Go slowly, glacially, effortlessly and gallantly—but go! Eating more fruits and veggies everyday will put pep in your step and a zip in your trip. Eating from *The Raw Truth To The Fountain Of Youth* will transform you from physicality to spirituality to originality, so you can begin healing and dealing in reality. Remember, rejection is the Universe's protection and redirection, and direction is more important than speed; the ocean is always in motion; stay in action or detour into destruction; energy flows where attention goes. So go now! Go out on a limb again, that's where the fruit is. Eat fruit and stay cute!

I want you, America, to get healthy now; I'm showing you how. Try these high frequency vibration treats of mine, they work all the time. If you can't find, or are nervous about trying, any of the ingredients, simply substitute it for something you like that is similar in taste and texture or just leave it out. The most important thing is to have fun trying something new, enjoy the process and eat your rewards! It's time to start eating more fruits and shoots. The real health food section in the supermarket is found in the fruit and vegetable aisle. So shop around the outside aisles of the market. I call it the Raw track! The rest is junk—except the toilet paper. Food in, food out.

You don't have to be a professionally trained chef to prepare these recipes. Look at me: I am a raw, veggie, vegan diva with a rawsome awesome imagination for the possibilities of rawlicious sensations, while making creations without limitations. Now, I've become an amazing raw chef. For your own delicious, raw living, please add or subtract anything in these recipes or food plan that you need to if it is not available, or not in your best health interest.

Get creative with your food, and get creative with your life. Remember to always use raw vegan organic ingredients, and fresh ripe, whole, raw organic fruits and vegetables whenever possible. Always select from the garden of vegan. These recipes will treat you with a brain full of working knowledge, not a belly full of junk.

Be a vegetarian and be a survivor. Survivors always win, when you survive one thing, you survive everything.

Viva Las Vegan!

Dip It & Whip It

Raw On-the-Roll Hummus and Wrap-in-a Snap, All in One

★★★★★

This one gets my Merrill Magic 5-star rating!
The ultimate raw meal deal. Serves 4.

—— Ingredients ——

½ c. raw macadamia nuts

2 c. raw sprouted garbanzo beans or 2 c. raw, soaked and sprouted soybeans

4 T. raw soaked sesame seeds

2 T. raw sesame tahini (plain or black)

2 T. raw organic olive oil

1 tsp. Celtic sea salt (optional)

2 cloves garlic
   juice, squeezed from ½ a lemon

1 bunch parsley
   cayenne pepper, to taste (optional)
   cilantro, to taste (optional)

Blend all ingredients in a food processor for 2 minutes, until smooth. Add sundried tomatoes, dried cranberries or goji berries (optional). Drizzle olive oil on top, sprinkle with chopped parsley and a dash of cayenne pepper and enjoy with fresh, raw vegetables

or your favorite dehydrated crackers. Spread on raw nori sheets with your favorite sprouts, cucumbers, scallions and raw, sprouted buckwheat kernels to make a Raw-On-the-Roll sushi. Eat the sushi with your hands and enjoy. Remember, God gave us hands for eating and picking and a brain for planting. This dish is lip-smacking, eviliciously delicious. It's very substantial and hearty, great to serve at a party. It's one of my favorites when I'm really hungry and have to be very active. You can also place above spread (hummus) on a raw, organic collard leaf with your favorite sprouts, organic raw black Peruvian olives, cucumbers, scallions, cut-up broccoli crowns and sprinkle with raw buckwheat kernels. Roll into a wrap in a snap and get ready to dip this into my *Dip-in-a-Whip* (see next page).

"Heaven must have sent me an angel with this wish of a dish."

Dip-in-a-Whip: Garlic the Great, Curry in a Hurry Sauce

Great replacement for those days when you crave Thai, Chinese, Japanese or Indian food, which are all cooked and high in unhealthful fats and oils, animal flesh, chemicals, preservatives and sugar. You're going to double your pleasure with this great dip. It's still a treat not to eat meat. Serves 4.

—— Ingredients ——

1 c. sesame seeds, soaked and sprouted
¼ c. raw tahini
1 T. pink Himalayan sea salt (optional)
4 T. olive oil
1 T. curry powder (medium)
2 cloves garlic (optional)
2 T. juice squeezed from one lemon
2 T. raw yellow miso (optional)
1 tsp. cayenne pepper
   parsley and dill, to taste
1 slice of ginger

Mix all ingredients in a food processor, blender or bowl, add a little water to liquefy (if using as a salad dressing or sauce). I like it thick as a brick for a dip in a whip with my wrap in a snap (you can also pour the dip on the wrap as a sauce before you wrap it). This dip makes a great salad dressing and a great spread for crackers or dip for veggies. You can also add into green soup or spread onto pears or apples. Who made the dressing? You did, in a New York minute.

Debbie's Spritty Spirulina Spread

★★★★★

This one gets my Merrill Magic 5-star rating!

This rawsome, nutritious, delicious spread is a great replacement for peanut butter, store-bought spreads, cooked green powders or pills, pasteurized and flash-processed juices, smoothies and drinks. It is loaded with vitamins, antioxidants, B12, magnesium, vitamin C, lysine, calcium, loaded wit, chlorophyll, RNA, DNA, beta-carotene and protein. It improves mental clarity, improves symptoms associated with menopause, improves sense of well-being, energy and stamina and is a hormone balancer and fertility enhancer. Promotes detoxification, especially heavy metal excretions. (See "Have a Green Party" for additional benefits of spirulina). Serves 3.

—— Ingredients ——

½ c. raw Hawaiian Spirulina (optional to also add chlorella, or blue-green algae)

⅛ c. maca powder (optional)

⅛ c. tocotrienols (optional)

⅛ c. mesquite powder (optional)

2 T. raw lucuma powder (optional)

⅛ c. raw carob powder or cacao powder

1 tsp. sweetener to taste (raw honey, agave or yacon syrup)

¼ c. raw cacao nibs (optional)

2 T. raw bee pollen (optional)

1 raw organic vanilla bean pod or 1 T. raw organic vanilla liquid (without alcohol)

2 freshly squeezed oranges or ½ cup water or your favorite freshly squeezed green or fruit juice can be added to desired consistency

1 fresh squeeze of fresh lemon juice

1 tsp. cinnamon

1 tsp. turmeric (optional)

⅛ tsp. cayenne pepper (optional)

Mix all ingredients into a paste. Add a little filtered water or more juice if needed to reach the desired consistency. Eat by itself with a spoon or spread on your favorite fruits, veggies like zucchini, celery, broccoli or radishes, or my raw, dehydrated crackers. You can spread on kale or collard leaves and then roll up like a burrito and put some figs, bananas, dates, pears or persimmons inside. Or try spreading a layer on raw nori sheets, topped with avocado, sprouts and veggies, roll and eat for a treat.

I have this twice a day—in the morning with my fruits or vegetables and at night with my fruit dessert. It's so satisfying and energizing, it gives me that feeling of euphoria. What I can do in heels I can do on wheels. It keeps in the refrigerator for days in glass jars, so you can make a big batch of it and have it for fast food to go. Play with this. It takes a few times to get it to your desired liking. I like it pasty in the morning on fruit and more liquidy for salad dressings and toppings and dips. This spread is very nutrient dense and rich.

"If at first you don't succeed with this one,
try not to hide your astonishment."

Bon Appétit!

Raw Bites

- *These recipes will treat you with a brain full of working knowledge, not a belly full of junk.*

- *Green is clean, however, be careful in making this, it can be messy. Green stains everywhere. Carry the message, not the mess—and don't make one.*

- *Remember, the higher the nutrients in the food, the less amount of food you need to eat, equaling weight loss and maintaining proper body weight.*

- *This* Spritty Spirulina Spread *will keep you fearless in flight, eating less and feeling light, sleeping right through the night.*

- *This raw treat will clean your insides, so your outsides and everything about you shines inside out.*

- *Enjoy that easy flow and glow to go with this fast easy-to-make Spritty Spirulina treat.*

- Spritty Spirulina Spread *gives you vibrant energy and beauty. Eat it and you'll look like me—a cutie with a booty.*

"Enjoy! A feast without the fuss."

Titillating Tomato Sauce Supreme
(3-in-1 Variation)

Also makes ketchup, tomato paste and salsa. Get with this saucy sauce. It's loaded with lycopene, vitamin C and fiber. Makes 1 cup. Serves 1-2.

—— Ingredients ——

1 c. organic sundried tomatoes (heirloom tomatoes are the best)

2 c. fresh organic tomatoes (heirlooms are the best. You can use roma, beefsteak or on the vine as well)

3 T. agave or raw honey (optional)

1 papaya (add for salsa only)

2 cloves garlic

1 tbsp. Celtic sea salt (optional)

1 jalapeño or chipotle pepper, chopped (optional)

½ tsp. minced raw ginger (optional)

2 T. raw apple cider vinegar (add for salsa and ketchup only)
filtered water for desired consistency (thick is better for paste, ketchup and salsa. Use more for sauce)
parsley, to taste
oregano, to taste

¼ c. olive oil
a red onion, chopped for salsa and tomato sauce (optional)

જ✢જ

1. **For tomato sauce/tomato paste:** mix heirloom tomatoes, olive oil, garlic, oregano, parsley, Celtic sea salt (optional)

and water to desired consistency. (Add sweetener if desired.) Mix all ingredients in a blender or food processor and serve over fresh veggies or sprouted beans, or use on my Raw Pizza Pizzazz. A sauce with a consciousness—no need to eat the meat and the ball because this sauce has it all! It's still a treat when there is no meat to eat.

2. **For salsa:** mix tomatoes, papaya, ginger, chipotle peppers or habanero peppers, and red onions. Add parsley, cilantro and a little raw apple cider vinegar. Blend in a blender or food processor or salsa maker and enjoy with my great Crunchy Cracklin' Crackers, Elvira's Enchiladas, raw veggies, Italian Stallion Salad or whatever floats your boat.

3. **For ketchup:** Mix tomatoes, sundried tomatoes, dates, Celtic sea salt (optional), apple cider vinegar, and your favorite herbs. I like Dill. Mix in blender and enjoy as an addition to all your favorite dishes especially my squash jerky fries.

I love this sauce. Use it here, use it there, use it everywhere. The truth is in the sauce. Who made the sauce? You did. You are becoming a master and a boss. Salute your sauce.

> *"Life is limiting, fun is not. Fun is limitless.*
> *Be more fun, fun is health and food is fun."*

Crunchy Cracklin' Crackers

Chocolate Chip Soy-Goji Crackers (Dehydrated)

These yummy crackers are sweet and a great substitute for the S.A.D. diet staples like bread, crackers, granola, croutons, cookies and "health" bars. These crackers are loaded with protein, fiber, vitamin C, magnesium, amino acids, antioxidants and many other vitamins and minerals. Serves 4-6.

—— Ingredients ——

1   organic vanilla bean, diced
2   organic bananas or plantains, thinly sliced
6   figs (fresh or dried), diced
2   apples, diced
½ c. hemp, sesame, sunflower seeds or pumpkin seeds (soaked and sprouted overnight)
2 c. quinoa, oat groats or raw buckwheat (soaked and sprouted overnight)
2 c. raw non-gmo organic soybeans (soaked and sprouted overnight)
1   T. cinnamon
¼ c. raw carob or raw cacao powder
¼ c. maca powder
1   tsp. stevia, honey, agave or yacon syrup (to taste)
1   c. cacao nibs
1   c. goji berries, mulberries or Incan berries

⅛ c. tocotrienols (optional)

⅛ c. lucuma (optional)

Reserve ½ cup of the goji berries and ½ cup of the cacao nibs to sprinkle on top of crackers. Choose three types of fruit, or use smaller quantities of all four and blend in a blender or food processor. Add remaining ingredients one at a time and continue blending. You can also use in-season fruits you love. Spread on tray and dehydrate for 24-36 hours at 115 degrees. After the first 12 hours, turn the crackers over and top with remaining goji berries and cacao nibs. Break or cut into crackers, small or large.

Enjoy the crunch and munch! These crackers are great for lunch and add a punch when you eat a bunch! Crunch out, veg out and get out. Polly want a cracker? I do! And so will the kids. Use my Spritty Spirulina Spread, nut butters, salsa, Heavenly Coconut Butter Spread or chocolate and maple sauce to spread on these crackers. You can also dunk them in my Mocha Choca Toca Maca Chino Tea or smoothies. Also enjoy them with salads and make them into a sandwich or use for croutons. These are a healthy replacement for the cookie and cracker craving.

"Life comes without instructions. Seek education, enthusiasm, envisionment and great recipes in your life."

Quinoa Goji Crackers (Dehydrated)

The quinoa gives a nutty flavor and the berries give sweetness. This cracker is loaded with protein, Vitamin C, B12, amino acids, iron and fiber. It's also a great filler-upper and a good substitute for bread, store bought, over-processed preservative-laden crackers, cookies, bars and muffins. And, they are 100% raw, organic. So don't panic. Serves 3-4.

—— Ingredients ——

½ c. soaked and sprouted sesame seeds (sprinkle on top when cracker is turned over)

½ c. soaked and sprouted sunflower seeds

½ c. hemp or chia seeds, optional (sprinkle on top when cracker is turned over)

½ c. soaked and sprouted macadamia nuts

2 c. quinoa, soaked and sprouted overnight

1 c. raw, organic goji berries, Incan berries or mulberries (save some to sprinkle on top when cracker is turned over)

1 organic banana or plantain

1 medium apple

1 mango or 3 persimmons (hachiya or fuyu)

1 tsp. cinnamon, to taste

1 organic vanilla pod, to taste
Celtic sea salt, to taste, optional (sprinkle on top when cracker is turned over)

⅛ tsp. cayenne pepper (optional)
sliced fresh ginger (optional)

᪥

Blend all ingredients (including sprouted seeds) in a blender. Spread onto a dehydrator tray at 115 degrees until firm (24 hours) for crunchy crackers. Turn over after first 12 hours and top with dried goji berries and seeds. If you prefer a chewy cracker, leave on the tray for a shorter time. Put in the fridge after dehydrating for a more crunchy, munchy, firm cracker. These crackers are great for sandwich making, spreads, dipping or crunched up in cereal, or used as a crouton for salads. I love to just plain munch a bunch for lunch. They give me my Merrill punch, so enjoy a bunch.

"Eating raw will give you joy to eat. Then eating to give you joy."

Soy Goji Crackers (Dehydrated)

Yummy, yummy, yummy in my tummy, tummy, tummy. Lots of protein, Vitamin C, fiber in these berry babies. Serves 3-4.

—— Ingredients ——

½ c. macadamia nuts or nuts of your choice

2 c. sprouted soy beans, soaked overnight (if soy sensitive, use other sprouted beans or sprouted greens)

1 c. goji berries (add to mixture and sprinkle on top when crackers are turned)

1 T. sweetener (stevia, raw honey, agave or yacon syrup)—add more if you like it sweeter

1 T. cinnamon

1 organic vanilla pod

¼ tsp. Celtic sea salt, optional (spread on top when crackers are turned over and add some to mixture

¼ cup sesame seeds, soaked and sprouted (to add to mixture; save some to be sprinkled on top when the crackers are turned over after 12 hours)

❧

Blend all ingredients (including sprouted beans, seeds and nuts) in a blender. Spread onto a dehydrator tray at 115 degrees until firm (24 hours). If you prefer a moist, chewy cracker, remove from dehydrator sooner. For a crunchier, crispier cracker, let it remain in the dehydrator, then, when done, place in the refrigerator for 2 hours or overnight. (Note: When dehydrating crackers, flip over after the first 12 hours, then you can sprinkle the goji berries, sesame seeds, and sea salt on top.)

Enjoy with your favorite nut butter, fruits, berries, my hummus, soy yogurt, persimmon smoothie, serenity salad, sprouted lentil salad, chocolate pudding, nutmilk or whatever flirts your skirt. They are awesome. I keep them handy and eat them like candy. They're easy to eat, carry and travel with. Chewy, moist, soft or crunchy. A great replacement for brownies, rice cakes, crackers or processed desserts. For all you chocoholics—add raw cacao nibs on top for the extra pop. Great for the holidays--have nutrition, will travel.

"Talk slowly, eat slowly, but think quickly."

Nutritious and Rawlicious

Banana and Kabocha Squash Jerky/Fries

I love jerky as a raw fast-food snack; it gives me lots of chewing time and it's easy to carry—just grab and go! It's full of vitamins, beta-carotene, A, C, fiber and minerals, and because it's chewy and filling, it really satisfies your hunger. Mmm, good! You can eat and enjoy as is or cold in salads, wraps, trail mixes, soups and cereals. Jerky can be rehydrated by soaking it in water or juice. Serves 4-6.

—— Ingredients ——

1   whole banana squash, cut into thin strips (remove seeds and dehydrate them as well for eating later)
1   whole kabocha squash, cut into thin strips
½   c. olive, hemp, flax or Brazil nut oil
¼   c. spirulina
½   c. lucuma powder
¼   c. maca powder
¼   c. mesquite
     juice of 1 lemon
¼   c. honey, stevia or agave
¼   c. thyme or basil, rosemary, dill or kelp
1   tsp. cinnamon
¼   tsp. sea salt

⚛

Roll squash strips in the oil mixture, and then blend together Spirulina, lucuma powder, maca powder, cinnamon and mesquite and roll strips in powder mixture (like a breadcrumb mixture). Drizzle with the juice of one whole lemon and sprinkle with thyme, basil, rosemary, dill, oregano or kelp. Lay strips on dehydrator tray and dehydrate for 24-36 hours at 115 degrees or until desired consistency. Turn squash over after 12 hours to oil, herb and powder the other side and keep dehydrating for another 12 hours. I remove mine a little earlier because I like them chewy and moist like licorice sticks or fruit wraps. Add a little more oil, herbs and sea salt on top and you've got squash fries. You can also warm these in the dehydrator for five or ten minutes before eating to enjoy warm with my Titillating Tomato Sauce Supreme, Ketchup. and salsa.

With their vivid orange color, you'll start eating these fries with your eyes and be in for a surprise. This is definite earthquake and hurricane food. It lasts a long time when kept in glass jars in the refrigerator.

They're chewy, ooey and gooey, delicious and nutritious. Eat them up and then brush your teeth! Then there's more for tomorrow.

"You will achieve more if you don't mind who gets the credit"

Coconut Corn on the Cob

This sweet treat is one of my savory favorites and is a delightful substitute for cooked corn on the cob, popcorn, creamed corn, corn tortillas or any other corn cravings. This high vibe dessert or meal is rich in vitamin C and fiber and contains alpha-linolenic acid, omega 3s, PEA, chromium, magnesium, anandamide, protein, zinc, vitamin E, antioxidants, enzymes and coenzymes, 28 minerals and medium- and long-chain fatty acids. Serves 4.

—— Ingredients ——

4   ears raw, sweet, yellow or white corn
½   c. coconut butter
2   tsp. Celtic sea salt (optional)
    stevia, honey or agave, to taste
½   tsp. cinnamon
½   tsp. organic raw vanilla pod
⅛   tsp. cayenne powder
2   T. raw bee pollen (optional)
4   T. raw hemp, sesame seeds or chia or all

Mix coconut butter, sea salt, sweetener, cinnamon, vanilla, cayenne powder and bee pollen in a bowl. Brush mixture directly on corn, then roll in hemp, sesame seeds or chia seeds or all and eat. Keep spreading on the coconut butter for more flavor. It's a sweet treat for all to eat, and provides lasting energy and that raw food glow to go! Eat to live great now. This is a corn-a-copia of taste! Let's get wicked and kick it. Kick the crap habit now. Corn is not just for chickens and birds anymore.

"One is ready when one is willing."

Debbie's Power Wrap-in-a-Snap

This is delicious with my Dip-in-a-Whip. Serves 1 or 2.

—— Ingredients ——

1 avocado, sliced

¼ mango or papaya sliced (optional)

4 black organic Italian olives, sliced

¼ c. red onions, chopped

½ bunch cilantro, parsley or dill, chopped (to taste)

2 raw Jerusalem artichokes, cut up (or try broccoli spears, zucchini or cucumbers)

2 handfuls of sunflower sprouts, alfalfa, broccoli, clover or your favorite sprout

1 tomato, sliced and/or ¼ c. sundried tomatoes, soaked and diced

1 tsp. red powdered dulse

½ chipotle pepper, ½ red or green chili pepper, chopped, to taste (optional)

2 large collard green or kale leaves, or 2 raw nori sheets

3 T. olive oil or favorite oil

Layer all ingredients on one side of collard green leaves, kale leaves or nori sheets, drizzle with olive oil, roll and eat! Open wide and have a rawsome, awesome snack attack! Enjoy with any of my dip in a whips or sauces. Great replacement for sushi. Get creative. Add other foods you like for that raw on the roll, roll it and eat it, get up and go flow.

Debbie's Dip-in-a-Whip

This dip is the perfect complement to my Power Wrap-in-a-Snap! Serves 3-4.

—— Ingredients ——

¼ c. sesame seeds soaked overnight and sprouted
¼ c. tahini
1 T. Celtic sea salt
¼ c. olive oil
   parsley, cilantro or dill, to taste
1 tsp. curry powder
2 cloves garlic (optional)
1 tsp. lemon juice
4 T. raw cacao nibs (optional to sprinkle on top of dip)
   filtered water

๑๏๑

Blend all ingredients in a blender or with a spoon until smooth. Add water to achieve desired consistency, thicker for a dip and thinner to make a tasty salad dressing. Enjoy with a yummy wrap, fresh veggies, dehydrated crackers or poured over salad.

This Wrap-in-a-Snap and Dip-in-a-Whip will add some pep to your step. This will help you sway your hips and jump your flips while you smack your lips.

"Winners do what losers won't."

Debbie's Raw on the Roll High-Energy Trail Mix

★★★★★

These get my Merrill Magic 5-star rating!
Heaven sent! Serves 2-4.

—— Ingredients ——

1   c. raw, organic goji berries, Incan berries, mulberries, loganberries or all four

½ c. dried, organic persimmons, or mangoes, or figs, or yacon strips, or mix some or all

½ c. raw, organic cacao nibs or beans

¼ c. raw chia seeds

½ c. raw pumpkin seeds*

¼ c. raw hemp seeds

½ c. raw sunflower seeds*

¼ c. Brazil nuts, cashews, almonds, or all three*

1   tsp. pink Himalayan crystal sea salt (optional)

☙❧

*Soak and sprout overnight then dehydrate overnight at 115 degrees for a crunchier texture.

Mix all ingredients together and season with pink Himalayan crystal sea salt. Enjoy by the handful, eat with a spoon, sprinkle on *Chocolate Coconut Ganache*, and add to my Skate Great Breakfast Cereal, smoothies, salads or scoop up with celery sticks so you can enjoy all the seeds. Then go get fit not fat.

"Get back on the road if you slip and fall.
See it as an interruption not a failure."

Debbie's Zip in Your Trip Concoction

Decadently divine anytime. This decadent snack to the future is globally sent. This is to live for. You will want more, but one is enough.

Mix my Raw on the Roll High-Energy Trail Mix with two tablespoons of your favorite raw nut butters. Try pecan butter, Brazil nut butter, almond butter, hemp butter, or cashew butter or one T. raw coconut oil or butter. I love Rejuvenative Food's nut butters. Top with a spoonful of cacao nibs. Eat with a spoon and right out of the cup. You won't come in for a landing until dinnertime with this one. Packed full of energy, satisfaction, flavor, sweetness and crunch, this treat sticks to your ribs. I get requests for this one all the time when I present in classes across the country.

"Indulge without the bulge!"

Debbie's Raw Pizza Pizzazz

★★★★★

This gets my Merrill Magic 5-Star rating!
Almost as good as a trip to Italy. This tempting, titillating, tasty treat is a great replacement for cooked pizza, tacos, chips and salsa, tostadas, sandwiches, lasagna and cooked pasta. This tomato-y treat is spicy, saucy and sensual! It's my favorite because it's fatty, filling, fun and Italian. It's loaded with calcium, iron, vitamin C, lycopene, plant fats, protein, minerals and calcium. It's great if you are transitioning from cooked food to raw food because it is not only satisfying, but also tastes just like the real thing. This dish is my winner—better than my mama's Thanksgiving Day dinner. Mangiare, Mangiare! (Eat, Eat!) Serves 2.

—— Ingredients ——

4   sprouted Gratitude Groat or buckwheat crackers
½ c. Debbie's Titillating Tomato Supreme Sauce or paste
1   c. soaked and sprouted macadamia or pine nuts
     (blend nuts with a little water in a food processor to a
     cheesy consistency, thick and spreadable.)
¼ cup red onion, finely chopped
1   clove garlic, finely chopped
¼ c. organic sundried tomatoes, chopped
     soaked arame, dulse, kombu seaweed (optional)
8-10 raw, black Italian or Peruvian olives, sliced
4   T. olive oil
1   tsp. Celtic sea salt
     dash cayenne pepper
     fresh parsley and dill, finely chopped

❦

Spread crackers with **Debbie's Titillating Tomato Supreme Sauce**, and then add nut cheese. Top with more tomato sauce, onions, garlic, sundried tomatoes, seaweed and olives. Drizzle with olive oil and sprinkle with sea salt and a pinch of cayenne pepper. Garnish with parsley and dill to taste.

—— Optional ——

Top with mango slices, papaya slices, diced pineapple, fresh persimmons, or figs for a tropical pizza pizzazz.

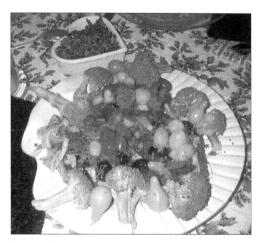

Pizza Pizzaz, my favorite Sunday dinner. This dish is a real winner, better than my mama's Thanksgiving day dinner.

Now that's Italian—crunchy, spicy and filling! This is my Sunday dinner and it replaces my Mama Mia Sunday dinners of cooked lasagna or macaroni and meatballs. Every bite is bursting with a variety of flavors. Nothing tastes as good as this raw dish feels. I feel like I'm back in Little Italy or my Mama Mia's kitchen, ditchin' and twitchin' the sauce for the boss—my dad. This garlic tomato flavor lingers in your mouth in a good way long after the lip smackin' ends. When I finish this, I always want to go dancing. I am happy, content, and full of energy.

"Believe in love at first bite and sight."

Durian Yogurt

This yogurt will keep you going all day without any delay and lots of play. You won't come in for a landing until dinner time. Durian is the only fruit that contains protein, fat, sugar and fiber. It is a detoxifier and aids in cleansing. It is so satisfying you won't want or need to eat anything else or anything with it. Excellent eaten alone. This is true food, enjoyment and flavor. It's such a good vibration and such a sweet sensation, take the durian vacation. Serves 2.

—— Ingredients ——

4   durian pods—remove the seeds
1   tsp. cinnamon
1   organic vanilla pod or 1 tsp. organic vanilla liquid (no alcohol)
¼   c. cacao nibs or powder (optional if you want chocolate Durian Yogurt)
2   tsp. raw shredded coconut or coconut butter (optional)

Stir the first three ingredients in a bowl or blender and eat right off the spoon like pudding, ice cream or yogurt. Sprinkle with cacao nibs and top with raw shredded coconut or coconut butter if you like. Can be frozen and eaten like ice cream.

Simply delicious. Simply organic. Durian Yogurt is versatile and delicious and mouthwatering. A great morning breakfast has never been easier. Dip it, whip it, lick it and get wicked. Spread it and do whatever you like, it adds the spike. I love it with my Skate Great Breakfast Cereal, and for a little extra protein, you can add your favorite nuts, seeds or hemp seed powder.

In Thailand they say, "When the durians fall, so do the sarongs." They also say durian gives you fire in the eyes and soul. Catch this one, enjoy it now.

Durian can be found in certain health food markets like Erewhon Market in Los Angeles, in some Whole Foods markets, Asian markets and some farmer's markets, and countries like Thailand and Indonesia.

"Let your heart's fires become your desires."

Elvira's Enchiladas

I named this dish after my fabulous loving mother Elvira; she was a master chef and baker, creating amazing combinations of flavors, spices and textures. This recipe is a cheesy, chewy, mouthwatering bite of goodness! You can give up the cheese and there won't be much left to squeeze on you: accept this dollop of pleasure and feel the "south" in your mouth. Serves 2.

—— Ingredients ——

1 c. mixed almonds, walnuts and cashews, soaked and sprouted overnight (this will be your nut cheese)
1 chili pepper, jalapeño pepper or chipotle pepper
2 cloves garlic
1 small red onion, chopped
2 collard greens
1 c. red and white cabbage, shredded
1 c. romaine lettuce, chopped
1 c. Debbie's Titillating Tomato Supreme Sauce
½ cup raw organic Italian or black Peruvian olives

֍

Prepare nut cheese by combining nuts, peppers, garlic and onion in blender. Spread the nut cheese on the collard green (your tortilla) and then smother with cabbage, romaine lettuce and more chopped onions. Roll up and top with my *Titillating Tomato Supreme Sauce* and drizzle more nut cheese on top, add sliced Italian or black Peruvian olives. Voilà!

You'll put a mile of a smile on Elvira's face when you enjoy this treasure of pleasure. *Viva Elvira!*

"When you say I love you, mean it."

Raw on the Roll Energy Balls

★★★★★

This gets my Merrill Magic 5-star rating!

These great balls of fire will allow you to take your knowledge, energy and power even higher and enjoy your food without the fire. Energy treats that are guaranteed to put pep in your step, zip in your trip and more raw in your drawer! All of these greens are superfoods, because they're super for you. The balls contain crystal manna (wild blue-green algae), blue manna, Spirulina. Crystal manna contains phenylethylamine for the brain/memory, concentration, alertness, functioning, clarity and focus. Blue manna is good for brain and joint support and is high in chlorophyll. It contains fiber and is antioxidant rich, it detoxifies and cleanses and is loaded with DNA and RNA, which support gene functioning. Spirulina is the world's richest source of B12 and a highly absorbable organic iron. It is a rich protein source and contains beta-carotene. Makes about 12-16 balls.

—— Ingredients ——

¼ c. spirulina, sun chlorella or crystal blue manna or blue-green algae (or use equal parts of all four)

1 c. raw coconut oil

1 c. goji berries, loganberries or mulberries (or use 1/3 c. of each)

½ c. raw cacao nibs

½ c. raw cacao powder or raw carob powder

3 tsp. cinnamon

2 fresh vanilla beans, cut up or 2 tsp. of raw organic vanilla extract (alcohol free)

⅛ c. lucuma powder (optional)

⅛ c. tocotrienol powder (optional)

⅛ c. mesquite powder (optional)

⅛ c. maca powder (optional)

2 T. dulse

1 c. hemp seeds, sunflower, seeds or sesame seeds (use all or one; soak and sprout overnight, sunflower and sesame seeds)

½ c. flaxseed (soaked and sprouted overnight) or flaxseed powder

½ c. raw buckwheat kernels soaked and sprouted and dehydrated overnight

½ cup raw organic shredded coconut flakes (optional) stevia, yacon syrup or raw honey (optional to desired sweetness)

☙❦❧

Blend all ingredients together by hand in a large bowl. Roll into balls and then roll balls in raw carob or cacao powder, then sprouted seeds, cacao nibs, dehydrated buckwheat kernels and raw organic shredded coconut. Put in refrigerator to harden or eat soft. Place in freezer to have a frozen energy ball buzz. You can also add E 3 Live® into mixture for an eternal energy lift and have a Skate Great Raw on the Roll day! They are great before a workout. They give you tons of energy.

"You will be shooting for the moon and if you don't make it, at least you will wind up among the stars with these great balls of fire."

Skate Great Breakfast Cereal

"Only dull people are brilliant at breakfast."
—Oscar Wilde

Flavor, fun, nutrition and tradition. Replaces the commercial cereals that are loaded with white flour, sugar, fat, preservatives and dead shelf life. (No enzymes) Serves 2.

—— Ingredients ——

1   c. soaked and sprouted buckwheat, quinoa, kamut or oat groats—or all four (Dehydrate overnight in dehydrator at 115 degrees or less.)
2   T tsp. maca powder (optional)
2   T. lucuma powder (optional)
2   T. tocotrienols (optional)
½   tsp. cinnamon
1   durian pod (if available) or your favorite fruit (optional)
½   c. goji berries, mulberries or Incan berries
¼   c. soaked and sprouted hemp, pumpkin, flax or sunflower seeds (sprouted and dehydrated at 115 degrees overnight for a crispy crunch)
2   T. coconut butter (optional)
4   T. raw cacao nibs or cacao beans
    stevia, raw honey, agave or yacon syrup to taste (optional)

Mix all ingredients together and eat alone or add coconut water, my Mocha Choca Toca Macha Chino Tea, your favorite warm tea, my macadamia or almond nut milk. This energy-packed cereal will jump-start your day! Raw, fast food—simply simple.

Good morning or good night, this snack always feels just right.

"Eat breakfast like a King or Queen,
lunch like a Prince or Princess and dinner like a pauper."

Satisfying Salads and Dreamy Dressings

Debbie's Italian Stallion Salad

This hearty salad is one of my favorites. As always, use organic produce whenever possible. This enjoyable dish is full of fiber, chlorophyll, protein, minerals, vitamin C, calcium, iron and it's all raw and very filling. Great for lowering cholesterol. Serves 3-5.

—— Salad Ingredients ——

1 head of kale or collard greens, torn into bite-size pieces
1 large bag of baby greens
1 bag of sunflower sprouts
1 bag alfalfa, broccoli, radish or clover sprouts
2 heads of raw broccoli crowns, chopped
2 red bell peppers, diced
4 stalks celery, diced
3 Persian cucumbers, diced
1 red onion, diced
1 spear of raw burdock root, diced (optional)
20 raw black Peruvian olives, pitted and sliced
2 cloves garlic, finely chopped
4 yellow or green raw zucchini, chopped, sliced or spiraled
1 c. sundried tomatoes, soaked and diced or 4 fresh tomatoes, sliced (I love organic heirloom, on-the-vine, cherry or grape tomatoes)

1 cup sprouted raw green peas, snow peas, garbanzo beans, soybeans or mung beans (optional)

2 avocados diced and sliced

—— Italian Stallion Dressing Ingredients ——

1 c. raw organic olive oil

¼ c. water, lemon juice or Bragg® raw apple cider vinegar to add to oil if you prefer a thinner dressing

1 bunch fresh parsley, chopped

1 bunch fresh oregano, chopped

1 bunch fresh dill, chopped

⅛ cup fresh rosemary, chopped

1 tsp. cayenne pepper

1 T. pink Himalayan crystal sea salt (optional)

2 cloves chopped organic garlic (optional)

⅛ cube ginger, diced or grated

2 T. dulse powder

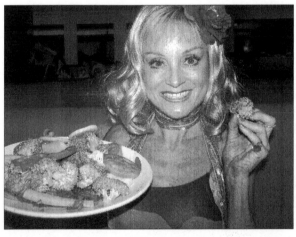

I eat my Italian Stallion Salad *twice a day to keep ill health at bay.*

๑๖๐

Toss all salad ingredients in a large bowl. You can prepare the salad a day ahead to save time. In a small bowl, whisk olive oil, herbs, cayenne pepper, sea salt, chopped garlic, ginger and dulse powder until blended. Toss dressing and salad in large bowl and serve.

Eat light, right and take off in flight. Rejoice in this edible, tasty, delectable salad feast. Have a pleasant meal. Eat to live great. Follow me America, let's eat healthy now while I'm showing you how. Salad is a traditional famous dish; they even named a fork after it.

*"If you eat more foods that grow on trees and plants
you will eat less foods that are manufactured in plants."*

Japanese Salad Dressing

A light and tasty dressing that's easy to make. Japanese Salad Dressing is versatile, subtle, and secretly lends a delectable richness to veggies, salads, soups, sauces, crackers, wraps, dips and sushi rolls. This dressing replaces all store bought, preservative and chemical-filled dressings. Serves 2-3.

—— Ingredients ——

½ c. raw sesame oil

1 tsp. Celtic Sea Salt

1 T. raw miso (I like yellow miso)

2 cloves of garlic, finely chopped

2 T. ginger root, finely chopped

¼ c. raw sesame seeds

⅛ cup raw apple cider vinegar, to taste

๏⚜๏

Add all ingredients to blender and blend on medium speed or whisk in a large bowl. This dressing is great on salads, fresh vegetables and greens, or drizzled over my warm or cold dehydrated goji, quinoa, buckwheat and oat groat crackers and can also be added to my Green Soup recipe or to my *Spritty Spirulina Spread.* I also like it with my *Wrap-in-a- Snap* for a *Dip-in-a-Whip.* Try it as a dipping sauce for squash fries or jerky, it's pure bliss. *Viva Japan! Arigato!*

"No matter how you feel, dress up, get up and show up."

Spirulina Salad Dressing: Italian Style

This zesty dressing packs an Italian-style punch, just like me!

—— Ingredients ——

1   c. olive oil
2   T. raw Hawaiian Spirulina
1   clove of garlic, finely chopped (optional)
1   tsp. Celtic sea salt, dulse granules or Bragg® liquid aminos
    (optional)
⅛   tsp. cayenne pepper (optional)
¼   c. Bragg® raw apple cider vinegar (optional)
    fresh chopped parsley, dill or oregano, to taste or
    combine all

Add all ingredients to blender and blend on medium speed or whisk in a large bowl. This dressing is great on salads, fresh vegetables and greens and is also used in my Green Soup recipe. Liven up your day with this nutritious dressing and you'll be getting more chlorophyll, vitamin B12, minerals and protein in your day, even if the rest of your diet is not totally the way you want it. Even a mosquito doesn't get a pat on the back until it starts working. Get your mojo working and get your groove on with this dressing. It's smart, smooth and tasty. Life is too short to waste time eating bottled salad dressing. *Viva Italia!*

"Fast food takes your money fast."

Debbie's Sprouted Lentil Salad

★★★★★
This gets my Merrill Magic five-star rating!

Sheer bliss you won't want to miss, bursting with freshness and flavor. Get raw and regular with this fun-filled fantasy. This dish is a great replacement for chicken and other meat-based dishes because it is rich in protein, fiber, calcium, vitamins A & C, minerals and EFAs. I ate this dish every day for seven years when I was first going raw. It's a great transitional dish to give you the protein you need and replace the craving for animal protein. It also gives you the crunch of chips, fried chicken, bread and crackers. The munch and crunch makes for a great lunch with a punch! You can add different fruits and nuts according to the season and eat this dish all year 'round. The lentils sprout in one hour, so it's fast, easy and quick. When I was in Brazil, I sprouted lentils in my hotel room in a teacup filled with water and they were ready to eat in an hour. I did this for a whole month. That's how I went raw. So there is no excuse not to eat raw when you travel. I went to any lengths necessary and as a result I have stayed raw for 18 years after that trip. If I can do it, you can do it. That's why I love these lentils. They were my life preserver, my angels to lift me into the raw lifestyle. Serves 4-6.

—— Ingredients ——

4-6 c. sprouted and soaked red lentils
½ c. sesame seeds or hemp seeds or both
2   red peppers, chopped
1   bunch cilantro, chopped

2   c. broccoli tops, cut up
2   c. Persian cucumbers, diced
1   red onion, chopped
1   c. sesame, olive, flaxseed or hemp oil (your favorite)
¼   c. raw apple cider vinegar
4   T. Celtic sea salt (optional)
1   whole mango, sliced or 4 fuyu persimmons (depending on the season)
8   fresh figs, dried mission figs, or calimyrna figs, sliced
16-24 raw black Peruvian olives, pitted and chopped
1   bunch parsley, chopped

After soaking and sprouting lentils overnight, place in a large metal or wooden bowl with peppers, cilantro, broccoli, cucumbers, onion, oil, vinegar and sea salt. Mix well. Decorate with mango, persimmons or figs. Sprinkle with sesame or hemp seeds and top with black olives, parsley and cilantro. Then drizzle oil over top. This is a mouth-watering masterpiece. Serve with broccoli spears, slices of zucchini, slices of yam, sweet potato, or Debbie's raw crackers. This can also be poured over my Italian Stallion Salad, sprouted buckwheat, quinoa, teft or kamut.

You have now created a raw casserole for the soul. There is no thrill quite like the flavor, crunch and munch of this rawsome kaleidoscope of taste. When I serve this dish at parties, Thanksgiving and other holidays, the bowl is empty in about 15 minutes. People are begging for more. This dish is loaded with flavor, fiber, fruit and color. Eat this dish first with your eyes and you'll be in for a surprise and totally mesmerized.

"No one is in charge of your happiness in eating except you.
Eat colorful food, have a colorful life."

Smoothies, Shakes and Delicious Drinkables

Green Keen Lean Machine Soup or Cocktail

★★★★★

This gets my Merrill Magic 5-star rating!
*This is delicious and satisfying, perfect for those "hungry"
days. "GO GREEN, GET CLEAN." Serves 3-4.*

—— Ingredients ——

2 heads broccoli
2 zucchini
1 bunch kale, collard greens or any leafy green
1 bunch parsley
1 bunch cilantro
1 large cucumber
4 celery sticks
¼ head red cabbage
1 red pepper
2 T. spirulina, chlorella, blue-green algae or your favorite
   green powder formula
1 cube ginger
4 T. raw, cultured sauerkraut

½ cup olive, flax, sesame oil, borage oil, Brazil nut
  or coconut oil
2 T. maca powder
1 tsp. dulse
1 small red onion, to taste (optional)
2 cloves garlic, to taste (optional)
1 carrot, 1 beet or 1 green apple (optional)
  pinch of cayenne pepper
  pinch of Celtic sea salt
  add any other veggie or green food you like

Blend all ingredients in a blender until liquefied. You can serve
it slightly thick for a stew-like soup or completely liquefied for
juice. For soup, serve immediately as it will be slightly warm from
the blender. Sprinkle with sprouted buckwheat kernels, hemp
protein powder, spirulina, blue-green algae or favorite green powder
formula. Top with raw, cultured sauerkraut if desired or add a swirl
of olive or your favorite oil to the top if you like. Eat with a spoon
or dunk with raw veggies or dehydrated crackers and enjoy.

Eat green, stay keen, clean, lean and serene. The greens will
keep you going. The soup will fill you up. The nutrients will calm
you down. This green soup will give you the stamina, strength and
energy you need for the day to flow, glow and go it your way.

*"With this soup you will smile and laugh all day
and keep the energy vampires away."*

Durian Tea

Three meals a day with life in between—this tea is life. This tasty brew infuses sweet and creamy with character and zing. It's a vacation in a cup. You can give up the cow now, with this durian kapow. It will energize you now, and start your day with a grateful wow! Serves 1.

—— Ingredients ——

1 bag of your favorite tea (mate, pau d'arco and green tea are my favorites, or try my Mocha Choca Toca Macha Chino Tea)
1 durian pod, including pit
1 tsp. cinnamon
1 vanilla bean
2 T. raw cacao nibs
2 T. raw carob powder or cacao powder
1 tsp. desired sweetener
1 tsp. tocotrienols (optional, if available)
1 tsp. maca powder (optional, if available)
1 tsp. mesquite powder (optional, if available)
1 tsp. lucuma powder (optional, if available)
1 tsp. raw bee pollen (optional)

Steep tea bag in warm, not boiling, water (under 118 degrees). Add durian pod with pit, then add cinnamon, vanilla and sweeteners then add powders, stir well and top with cacao nibs. I sip this with a straw every morning so the cacao nibs surprise my taste buds. Mmmm, delicious and nutritious. Drink up, fill up, get up and get rolling! Start off your rawsome day the durian way!

"Time heals almost everything, give time time.
Make time for tea time."

Mango Smoothie

My Tahiti Sweetie—a tropical good night delight. I love this banquet full of flavor for my late night goodnight! After dancing and singing or working out. Light, bright and hits the spot just right. Serves 1.

—— Ingredients ——

1 mango
1 banana or plantain
1 cube ginger
1 T. squeezed lemon juice
1 T. sweetener, if desired

—— Optional Toppings ——

goji berries
mulberries
shredded coconut, coconut butter or coconut oil
cacao nibs
pomegranate seeds
raw, sprouted buckwheat kernels

Blend ingredients in blender for a minute. Pour in champagne glass or parfait glass and top with your choice of goji berries, mulberries, shredded coconut, coconut butter or oil, cacao nibs, pomegranate seeds or buckwheat kernels.

This is pure decadence for me and this also makes for a great snack. Whip it up anytime. Eating small, healthy snacks helps control weight gain and sustains energy. Great replacement for ice cream, yogurt and heavy fat and sugar-laden smoothies on the market that are loaded with chemicals, preservatives, additives, fat and sugar powders. Another vacation in a glass. Here's to my Tahiti Sweetie! It's time to tango with mangos.

> *"Get rid of anything that isn't useful,*
> *beautiful or joyful in your life."*

Mocha Choca Toca Maca Chino Tea

★★★★★
This gets my Merrill Magic 5-star rating!
My morning heart starter.

—— Ingredients ——

1   bag of Yerba Mate tea, green tea or your favorite tea
1   tsp. raw, organic maca powder
1   tsp. raw honey, agave, stevia or yacon syrup
¼   tsp. turmeric (optional)
1   tsp. cinnamon
⅛   tsp. cayenne pepper (optional)
1   T. raw cacao nibs
2   T. raw cacao powder or carob powder
1   organic vanilla bean pod, sliced open or vanilla liquid
    (no alcohol)

—— Optional Ingredients ——

1   tsp. raw bee pollen
1   tsp. tocotrienols
¼   c. raw almond, coconut, or macadamia nut milk
1   tsp. lucuma powder
1   tsp. mesquite powder
¼   tsp. sliced raw ginger

Heat filtered water slightly (just under a boil) to make tea. Or, if you have the time, make sun tea. Stir all ingredients into the tea after it brews a few minutes. Or, you can also mix all ingredients (including brewed tea) in a blender on frappe setting. Pour into a glass and top with cacao nibs. Sip through a straw and enjoy the cacao nibs as they secretly come through for you! This drink is better than a frappaccino, it's a Mocha Choca Toca Maca Chino Tea.

You can also add some tocotrienols, raw almond, macadamia or coconut milk. Dropping some goji berries in will also give you that extra sweetness. One sip to your lip won't mean forever on your hip; this tea will take you on a rawsome trip. Enjoy, from me to you. Here's to your health.

> *"Under certain circumstances there are few hours*
> *in life more agreeable to the hours dedicated to the*
> *ceremonies known as afternoon tea."*
> —Henry James

Nano-Banano Sapote Smoothie

This gets my Merrill Magic 5-star rating!

This rawsome awesome treat is a reason to give up sugary sweets! Serves 3.

—— Ingredients ——

2   bananas
3   sapotes (a seasonal fruit found in tropical markets)
1   pod vanilla (organic and raw)
¼   tsp. cinnamon
2   T. raw, organic coconut butter, coconut oil or shredded coconut (optional)
    cacao nibs (if desired)
1   T. maca root (optional)
1   T. tocotrinenols
1   T. raw honey, stevia or agave (optional)
⅛   slice ginger (optional)
¼   cup water or coconut water, if you like liquidy texture

Blend all ingredients until smooth, pour into champagne or parfait glasses, garnish with a fresh mint leaf, cinnamon, cacao nibs, shredded coconut, coconut butter or coconut oil. You can also cut up banana and sapote slices and garnish around the smoothie. Serve and enjoy! This one I named after my dad, Nano. I used to make him a banana split every night. I substitute this for a split and it's a perfect fit. Scrumptiously, eviliciously, deliciously divine. Have fun with this one.

"Don't take yourself so seriously. No one else does."

Nut Milk Drink/Spread

Get nutty on nuts! Make this delicious, soothing milk using your favorite sprouted nut or sprouted seeds. I like to use macadamia nuts, almonds, cashews, Brazil nuts or combine them to your liking. Serves 2-3.

—— Ingredients ——

1 c. raw soaked and sprouted nuts, seeds (almond, cashew, macadamia, Brazil) or soaked and sprouted seeds (sunflower, sesame or pumpkin)

2 c. coconut water, filtered water or tea

1 tsp. cinnamon and/or nutmeg (optional)

2 T. tocotrienols

3 tbs. agave, yacon syrup, raw honey, stevia, or dates to taste (adjust amount to taste)

2 T. maca powder (optional, adjust amount to taste)

2 T. lucuma powder (optional, adjust amount to taste)

1 stick organic vanilla bean

¼ c. raw cacao powder or carob powder or carob nibs, optional for "chocolate" milk

1 tsp. sea salt, to taste (optional)

2 T. of coconut butter (for Nut Milk Spread)

❧

Blend all ingredients in a blender until frothy and smooth. If desired, strain the liquid through a nut milk or sprout bag into another container. Add to my Mocha Choca Toca Macha Chino Tea, Skate Great Breakfast cereal or drink plain for a filling, soothing energy treat! Enjoy with Nano's Fig Neutrons for an alternative to traditional milk and cookies or add ice to make a delicious nut milk frappe or add less water to make a smoothie. Add coconut butter for Nut Milk Spread. Store unused milk/spread in the refrigerator in a glass jar for a few days. You can add your favorite fruit (i.e., bananas, strawberries, blueberries) to this mixture to make a nutty fruit milk. Top with cacao nibs, cinnamon and a mint leaf.

This drink is voluptuous, sensuous, frothy, flavorful and filling. I love to sip it, lick it, spread it and smudge it on my lips. A salute to the day.

> *"Live life with the five E's: energy, enthusiasm, excellence, education and empathy."*

The Merrill Magic Durian Persimmon Smoothie

★★★★★

This gets my Merrill Magic 5-star rating!
One of my favorites, I call it the best aphrodisiac in the
world. This is Heaven's angel food, to put you in the mood.
This drink is liquid love.

—— Ingredients ——

4   pods of durian fruit, pits removed
4   persimmons (hachiya preferred—soft and ripe or fuyu
    hard or soft)
1   tsp. cinnamon
⅛   of an organic vanilla bean
2   T. raw cacao powder or raw carob powder, if you want a
    chocolate flavor
    cacao nibs, shredded coconut, coconut butter or coconut
    oil to taste for topping of smoothie (optional)

ॐ

Blend all ingredients in a blender until smooth (about 30 sec.).
Top with cacao nibs, shredded coconut, coconut butter or coconut
oil. You can also decorate the side of the glass with slices of fuyu
persimmons, great for dipping too! Or, for a frozen treat, freeze
the mixture before adding garnish to make a delicious, nutritious
dessert—just like ice cream. I scream, you scream, we all scream
for Merrill Magic Durian Persimmon Ice Scream.

"You'll get a mile of smile from this treat."

Succulent Sweets

Chocolate Sauce

This sumptuous treat contains magnesium, protein, Vitamin C, B vitamins, essential amino acids, theobromine, fiber, lysine, vitamin E, unsaturated alpha lipoic acid and fatty acids, phosphorus and potassium. Your tummy will definitely tell you if what you ate is working for you after this chocolate fantasy.

—— Ingredients ——

1 c. raw cacao powder
4 T. lucuma powder
¼ c. tocotrienols
⅛ c. mesquite powder
   water or coconut water to create desired consistency
4 T. bee pollen (optional)
   add agave, raw honey, stevia, or dates to desired sweetness

Blend cacao powder, lucuma powder tocotrienols, water, mesquite and bee pollen in a blender to make a healthy, delicious chocolate sauce. You can eat the mixture as is or freeze overnight and enjoy the next day as a frozen chocolate bar treat or pour sauce over CoComoco Corn Chewies.

This sauce can also be used over fruit, in tea, on my buckwheat cereal or raw crackers, or just eat it right off the spoon. I love to mix it with organic nut butters, such as chunky almond butter, cashew, pecan and hemp butter. This sauce is deviliciously delicious. You may add warm water if you want a hot fudge sauce! Mmmmmm. Great on raw ice cream, fruit salad and puddings. Have a "chocolate" fiesta. Eat chocolate, spread chocolate, drink chocolate, love chocolate!

"When you feel your worst, try your hardest."

Debbie's Edible Raw Bites

Melt in your mouth smoothness. This tasty treat will give you a memory blast from the past! They remind me of Reese's Pieces.® Serves 2.

—— Ingredients ——

¼ c. raw cacao butter, cut up into small pieces
½ c. raw cacao nibs or beans
½ c. raw jungle peanuts, walnuts, almonds or Brazil nuts (or combine all)
 dash cinnamon (optional)
 Celtic sea salt (optional)

Place first three ingredients in a baggie. Add a dash of cinnamon and Celtic sea salt, shake it 'til you make it, and eat it by the handful.

This snack is so simple, so satisfying, so delicious and nutritious. Easy to keep on hand in glass jars all the time. Being raw is never compromising. No need to eat candy and candy bars when you have this rawsome snack for that hunger attack. Pain is natural. So is the cure. When the pain of where you're at is greater than where you are going, you move. Move to a raw food diet and you can alter your life by altering your food. You will be an alteration for the next generation. Lead by example. And you get to enjoy rawsome Edible Raw Bites. Yay for this day!

"Share with friends and family, be generous everyday, and call your family often."

Debbie's Raw CoComoco Corn Chewies

This is a wonderful replacement for those crisy, chewy rice treats, brownies, cookies, candy bars, and popcorn. It contains magnesium, serotonin protein, antioxidants, good fats, theobromine, fiber, lysine and B vitamins. Serves 1-3.

—— Ingredients ——

2 c. dried or dehydrated purple corn, soaked until softened, then dried with a cloth

½ c. raw jungle peanuts, cashews, macadamia, walnuts or Brazil nuts (or mix all together)

½ c. raw cacao nibs

¼ cup white cacao butter, cut up into small pieces

¼ c. goji berries, mulberries or Incan berries (optional)

Mix all ingredients in a large bowl and it's ready to enjoy. Munch on it like popcorn or eat anytime you have a snack attack to give you that rawsome awesome energy back. It's great to eat before or after exercise. Add to salads or desserts, or create a trail mix. Chew-Chew the Chewies!

"Make peace with your past so you won't chew away your present."

Divine Sapote Pudding

★★★★★

This gets the Merrill Magic 5-star rating!
*Raw, organic goodness. This orgasmic dessert is one of my
favorites. Serves 2.*

—— Ingredients ——

4   sapotes, ripe, soft and pitted
½ c. durian or 1 banana or both
3   tsp. raw cacao powder, carob powder or cacao nibs
    (optional if you want a chocolate sapote pudding)
3   T. tocotrienols powder (optional)
2   T. raw lucuma powder (optional)
2   T. organic raw coconut butter, coconut oil or young
    coconut meat (optional)
    cinnamon, to taste (optional)
    vanilla, to taste (optional)
2   T. raw, chopped pecans or cashews to sprinkle on top
    afterwards
2   T. raw shredded coconut to sprinkle on top afterwards
¼ c. water or coconut water, if you like it more liquidy
1   apple, slice (optional)

❧

Blend all ingredients in a blender until smooth. Serve with raw
apple slices; dunk and delight in the fantastic flavor. Sprinkle chopped
pecans or cashews and shredded coconut on top.

This Divine Sapote Pudding has a pronounced taste and creamy
texture. Perfect for sipping and dipping. It reminds me of fresh-
baked banana cream pie right from my mama's kitchen. Trick your

taste buds with this realistic rendition of banana cream pie that will leave you with a sweet, satisfying, aftertaste of contentment. The thicker the better. Delicious as a pudding or frozen ice cream treat. This organic goodness is a delightful way to enjoy the unique flavor of sapotes.

"Life isn't fair, but it's still good." This treats make it even better.

Heavenly Coconut Butter Spread

★★★★★

This gets my Merrill Magic five-star rating!

This is my morning pick-me-up with veggies or fruit, or my midnight snack as a fruit paste. It's loaded with vitamins, minerals and nutrients so it's a great, delicious way to get them into your diet. It's great on salads, sprouted grains, crackers, and is delicious with fruit wrapped in collard greens, or just plain fruit alone. You can also add to smoothies and my Spritty Spirulina Spread *or use as a salad dressing. Serves 2-4.*

—— Ingredients ——

4   T. raw organic coconut butter or coconut oil

1   c. raw, organic, Tibetan goji berries, mulberries or Incan berries

¼   T. raw organic cacao nibs or beans

1   tsp. cinnamon

1   tsp. Celtic sea salt (optional)

2   T. raw carob powder or cacao powder (optional if you want a chocolate spread)

1   organic vanilla bean, sliced in small pieces or liquid vanilla- no alcohol

Stevia, yacon syrup or agave (optional to desired sweetness)

4   T. spirulina, chlorella or green powder formula, optional (I prefer Spirulina in this recipe)

1   tsp. maca powder

1   T. tocotrienols

1   tsp. lucuma powder

1   tsp. raw hemp seeds or chia seeds

❧

Mix all ingredients thoroughly in a large bowl until smooth. If you like it hard, refrigerate; if you prefer a soft consistency or oil, do not refrigerate. Spread on fruit, crackers, vegetables, add to my *Skate Great Breakfast Cereal,* my *Green Keen Lean Machine Soup and Cocktail,* smoothies or grab a spoon and just lick it and get wicked! This Heavenly Coconut Butter Spread will make your heart sing. You won't believe it's raw vegan.

It's a perfect, buttery consistency, soft and satisfying. Meets the mouth with a variety of tastes and a smooth texture. I love butter and this replaces the butter craze for me. This coconut butter keeps me satisfied, happy and fulfilled. Coconut heals and serves mankind.

Coconut Lore

A coconut/palm tree can live 100 years, during which it can yield thousands of coconuts. In Sanskrit, coconut/palm translates to "tree, which gives all that is needed to live." This refers to the fact that virtually all parts of the tree can be used in some way—from food and drink to fuel, furniture and shelter.

"No matter what your lot in life is, build something on it."

Holy Persimmon Pope-sicle

*This cold treat is guaranteed to bring you closer to God:
<u>G</u>ood <u>O</u>rderly <u>D</u>irection or <u>G</u>ood <u>O</u>ut <u>D</u>oors or <u>G</u>roup <u>O</u>f
<u>D</u>ynamos. Persimmons are high in vitamins A and C and
fiber, and your favorite topping will give you extra vitamins,
minerals, enzymes and nutrients. Serves 2.*

—— Ingredients ——

1   c. of your favorite water
¼   c. raw coconut oil
2   hachiya or fuyu persimmons
2   popsicle sticks
    raw cacao nibs or powder, goji berries, shredded coconut
    or chopped nuts (cashews, walnuts, macadamia nuts), to
    taste (optional)

Insert popsicle sticks into the persimmons of your choice (they
can be ripe or unripe) and dip in water to moisten. Set on wax
paper and freeze overnight. When you take them out, they will
be ripe, sweet and ready to eat. (Freezing them will ripen them
quicker.) To maximize your pleasure, dip in raw coconut oil and
sprinkle with raw cacao nibs, cacao powder, shredded coconut, goji
berries, nut pieces or all.

Enjoy your toy and pray for health while you eat. Have fun; you
won't be able to stop at one. You will be too blessed to be stressed.
This pope-sicle is better than a candied or caramel apple on a stick,
which was my favorite treat as a kid. Let's get down and chow
down on this one. This pope-sickle is a great way to get kids to eat
their recommended fruits of the day but feel like they're eating

candy. Here's hope for the pope-sicle. This treat is your organic line of defense against the offense of sugar and fat.

> *"Candy is dandy, liquor is quicker,*
> *but raw is Mother Nature's law."*

Merrill Magic Creamy Maple Sauce

This delicious sauce tastes just like butterscotch or maple syrup and is the perfect topping for cereal, fruit, raw ice cream, my Apple Debbie, crackers or add to my favorite Spectacular Splendid Persimmon Pudding/Ice Cream/ Smoothie. *I love freezing it and making maple squares. Serves 2-3.*

—— Ingredients ——

1 c. to 1 ½ c. warm filtered water or coconut water
¼ c. lucuma powder
¼ c. tocotrienols
¼ tsp. cinnamon
¼ c. raw cacao nibs (optional)
¼ c. raw cacao or carob powder (optional)
1 organic vanilla pod
1 dash cayenne pepper (optional)
1 tsp. sweetener (stevia powder or sweetener of your choice)
1 tsp. organic maple or butterscotch flavoring (no alcohol)

Blend all ingredients in a bowl with warm filtered water or coconut water (not heated or boiled). Adjust liquid to achieve desired consistency. Sprinkle with cacao nibs or add nibs into mixture.

This sauce is organic, instamatic, automatic and vibrantly volcanic. This will give you the magic to remove tragic in your life. Appetite comes with eating. Eat raw and your appetite for raw increases from raw to richness. *Bon appetit.*

"Make one person happy every day, even if it's yourself."

Nano Banano on a Stick

Named after my dad, Nano. This was his favorite: bananas and peanut butter. So I mixed it and fixed it and now I am giving it to you. This lip-smacking, evilicious, sensualicious treat, is a great replacement for that sugar craving and can be enjoyed au naturale, or frozen. This recipe contains lots of potassium, magnesium and protein. Serves 2.

—— Ingredients ——

2 organic bananas

¼ T. cashews, almonds, jungle peanuts, walnuts, sesame seeds, or hemp seeds, finely chopped or crushed, soaked and sprouted

2 T. raw nut butter (cashew, macadamia, almond, pecan or hemp)

¼ c. raw carob powder or cacao powder

4 T. raw cacao nibs

1 tsp. cinnamon

1 tsp. Himalayan sea salt (optional)

2 popsicle sticks

shredded coconut, to taste

Insert popsicle stick into peeled banana and smother on 1 T. nut butter of your choice. Roll banana in carob or cacao powder, sprinkle with cinnamon, crushed nuts, seeds and cacao nibs. Shower with shredded coconut. Eat as is, or freeze and enjoy later.

This is an extraordinary, delicious sensation that is very filling and sweet. The flavors will burst in your mouth at different times, and stay in your heart to give you a banana, coconut, chocolate nut essence of presence. It's beautiful. It's also a great replacement for sugary, fatty, cholesterol-filled ice cream bars, sundaes, frozen yogurt treats, sweet desserts, cakes and pies. Nano's gift from me to you.

"Close your mouth, open your heart.
You can even eat just half, that's a start!."

Nano's Raw Fig Neutrons

These cookies are named after my father's favorite cookie. (I thought I was!) They are better than store-bought Newtons! Nano's Raw Fig Neutrons hit the spot to the raw bone. They are a great substitute for any cookie, muffin or processed dessert because they're loaded with iron, minerals and magnesium. I serve them as acceptance appetizers at parties. Nano's Neutrons are good for everything that ails you and they'll keep you as regular as rain. Serves 4.

—— Ingredients ——

4   fresh or dried figs soaked (calimyrna or black mission are best)

1   T. coconut butter or coconut oil

1   T. dried coconut, shredded

¼ tsp. cinnamon

⅛ tsp. Celtic sea salt (optional)

1   tbsp. raw cacao nibs or powder/or carob powder or all three

⅛ tsp. organic vanilla (either liquid or pod—no alcohol)

2-4 dehydrated crackers (your favorite kind or try my Oat Groat Crackers, buckwheat, soy goji or quinoa crackers)

Soak dried figs for 3 hours to soften or use fresh figs in season. Spread a layer of coconut butter, shredded coconut, cinnamon, sea salt and cacao nibs or powder on cracker. Add liquid vanilla or scrape vanilla pod to top. Press fresh or soaked figs on top of cracker and coconut mixture. Enjoy open-face or press another cracker on top to make a fig Neutron sandwich. Sometimes I add

Raw Rejuvenative nut butters on top before I sandwich it, such as pecan, cashew, almond or hemp for extra protein and energy. This is definitely a meal in itself—a raw meal deal. Get creative. You can add other ingredients as well and have an opulent feast here. Enough is a feast.

These Neutrons help me kick up my heels and get on my wheels to glide with pride and work my rawhide. The figs will pick you up, the cacao will fill you up, and the crackers will help you chow down. This Neutron is rawlicious. Don't be shy of finger lickin' good.

"Read this book, feel good; eat raw foods, feel great."

Spectacular Splendid Persimmon Pudding/Ice Cream/Smoothie

★★★★★

This gets my Merrill Magic 5-star rating!
Another three-in-one—less work and lots of fun. A colorful holiday treat! I serve it in a goblet or parfait glass to create a great treat for the eyes as well as the tummy. Kids love it as much as adults. Serves 3.

—— Ingredients ——

6   persimmons, seeded (hachiya or fuyu, very soft and ripe)
½   cup chopped macadamia nuts
1   stick of organic vanilla bean
1   tsp. cinnamon
¼   cube ginger, diced
1   c. pomegranate seeds to sprinkle on top, if in season
½   kiwi, diced
2   T. coconut butter or coconut oil to dollop on top
1   T. bee pollen (optional)
2   T. tocotrienols (optional)
2   T. cacao nibs to sprinkle on top
2   T. raw cacao or raw carob powder to add to mixture if you
     want a chocolate-persimmon pudding
     filtered water or coconut water from young Thai organic
     coconut

෴

Blend all ingredients in a blender until smooth. Add water to adjust the consistency; add a small amount for pudding and more for a smoothie or ice cream-like texture. Spoon pudding into parfait glasses or goblets and top with cacao nibs, macadamia nuts, coconut butter or coconut oil and pomegranate seeds. For a festive look, alternate layers of kiwi slices, strawberries and/or blueberries with dollops of persimmon pudding. Add a mint leaf for decoration and you've got the perfect holiday treat. You can also freeze this and eat like ice cream.

This blended, scrumptious, sensational dessert is a meal, a feast and a banquet of taste and flavor. It makes for a great, festive holiday dessert or aperitif. This persimmon smoothie is an abundance of nutritious sensation, color, joy and satisfaction. It is my favorite food in the entire world. I can eat it every day, three times a day, 365 days a year and never get tired of it. From me to you, enjoy this fabulous treat that's ever so sweet. You can now have it all! All the nutrition this dish has to offer.

"If you don't take a stand for something, you'll fall for anything."

Raw Apple Debbie

An apple a day keeps ill health at bay. I eat to look and feel great. Serves 1.

—— Ingredients ——

1 Rome apple (or other apple of your choice)
2 T. tocotrienols
½ c. warm coconut water, warm sweetened tea or your favorite nut milk
¼ c. seed mixture (hemp, flax, sunflower)
2 T. goji berries
2 T. cacao nibs
2 T. raw cacao or raw carob powder
¼ tsp. cinnamon, raw honey, agave or stevia (optional)
1 T. dehydrated buckwheat kernels to sprinkle on top

Core apple, place tocotrienols in center and then pour warm liquid on top and stir. Add seed mixture, goji berries, cacao nibs, cinnamon and sweetener, and buckwheat kernels. Simply delicious and nutritious! Eat in this direction for breakfast or dessert and you will flow in perfection. I ate this everyday for breakfast the first seven years of transitioning to a vegetarian/vegan lifestyle. It sustained me and filled me up until dinner time. Direction is more important than speed. An *Apple Debbie* a day keeps your colon OK.

> *"Eating a nutritious breakfast helps us focus on healthy eating habits all day."*

Sweet Chocolate Dip, Spread or Sauce

Set it and forget it. Go exercise and come back to fantasize with this choc-full of flavor. This sweet chocolate delight is great on fruit, crackers, cereals and smoothies. It's low in fat and a perfect late-night snack, afternoon pick-me-up or morning breakfast! Serves 4.

—— Ingredients ——

¼ c. raw carob powder or cacao powder or both

¼ c. goji, Incan, mulberries or pomegranate seeds for topping

1 T. ginger, finely chopped

2 T. raw bee pollen (optional)

2 T. raw lecithin granules (non-gmo)

2 tsp. Celtic sea salt, optional

2 T. cinnamon

stevia, honey or agave, to taste

½ c. raw cacao nibs or cacao beans for topping

raw jungle peanuts or any nut can be added for extra protein and flavor to sprinkle on top

⅛ c. raw mesquite powder (optional)

⅛ c. tocotrienols (optional)

⅛ c. lucuma (optional)

½ organic vanilla pod or vanilla flavoring, no alcohol (optional)

1 c. coconut water, filtered water or warm tea makes for a warm sauce (optional)

¼ c. soaked, sprouted and dehydrated buckwheat kernels

❧

Blend all ingredients in a blender until smooth. Add coconut water, filtered water or warm tea for a thinner consistency. Serve as a pudding, a dip, a spread or serve with apples, my smoothies, or any fruit. It's also great as a sauce for my Skate Great Breakfast cereal, fruit salads, my crackers, sprouted grains or raw ice cream. Top with sprouted dehydrated buckwheat kernels, raw cacao nibs, pomegranate seeds or berries. It tastes like hot fudge sauce or English toffee. You can also freeze it in ice cube trays or cups for a frozen chocolate fiesta.

This recipe is a delicious comfort food to get you in the mood. Versatile, subtle, sweet, this chocolate lends a delectable richness to everything it touches, even you. Go from raw to richness now with this fabulous treat. This virtually fat-free sauce holds its own to any cooked chocolate sauce. Turns any ordinary day into the best day. This is a good mood food. Enjoy the best and forget the rest.

"Love deeply and passionately, eat with embellishment.
You might get hurt, but it's the only way to live life completely."

Chocolate Coconut Ganache

This chocolaty, creamy treat is better than the real thing.
It is the real thing. Serves 4-6.

—— Ingredients ——

1 c. coconut butter or coconut oil

½ c. dried goji berries (save a few as garnish)

½ c. cacao powder

¼ c. cacao nibs (save a few as garnish)

1 tsp. organic vanilla powder, or 1 pod

1 tsp. cinnamon

½ c. raw shredded coconut (save some as garnish)

¼ c. raw honey, agave, yacon syrup or 2T. stevia (optional)

½ c. hemp seeds

ॐ

Blend all ingredients in a food processor until smooth. Serve at room temperature and garnish with goji berries, cacao nibs, shredded coconut, and buckwheat kernels. You can also roll into little balls, freeze, and eat like a truffle!

"If you are in love and joy, you will attract love and joy."

Decadent Coconut Mousse

This white creamy coconut treat will take you on a dream vacation.
Serves 4-6.

—— Ingredients ——

½ c. raw macadamia nuts or raw cashews

1 c. coconut butter or coconut oil

6 medjol dates, pitted

1 tsp. organic vanilla powder, or 1 pod

1 tsp. cinnamon

2 T. raw honey, agave, yacon syrup or stevia to taste (optional)

½ to 1 c. coconut water (if needed for desired consistency).

Blend all ingredients in a food processor until smooth. Enjoy as is by the spoonful, or as a spread on crackers or green leaves. Serve with blueberries, bananas or your favorite fruit.

"When I eat this, my heart sings."

Chapter 40

Notes, Quotes, Tips, and Tricks

"I quote others only in order the better to express myself."
—Michel de Montaigne

Some of these quotes and tips are of my own making; the rest are the wise words of others who have helped me on my journey. All have become words to live by in my rawsome, awesome road to happy bliss. These are my rules to never lose with your health. Keep these in your car, briefcase, on your mirror, refrigerator, computer or even in your recording device. They will support you in living a delicious life. Read these quotes at your leisure or read a quote for the day.

♦ The suggestions I give in this book are guides to progress, not perfection.

♦ Chew all your food well. Drink your solids, chew your liquids.

♦ Never eat late at night, before bed, or in the middle of the night.

♦ Real foods are found in two aisles of the supermarket: the fruit and vegetable sections.

♦ Fruit is a dessert.

◆ Support your local farmers by shopping at Farmer's Markets for organic raw fruits and vegetables. They are "rawsomely awesome."

◆ Do not eat fruit and vegetables together at the same meal except for pineapple, papaya, tomato, and avocado.

◆ Always sit when eating.

◆ Drink fresh squeezed vegetable juice and/or wheat grass juice every day.

◆ Prioritize your priorities.

◆ If you don't change your taste buds, habits, and addictions, it will cost you your health.

◆ Bless and put love in all your food.

◆ Spend as much time as possible in the good outdoors. Good Out Doors = God.

◆ Surround yourself with loving, conscious, committed and healthy people.

◆ Eat only FRESH, RIPE, WHOLE, RAW, ORGANIC fruits, vegetables, sprouted nuts, sprouted seeds and sprouted grains.

◆ Disease is formed in a non-oxygen environment. Raw fruits, vegetables, nuts, and seeds contain oxygen, enzymes, nutrients, and water to help the body remain healthy.

◆ Exercise. Do something you like for one hour a day, six days a week.

◆ Believe in, and spend time with, a higher force every day.

◆ Express yourself creatively and sensually in your work, fitness, and fun.

◆ Have fun everyday. Fun is limitless, life is not.

- Forgive yourself and everyone else. Please don't hold grudges. It eats at you, and you eat at it.

- The slower you go, the faster you know. Slow down and live. You're not livin' if you're driven.

- Not planning is planning to fail. Plan your meals, exercise, and spiritual time daily.

- Completion is perfection. Complete everything you start.

- Give to the world and the world will give to you.

- Share everything you know with others. You can't keep it until you give it away.

- Don't take advice from anyone who does not have what you want.

- Be a leader and a winner, not a follower and a loser!

- Don't deny it 'till you try it and apply it!

- Breathe, and put your fork down between bites.

- Pray before you eat. Prayer is medicine; your higher force is your doctor.

- ASAP = Always Say A Prayer. It helps.

- True disease is disorder in the body caused by overeating and under sleeping. The body needs time to digest the mess we create.

- How much of a bottom do you want to hit with your health? Your bottom may be six feet under.

- The Standard American Diet = S.A.D. Diet! Change your diet to the glad diet of raw, ripe, fresh, whole organic foods.

♦ Health is not just what we put in, but what we eliminate, assimilate, absorb, and digest.

♦ Eat more green foods for chlorophyll, oxygen, enzymes, vitamins and nutrients for your body.

♦ Live food = live energy. Dead cooked food = dead energy.

♦ Eating raw helps you cleanse, repair, maintain and heal.

♦ Eat more quality foods, and you will eat less.

♦ Habit hunger can be changed.

♦ More people die in the kitchen than any other room in the house!

♦ When fear knocks at the door, faith will answer. Just knock and it will open. Fear says don't look, and pride says you don't have to.

♦ You can't get indigestion from swallowing your pride.

♦ Raw fruits and vegetables are the best snack to get your energy back on track.

♦ You can take the elevator going down, but you gotta take the steps going up.

♦ My snack to the future is 2 oz. of wheat grass a day to keep sickness away. I haven't had a cold, flu, virus or sickness in 28 years.

♦ If you are messed up, fed up, given up, and shut up, then get up, get fit, get rolling and get raw now!

♦ Making time for yourself, friends, family and others is key to good health and well-being.

♦ Eat for humanity, sanity and vanity.

◆ Eat no pesticides, vermicides, fungicides, and herbicides. They all equal suicide!

◆ Normally, we overlook an issue or problem—we ignore it by eating and drinking it down, getting bigger around, then the truth of why we are eating can never be found.

◆ It's still a treat not to eat meat as long as you can have a great raw sweet! Try my Chocolate Pudding, Sapote Pudding or Nano Banano On A Stick, yum yum in my tum tum.

◆ What you believe, you receive. Receive the gift of health now.

◆ Our own thinking affects how we perceive other's behaviors. Positive thinking gives us positive results.

◆ Worrying is like a rocking horse. It never gets you anywhere.

◆ It's not what you're drinking, it's what you're thinking. Stinking thinking will destroy us.

◆ Keep the law of attraction alive with your health: be health, do health, have health.

◆ All sickness is a marker for a deeper problem: look within and begin the healing.

◆ The foods you eat affect the moods you greet.

◆ Be divaliciously, eviliciously raw—that's the law.

◆ Employ Mother Nature in your home; she is the best chef in the world.

◆ You can't change the wind, but you can adjust the sails.

◆ Progression, not perfection.

◆ Eating raw helps transform you from physicality to spirituality, while organically living in reality.

◆ Think it, ink it, thank it. Have an attitude of gratitude every day, all day.

◆ Shop locally and act locally, but think globally.

◆ Raw foods will put some pep in your step and some zip in your trip.

◆ Good food = good mood.

◆ Follow your heart's desire, and you will be on fire.

◆ Be like the ocean, always in motion—stay in action or detour into destruction.

◆ Focus on health and you will have health. Energy flows where attention goes.

◆ Setbacks are set ups for success. Progress to the next level, don't perfect the next level.

◆ The only time we begin something at the top is when we are digging a grave.

◆ Have a great treat, eat fruit as a sweet.

◆ The only time success comes before work is in the dictionary.

◆ Now is the time to see the impossible become the possible.

◆ Eliminate preservatives in your food and preserve your body.

◆ Get wicked and kick it. Kick the crap habit now.

◆ Have a raw Wrap in a Snap and a Dip in a Whip for lunch or dinner.

◆ Skating works the butt, legs, abs and thighs and when you're done, you will be so energized.

◆ Eat great, exercise great, energy great.

♦ Count your joys instead of your tears, count your courages instead of your fears.

♦ If something doesn't work out the way you'd like it to, look for something else good to come out of it.

♦ Drain your brain with writing every day. Write things right.

♦ There are 24 hours in a day, 60 seconds in a minute, three months in a season, and 12 months in a year. That's the reality of real time—there is no such thing as microwave or sitcom timing, or a quick minute. We cannot force things in our health process.
Practice + patience + persistence = permanence.

♦ When you are down to nothing, your higher spirit is up to something.

♦ Whether they fly, swim, trot or flap, they are animals. Please stop justifying the over consumption of eating animals.

♦ When you feel you have lost it with your health, don't lose the lesson.

♦ Remember the three R's—Respect for yourself, Respect for others, Responsibility for all your actions.

♦ Misery and poor health is a decision and a choice you make. You can decide on joy and extraordinary health instead.

♦ Move a muscle, change a thought.

♦ Anything valued above your health will be lost. You may have to lose your health to find your health. Lose yourself, find yourself.

♦ If you are too busy to work on your health, you are too busy. How sad is that?

- Do your best and forget the rest.

- Being famous in your life means: having Fun Among Many—Out in the Universe Serving.

- If your food is not organic, it's a waste of your chewing time.

- Failure is fertilizer for success.

- A master will always be a student.

- The only way out is through it.

- There is a difference between slipping, and living back in the problem.

- There are three laws to follow: 1) The laws of physics 2) The laws of the universe 3) Mother Nature's law and that is raw.

- Luck is the name losers give to failure.

- It is if I say so, and it's not, if I say it's not!

- The true problem with junk food is that we eat it because we are upset, and we are upset because we eat it.

- Fear is the first drug! Followed by cooked food, prescription drugs, alcohol, recreational drugs, nicotine, processed foods, sugar and the over consumption of eating animals.

- Green is clean.

- Share your health, let it be contagious.

- Where there were once walls, there will now be open doors.

- When you eat no junk, you have no junk thoughts.

- Get rid of the junk and gunk in your trunk, and put some raw in your drawer.

- Not exercising is not an option.

♦ Eating animals is not an option; if you choose it, you lose it (your health, that is).

♦ It's not age, it's rust.

♦ How you do anything is how you do everything.

♦ You can't do right wrong, and you can't do wrong right.

♦ Be interested in feeling good, not just looking good.

♦ Affirmation: My health is phenomenal—it should be, it will be, and it is.

♦ Shout it out, dance it out, write it out, talk it out, sing it out, skate it out, jog it out, stretch it out, speak it out, but get it out. Declare it out! GET IT OUT NOW!

♦ Don't believe all you hear, spend all you have, or sleep all you want, or take advice from anyone who does not have what you want.

♦ Believe in love at first sight, and your first vegan bite.

♦ Think about, thank about, and bring about.

♦ Leaders and healers don't ask us to believe in them. They teach us to believe in ourselves.

♦ Life came without instructions. Seek education, enthusiasm and envisionment in all areas of your life today.

♦ Maybe your food should be weighed and measured, not counted.

♦ No matter what your lot in life is, build something on it.

♦ Make one person happy each day, even if it's you.

♦ Raw foods will add life to your years as well as years to your life.

- Ask for forgiveness, not permission.

- Ability is what you're capable of doing. Motivation determines what you do. Attitude determines how well you do it.

- Be raw on the roll and out of control! Be off the charts and touch many hearts!

- Everything after "but" is B.S.

- Let go of thoughts of limitation, enjoy meditation and take an emergency vacation, for you are part of the creation.

- Be a natural born healer and add value to your life and the lives of those around you.

- I said it, I meant it and now I represent it. You can represent it too. Represent it in your life and the lives of those around that you love and come in contact with.

- Raw food saves lives, exercising revives lives.

- Listen to learn, learn to listen.

- When the insanity of craving hits, raw vegan food defends.

- "To keep the body in good health is a duty...otherwise we should not be able to keep our mind strong and clear."—Buddha

- You are what you eat.

- Foods should be eaten from the garden of vegan.

- When you feel your worst, try your hardest.

- When you do good, you never really know how much good you do.

◆ When you reach the end of your rope, tie a knot and hang on.

◆ To get what you never had, you must do what you've never done.

◆ Worry is an ironic form of hope.

◆ A man must be able to feed himself, fuel himself and fight for what he believes is his right to have dignity, power and health.

◆ Today is the tomorrow you worried about yesterday.

◆ Health is a state of complete physical, mental and social well being, and not just the absence of disease.

◆ TIME = <u>T</u>hings <u>I</u> <u>M</u>ust <u>E</u>arn.

◆ What lies behind us and what lies before us are tiny matters compared to what lies within us.

◆ Look how far you have come and look at where you are going—at least the end of this book!

◆ Only those who risk going too far will know how far they can go.

◆ A smile is contagious; be a carrier with a mile of a smile.

◆ "Hate is like acid. It can damage the vessel in which it is stored as well as destroy the object on which it is poured"—Ann Landers

◆ "The best thing to do behind a friend's back is pat it." —Ruth Brillhart

◆ It is easier to go down a hill than up, but best the view is from the top.

- "If you think you're too small to make a difference, you haven't been in bed with a mosquito."—Anita Roddick

- "Courage is contagious. When a brave person takes a stand, the spines of others are stiffened."—Rev. Billy Graham

- You are the only person on this earth who can use your ability.

- Happiness is like a butterfly. The more you chase it, the more it will elude you. But if you turn your attention to other things, it comes softly and sits on your shoulder.

- If there's no wind, row.

- Forgiveness is the sweetest revenge.

- The pain pushes until the vision pulls.

- You can't base your life on other people's expectations.

- "Do not follow where the path may lead. Go instead where there is no path and leave a trail."—Muriel Strode

- Make your life a mission—not an intermission.

- "The man who has no imagination has no wings."
  —Muhammad Ali

- "You may be disappointed if you fail, but you are doomed if you don't try."—Beverly Sills

- "The only people you should ever want to get "even" with are those who have helped you." John Honeyfield

- "Pride is tasteless, colorless and sizeless. Yet it is the hardest thing to swallow." —August B. Black

- Money will buy a pretty good dog, but it won't buy the wag of the tail.

◆ "The best bridge between despair and hope is a good night's sleep."—E. Joseph Coleman

◆ Love deeply and passionately. Eat with embellishment. You might get hurt, but it's the only way to live life completely.

◆ Eat slowly, talk slowly, walk slowly and think quickly.

◆ When someone asks you a question you don't want to answer, smile and ask them why they want to know.

◆ Seek your higher self early and often.

◆ Eat for longevity, health, fitness and beauty; if you do, you'll look like me, and be a cutie with a bootie.

◆ "I know God doesn't give me anything I can't handle. I just wish he didn't trust me so much."—St. Theresa

◆ Don't quit before the miracle.

◆ There's always room for improvement. It's the largest room in the house, and we all need to spend a lot more time there.

◆ Please don't spend your health chasing wealth, and then your wealth chasing health.

◆ Uncook or be cooked.

◆ When you eat organic, there's no panic. You're automatic, systematic and instamatic.

◆ Look within and you will win.

◆ A man wrapped up in himself is a very small bundle.

◆ Be a leader, not a follower. You know what happens when you follow the herd—you step in poop.

◆ When you realize you've made a mistake, take immediate steps to correct it.

- ◆ If opportunity doesn't knock, build a door.

- ◆ "The art of being wise is the art of knowing what to overlook."—William James

- ◆ You can make more friends in a month by being interested in them than in ten years by trying to get them interested in you."—Charles L. Allen

- ◆ Be kind. Every person you meet is fighting a hard battle.

- ◆ "Success seems to be largely a matter of hanging on after others have let go."—William Feather

- ◆ You can either complain that rose bushes have thorns— or rejoice that thorns have roses bushes.

- ◆ "It's better to do something imperfectly than nothing flawlessly."—Robert Schuller

- ◆ When in doubt, leave it out.

- ◆ It's ok to love myself and hate my bad habits.

- ◆ Please don't live as if the other shoe is going to drop. What if your higher spirit has only one foot?

- ◆ I can feel hunger and not act on the feeling.

- ◆ Success is when opportunity meets readiness.

- ◆ Fruit is raw fast food.

- ◆ Dress up and show up, and life will rush in to meet your every need.

- ◆ Eat raw, it's Mother Nature's law, bringing order to the body, mind and spirit.

- ◆ It's easier to stay in shape than to get in shape. It's easier to stay raw than to get raw.

♦ Proper planning prevents poor performance and problems.

♦ Animals trust us, every time we eat them, we violate their trust.

♦ Nobility is humility and fertility for well-being.

♦ Silence nourishes hope.

♦ Commitment is never an act of moderation!

♦ We are killing ourselves with our forks.

♦ What you don't eat, you don't crave.

♦ Not planning is planning to fail.

♦ Raw, living foods do not warrant unlimited consumption.

♦ Fast food takes your money fast.

♦ Bless you, Be-less-You.

♦ Be a survivor; survivors always win. When you survive one thing, you survive everything.

♦ Eat fruit, stay cute.

♦ See it, hear it, say it, write it and have it.

♦ While you are judging yourself by your thoughts, the world is judging you by your actions.

♦ "Things turn out best for people who make the best of the way things turn out."—Art Linkletter

♦ Be happy with who you are and what you do.

♦ The highest frequency you can be on is love and health.

♦ A vegan lifestyle provides protection against numerous diseases, including the three biggest killers: heart disease, cancer, and stroke.

♦ Stay true to your dreams, stay true to yourself.

♦ If the cure works, you probably have the problem.

♦ Be wise, exercise! Regular exercise makes you feel stronger, younger, more energetic, and alive.

♦ Eat raw, you'll pop and be non-stop.

♦ See yourself looking and feeling young, happy, vibrant and alive, and you will be it, do it and have it.

♦ When you get even, you get even sicker.

♦ Remember to have fun—the more you play, the more your health, and life works.

♦ Enjoy yourself = In-Joy-of-Self.

♦ A workout makes you better today than yesterday. It strengthens the body, relaxes the mind, and toughens the spirit. When you workout regularly, your problems diminish and your confidence soars.

♦ There is no thrill quite like doing something you didn't know you could do.

♦ The darkest hour is only 60 minutes long: you can endure it. Whatever it is now, it will be different in 60 minutes.

♦ Raw, living food is extraordinarily, ordinary.

♦ NO means: Next Opportunity.

♦ Raw foods are opening the gates of heaven to the fountain of youth.

♦ Eat more greens, have a green party, and invite yourself to it, or your mind will have a party, and invite negativity.

♦ When you are in health, you are in love, when you are in love, you are in health, when you are on this frequency, you will be healthy and attract health and attract love.

♦ Follow your bliss and where there were once walls, the Universe will open doors.

♦ Let's get wicked, kick it and lick the junk food habit now!

♦ Your health behaviors are the effects of your thoughts. Let your behavior be the cause of your thoughts. Think positive, loving thoughts of yourself and others.

♦ Be at the cause of your health, not at the effect of your thoughts.

♦ Please, for your health: adopt the raw vegan diet or vegetarian diet. Be a vegan, be alive, and thrive. There's nothing to it, but to do it!

♦ One in three children will develop diabetes; spread the message to your kids. Lead by example.

♦ You can't heal what you can't feel.

♦ What you are visualizing, you are materializing.

♦ Get up and get going, you'll keep growing, glowing and flowing.

♦ If you are in love and joy, you will attract love and joy.

♦ If you go there in your mind, you will go there in your body.

♦ Bring the mind and the body will follow, bring the body and the mind will follow.

♦ Going raw and losing weight is easy as long as you don't eat the cheesy.

♦ You were born to succeed, not to fail.

♦ We are living in the most powerful time the world has ever seen. Everything is at our fingertips.

♦ The power that is within you will draw it to you.

♦ Stop using food as an excuse for validation, gratification and recreation. Food is none of the above.

♦ Drug companies do not want you to be eating foods and supplements that will make you well, as that will have an adverse effect on their product sales.

♦ "Let food be thy medicine, let medicine be thy food."—Hippocrates

♦ We all want everything in microwave timing, we have to be patient or we will be a patient. Know it's a process, not an event.

♦ Let your dreams be your reality.

♦ When eating bread, there is danger ahead—and your energy is dead.

♦ The only way out is through it.

♦ Obstacles birth opportunities. Let your raw vegan, organic lifestyle be your opportunity, not an obstacle toward your health.

♦ More "We," less "Me."

♦ If you can't find a way, then make one.

♦ Lack of expression = depression.

♦ If you need a miracle in your health it's OK. There's a lot around you. If you don't believe in miracles, come and be one.

- It's better to feel better than look better. First feel better and then you'll look better.

- Misery and poor health is a choice and a decision you make. Choose great health.

- Being incomplete in your life, always displaces miracles.

- The only person you can change is you.

- Transition your behaviors to a healthier lifestyle now, it's the only time you've got.

- Opportunity knocks once, but temptation leans on the door-bell—so whatever you do, don't answer it when it rings.

- My raw food lifestyle has brought me from physical to spiritual. From non-belief to belief. From disconnection to connection. Uninspired to inspired and aspired. From lack of knowledge to intuition. From being dead to alive.

- Just pop the nuts, drink the grass and snack on fruit. That's how you'll keep in shape and stay so cute.

- By getting our health back, we get our power, brilliance, beauty and intelligence back.

- Always leave loved ones with loving words—it may be the last time you see them.

- Be an attraction not a promotion. Give to the world and the world will give to you.

- Pledge to go Veg!

- Right here right now that's where you are. That's where your feet are. That's where your higher spirit is.

- Be a source for global health, wealth and knowledge.

♦ When you eat raw it's easy. Easy on me and easy on you.

♦ Happiness is the fruit of success.

♦ "An ounce of action is worth a ton of theory."—Friedrich Engels

♦ Get back on the roll if you slip and fall—see it as interruption, not a failure.

♦ Raw foods are foods for life. Foods for eternal life.

♦ An extraordinary life is an expensive proposition for your health.

♦ Never laugh at other people's dreams. People who don't have dreams don't have much.

♦ A raw lifestyle will keep you forever young and helps you give up the urgency for plastic surgery.

♦ Talk slowly, eat slowly, but think quickly.

♦ To be all you can be, you must stop putting substances into your body that are deterrents to your body.

♦ The grass is greener on the other side but it's just as hard to mow.

♦ Get the raw WOW NOW!—Wake up, Open up, be Willing.

♦ "Champions keep playing 'til they get it right."—Billie Jean King

♦ "As a man thinketh, so he is." Proverbs 23:7

♦ Don't spend your health chasing wealth, and then your wealth chasing health.

♦ Let your hearts fires become your desires.

- To get the wisdom to go even higher, food is best eaten without the fire.

- A fault recognized is half corrected.

- RAW not WAR.

- "Do not bite at the bait of pleasure, 'til you know there is no hook beneath it."—Thomas Jefferson

- Share the message, not the mess.

- "We will never know the worth of water 'til the well goes dry."—Scottish proverb

- Go at your own pace. Keep your eye on the finish line, not the starting line.

- Eat for need, not for greed and speed.

- Green is the new gold.

- Great health is making time for you, making time for friends and family and giving time to others.

- Disease, sickness and disorders are a marker for a deeper problem. Look within and you will win.

- Imagine being fully satisfied with who you are.

- Learn meditation; learn self, learn health.

- "One cannot think well, live well or sleep well, if one has not dined well."—Virginia Wolfe

- Make one person happy each day, even if it's yourself.

- There are those who make things happen, those who watch things happen, and those who don't know anything happened.

- Fear less, fall less, fail less.

♦ When you lose, don't lose the lesson.

♦ Between God and Me, there is no between.

♦ Don't let a little dispute injure a great friendship.

♦ Marry a man or woman you love to talk to; as you get older conversational skills will be as important as any other.

♦ Don't believe all you hear, spend all you have or sleep all you want.

♦ When you say, "I love you," mean it!

♦ When you say you're sorry, look the person in the eyes.

♦ If I want what I've got, I have to keep doing what I'm doing.

♦ For every problem there is an opportunity.

♦ It works if you let it, do it, and work it.

♦ You don't have to like it, you just have to do it.

♦ Raw food is beautifully basic.

♦ Swallow your pride, it's not fattening.

♦ Eating raw will make you feel happy.

♦ Learn to say no—no is a complete sentence.

♦ Planning ahead in business is called a budget; in the middle of the night, it's called worry.

♦ Cooked food is like old news you can't use.

♦ Do what you love and you'll never work a day in your life.

♦ Pamper yourself with healthy food, don't punish yourself with food.

♦ Staying in action restores inspiration and motivation.

- Eating a raw food diet will allow you to fall so in love with yourself, you'll ask yourself out.

- Doing just a little will help a lot.

- Eat the fruit that allows you to spit the pit.

- Idle hands create way too much channel surfing, which leads to overeating and weight gain. Stay busy.

- A workout is a personal triumph over laziness and procrastination.

- A workout is a wise use of time and an investment in excellence.

- A workout is a key that opens the door to opportunity and success. Hidden within each of us, is an extraordinary force. Physical and mental fitness are the triggers that can release it.

- When you zip the lips, you narrow the hips.

- Action creates momentum and restores integrity.

- All health is an inside job.

- The less you carry around, the longer you are around.

- Keep the wisdom, lose the weight.

- Stick to it and it will stick to you, and you will stick out in the world and the world will be stuck on you.

- Stagnation is constipation and procrastination.

- Live to give; you can't take it with you.

- As you become weak in the ego, you become strong in organic intelligence.

- Power is the rate at which you make results happen.

◆ "Do not follow where the path may lead. Go instead where there is no path and leave a trail."—Muriel Strode

◆ What lies behind us and what lies before us are tiny matters compared to what lies within us.

◆ Close your mouth, open your heart.

◆ Make your life a mission, not an intermission.

◆ Raw foods offer you a fit body, a healthy mind, and a happy spirit.

◆ You will achieve more if you don't mind who gets the credit.

◆ Act "as if."

◆ Fake it 'till you make it.

◆ "Live your life and forget your age."—Norman Vincent Peale

◆ "If you don't like something, change it. If you can't change it, change your attitude. Don't complain."—Maya Angelou

◆ Life can be understood backwards, but must be lived forwards.

◆ Do this over time, not overnight.

◆ I'm too blessed to be stressed.

◆ When you speak defeat, you draw in defeat.

◆ Negativity is contagious—and so is positivity.

The opinions expressed in this book are strictly my own. My goal is that my *Raw on The Roll Success System* of simple solutions, suggestions, pics, tricks, tips, notes, quotes, skills, and drills will enhance your life, health, creativity and spirituality. Take what you like and leave the rest, or leave the rest for when you are ready.

Until we meet again on the rawkin' raw road of happy bliss, I send you a kiss! Good Luck and Good Health!

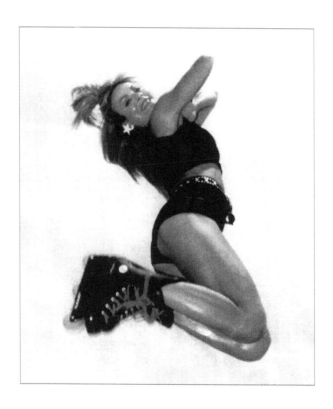

Testimonials

"Debbie has an infectious personality, knows and can relay her subject matter flawlessly. She is an incredible source of 'raw' information. Debbie and her new book helped me to understand where I went wrong in my diet and to get a more balanced diet in place."
—Mary Luciano, Athlete and Healthy Living Educator

"Debbie Merrill has a unique way of teaching people about the raw/ living foods lifestyle. She is full of raw energy that will inspire you to become part of the adventure of living a vibrant and healthy lifestyle."
—Rhio
Author of *Hooked on Raw*, www.rawfoodinfo.com

"A wonderful read, a page turner. Every chapter provides interesting material that will have you appreciating the importance of developing healthy eating habits. Debbie is a unique and special talent."
— Reg Clark, Ph. D.
Author of *Family Life and School Achievement*,
(University of Chicago Press), California State
University, Los Angeles, CA

"Debbie Merrill is a continuous source of wisdom about health and its connection to what we eat and how we live. As a TV news journalist and author, I have often relied on Debbie's advice to help me with diet and energy issues. She has shown me innumerable tricks and strategies for eating the optimal diet while still enjoying the food. Debbie will always be my health guru."
—Jane Velez-Mitchell
Author of *Secrets Can Be Murder*, (Touchstone)

"*Debbie Merrill is the most energetic person I know. She looks great and it is wonderful health. Her knowledge of health and fitness is the result and I highly suggest everyone use her advice to achieve the great health she has. Her new book,* The Raw Truth to the Fountain of Youth, *will show you how. I highly recommend reading it and get what she's got.*"

—Paul Nison
Speaker, Raw Food Chef and Author of *Health According to the Scriptures* (343 Publishing Co.), www.PaulNison.com

"*Debbie Merrill is a source of inspiration for the raw food community and the world beyond that is soon to become the raw food community. She offers us a living testimony to the vitality of a live food diet. Living boldly and radiantly, her life, her spirit and her work exemplify the principles of an aligned lifestyle. Her guidance along this ancient turned avant-garde path is relevant and valuable for those looking to live their true potential.*"

—Matt Amsden
Author of *Rawvolution* (Harper Collins), and Janabai of Euphoria Loves Rawvolution, Santa Monica, CA. www.euphorialovesrawvolution.com and Beauty and Wisdom, Santa Monica, CA. www.beautyandwisdomla.com

"*Who is Debbie Merrill? A dynamo, a lightning bolt, a photon of infinite possibilities, and a wise, pulsing inspiration for us all, and so is her book,* The Raw Truth to the Fountain of Youth.

—Happy Oasis
CVO Chief Visionary Officer, www.RawSpiritFest.com

"This book is great. Debbie Merrill does everything with style and The Raw Truth to the Fountain of Youth *is her gift to us in a "put-it-all-together and make-it-easy" format. This read will add years to your life and life to your years. I promise you won't be able to put it down."*

—Steve Meyerowitz, Sproutman
Author of *Wheatgrass Nature's Finest Medicine* (Book
Publishing Co), www.Sproutman.com

"Debbie Merrill is a remarkably talented and amazing woman. Her latest book, The Raw Truth to the Fountain of Youth, *is a must-read to anyone interested in pursuing the healthiest lifestyle. She's definitely an inspiration to us all!"*

—Jeff Popick
Author of *The Vegan Sage* and *The Real Forbidden Fruit:
How Meat Destroys Paradise and How Veganism
Can Get It Back,* (Vegan World Publishing)
www.Jeffpopick.com & www.therealforbiddenfruit.com

"We loved having Debbie on "Jimmy Kimmel Live!" Her energy was great and so was her subject matter. I'm sure her new book, The Raw Truth to the Fountain of Youth, *will benefit a lot of people."*

—Uncle Frank
Jimmy Kimmel Live!, www.ABC.com

"Debbie is an incredibly talented human being. Her fabulous rawsome energy is so contagious, on and off skates, from providing education and inspiration for anyone who meets her or reads The Raw Truth to the Fountain of Youth. *This book is a miraculous answer to the health issues of today. She lays it out so simply, she sings it, skates it, dances it, teaches it, lives it, shares it and promotes it. Ancient Sun loves her and her new success* The Raw Truth to the Fountain of Youth.

—James Tejada of Ancient Sun Nutrition
www.ancientsuninc.com

"Debbie Merrill is the wheel deal! Her love and artistry of skating is a victory to her health and fitness. Her fulfillment to every life she touches brings them closer to their goals. We supported her successful Learn to In-Line Skate DVD and her new book The Raw Truth to the Fountain of Youth *will be a wonderful addition to her enterprise. Debbie is out to transform life itself and all those rolling along with her."*

—Joe Olivas
Product Marketing Coordinator, Rollerblade USA
www.rollerblade.com

"When Debbie arrived at the studio to record her public TV show, I knew I was in for a treat. I found Debbie's energy and vitality contagious. Her enthusiasm for life and love inspired everyone around her. What I like about Debbie's TV program is that she entertains as well as educates everyone to the benefit of a healthy lifestyle. Her new book, The Raw Truth to the Fountain of Youth, *is a continuation of her TV program with detailed knowledge and perfection in an easy and fun way."*

—Mark A. McGuire
Television Director, Los Angeles, CA

"Debbie's view of life and food, and life as it relates to food, is totally refreshing and inspiring. Vita-Mix® is proud to be part of Debbie's journey The Raw Truth to the Fountain of Youth—she is an amazing example of the power of personal determination. Her positive attitude can't help but be contagious to anyone who reads this book!"

—Wendy Manfredi
Vita-Mix® Corporation, www.Vitamix.com

"Debbie's book is informative, and exciting to read. She is truly on target as to the health and emotional benefits that can be derived from going raw. I highly recommend this book to anyone looking to increase their energy, and expand their thinking in ways that could only be a boost to their overall good health."

—Bonnie Schachter
Publisher, Pocket Reference Journals,
www.PocketReferenceJournals.com

The Raw Truth to the Fountain of Youth *is the way Debbie inspires the world around her with her commitment and lust for life and health. We at Nutrex Hawaii are committed to the same excellence in our products as Debbie is in her health, well-being and diet. This book is a must read and just in time for the new rawvolution of green is clean and eco friendly."*

—A Prehn
Nutrex Hawaii, www.nutrex-hawaii.com,
Spirulina-Nature's Superfood (Cyanotech Corporation)

"We support and respect Debbie's endeavors with her lifestyle, food and fitness.

—Bruce DePalma
Co-opportunity, Santa Monica, CA,
www.coopportunity.com

"Debbie Merrill is a vibrant role model for great health and living in the moment. As an extension of Debbie, her book, The Raw Truth to the Fountain of Youth, *offers its readers the promise of that same natural high and quality of health for life."*
—Lisa J. Ensign
Nature's Rx Health Food Market and Café Totanaca,
www.naturesrxonline.com

"Debbie's commitment to health and the health of others is astonishing. She is an inspiration to all who aspire to an optimum level of life. She can skate circles around anyone half her age! We know she loves her greens and her E3live and we support her show and all her efforts. We are sure her book, The Raw Truth to the Fountain of Youth, *will definitely benefit anyone who reads it."*
—Tamera Campbell and Michael Saiber
CEO and President of E3live, www.E3live.com

Debbie Merrill, the raw guru to health-conscience individuals is helping people eat more joyous food, straight from mother nature's kitchen. Debbie exudes vitality, expertise, athleticism and youthful agelessness to those lucky enough to experience her. Debbie's engaging abilities to the public on behalf of Rejuvenative Foods continue to help new and repeat customers realize appreciate and understand the exciting array of Rejuvenative Foods. "Debbie Merrill Knocks em live." Thank you Debbie for your tremendous dilligence and energy.
—Evan Richards, CEO of www.rejuvenative.com

"Debbie has been such an inspiration to us all! Her energy is off the charts! She is the perfect spokesperson for the raw vegan lifestyle, a beautiful woman inside and out. Her book, The Raw Truth to the Fountain of Youth, *is truly a treasure—sure to inspire vibrant health and happiness to those who read it."*
—Jennifer Ferguson
Essential Living Foods, Inc., www.EssentialLivingFoods.com

"Debbie Merrill is a living foods miracle. She wants America healthy. Debbie's raw food lifestyle follows the laws of nature, simple and divine. With this book she extols the values of vibrant health and bounteous energy thru living foods as she teaches and inspires the world to do so as well!"

—Marlena Zaro of Rejuvenative Foods
Makers of raw sauerkraut, www.rejuvenativefoods.com

"We love Debbie and have supported her TV show throughout the years. All of Debbie's lectures, demos and efforts to promote healthy eating and shopping are amazingly educational and inspiring. She sends us all her health conscious friends and customers for the best in organic eating. Her work in the health and raw food movement is extraordinary and unstoppable. Just like her energy, compassion and love for human potential, her new book, The Raw Truth to the Fountain of Youth, *carries the same force and power as Debbie does, and will be a tremendous success."*

—Tony Welch & Marina Pensado, Store Managers, Wild Oats
Market, Santa Monica, CA, www.wildoats.com

"As owner/operator of one of the largest rental fleets in the USA, we at Perry's Cafe and Rentals have known Debbie Merrill professionally for many years. Debbie shares the beach with us in Santa Monica providing skating lessons for all with enthusiasm and genuineness. She is quite a character, full of energy, vitality, and, forever devoted to health and exercise. Full commitment to the raw lifestyle shows her passion to do it right. The Raw Truth to the Fountain of Youth, *her new book, is definitely doing it right. She lets us know that we can all take care of ourselves a little bit better.*

—Melody Chacker
President/Owner of Perry's Café and Rentals
www.perryscafe.com

"As an importer and proprietor of raw organic health foods, Navitas Naturals has loved working with Debbie. She quite simply gets it; understanding the value of these foods and has a wonderful ability to translate that so everyone can enjoy the secret of a healthy, diverse and satisfying diet. Her book, The Raw Truth to the Fountain of Youth, is a must read for anyone wanting to incorporate organic raw foods into their lifestyle."

—Zach Adelman
Founder of Navitas Naturals, www.NavitasNaturals.com

"I fell in love with Debbie's raw energy the first time I met her. Debbie exudes so much love, energy, appreciation and commitment to the raw food community and its message of vibrant health for everyone. Her book, The Raw Truth to the Fountain of Youth, has all of this in it as well. I always am excited to support Debbie because she exudes all the beautiful foods that she puts into her body. Her spirit is always so uplifting and dynamic, I encourage Debbie to keep shining and soar!"

—Nwenna Kai
Owner and Culinary Designer of Taste
of the Goddess Café, www.tasteofthegoddess.com

"Debbie Merrill has great energy. All of Debbie's lectures, demos and efforts to promote RAW FOODS and healthy eating is extraordinary along with her amazing focus on lifestyle. She inspires everyone to GET RAW and ROLL, with her new book, The Raw Truth To The Fountain Of Youth. I like to think of her as BONITA SENORITA, DEBBIE MERRILL."

—Juan Hernandez
Store Manager and Raw Food Event Coordinator,
Erewhon Natural Foods Market, Hollywood, CA,
www.ErewhonMarket.com

"I admire Debbie's beautiful spirit and her total dedication to her raw food lifestyle. Her cause to help others attain health and wellness is remarkable. This book will help a lot of people."

—Lillian Muller
Author of *Feel Great, Be Beautiful Over 40*
(Studdart Publishing), and Playboy's #1 Playmate
of the Year Cover Girl, www.LillianMuller.com

"When I met Debbie Merrill she was a shining light full of energy. I was so impressed with her talent and brilliance on and off skates. Her new book, The Raw Truth to the Fountain of Youth, *is the new revolution on the planet and for the raw food movement. Debbie's letting people know they can be ageless and full of vitality and health for their existence.*

—Robert Williams
www.UltimateSuperFoods.com

"Debbie is so inspiring to me. I love her commitment to the message of bringing raw foods, not just to her local community, but globally. Debbie loves our raw superfoods and her book, The Raw Truth to the Fountain of Youth, *is easy to incorporate, fun and a great resource on how to go raw."*

—JoAnn Cuddigan
Holistic Enterprises LLC, www.MSMSupplements.com

"Debbie Merrill has dedicated her life to creating the ideal relationship between you and your health and well-being. That devotion is fully reflected in her new book, The Raw Truth to the Fountain of Youth. *It's a must read for all for health and wellness."*

—Alan Heinze, CEO Imagelock West
Communications, www.usa-server.net

"Debbie's energy, creativity and passion has always been an inspiration to me. I believe her "rawsome" lifestyle, experience and knowledge has something for everyone, and I know anyone who reads her book, The Raw Truth to the Fountain of Youth, *will enjoy the ride!"*

—Caryn Rae Robin
Caryn Rae Travel, www.CarynRaeTravel.com

"When I first met Debbie at a Raw Potluck I thought, 'wow, this woman is a fire cracker! I must hear what she has to say.' Just coming back from a month on the road as a private chef I hadn't met anyone with so much energy, spunk and thriving on Raw Vegan diet! As with anyone I meet that stands out in my mind, I wanted to know more about how Debbie personally kept her figure, vibrant health and personality so electric. Months later, I was invited to come on Debbie's show to demonstrate some raw dishes. I had no idea what to expect. Swooping onto the set in her stars and stripes rollerblades, tassels swingin' and flags flying, I couldn't believe how much pure energy this lady had. Debbie has this spark and raw energy every day! I love it, you will want to read Debbie's new book, The Raw Truth to the Fountain of Youth. *It's just like the author. Anything she touches is electric baby!"*

—Chef Sweet Melissa "Mango"
Terra Bella Café, www.terrabellacafe.com

"Debbie Merrill is an enthusiastic, vibrant and talented woman. She is a dynamic TV host, skating expert, health advocate and now author. Her first book, The Raw Truth to the Fountain of Youth, *is a great inspiration for all of us who aspire to live a healthy, rich and energized life."*

—Angela Hartman
A. Hartman, Inc.

"Debbie Merrill, she is one of the greatest skaters of all time. When you get her love, you will fly to the sky. When you read her book, The Raw Truth to the Fountain of Youth, *you will be inspired even higher. One love, Debbie love. Keep healing the people."*

—Rawsheed
Alchemist of Raw Foods

"Debbie's vibrant, positive, fun-filled contribution to the health and well being of the planet and its people is exploding and irresistible. Her 100% dedication to the raw lifestyle makes this book an extraordinary, unstoppable success in the modern age, just like her."

—Mark Perlmutter
creator of "Raw for 30 Days," www.rawfor30days.com

"Debbie Merrill is an incredibly vibrant, wonderful testimonial to the raw lifestyle, and it's not just about the food. Debbie is a "maximum potential in every moment" person. She has woken up to the law of consequences and creates a healthy, happy and loving life with every bite, bend and breath."

—Rod Rotondi
Owner of Leaf Cuisine Raw Restaurant,
Culver City, CA, www.leafcuisine.com

Debbie is absolutely committed to her own health and personal growth, and equally committed to helping others achieve better health. She follows her own advice, and walks the walk. Her new book, The Raw Truth to the Fountain of Youth *is a powerful example of her being a leader in the movement to help transform the health of life itself. I have been inspired watching her."*

—Marsha Epstein, MD, MPH and vegetarian for 11 years

"Debbie Merrill isn't shy about sharing her views. She's even written a book about them! Read Debbie's book, The Raw Truth

to the Fountain of Youth, *and you'll know this Raw, Veggie, Vegan dynamo has succeeded in her pursuit to be the best she can be —fit, healthy and full of joy. And she wants her readers to achieve those goals as well!"*

—Victoria Giraud
Freelance Writer/Editor,
Author of *Melaynie's Masquerade* (Author House)

"My eclectic, electric student, Debbie Merrill, exemplifies the life-style of one who dines exclusively on raw food. The energy, youth and joy she brings to her work as a performing artist sets a standard for all of us to aspire to, and her book, The Raw Truth to the Fountain of Youth, *offers that same zest and electricity."*

—Gary Austin
Acting Coach to the Stars, www.GaryAustin.net

"This powerhouse of energy and rhyme stands on wheels as a true symbol of what a Raw Veggie Vegan Diva is and does. She wears many hats throughout a single day, gliding through with ease and vitality. It is always a pleasure knowing her and having her on my show, Rawkin' Radio. Her new book is the result of her power, catch it."

—Revvell P. Revati
http://Revvell.com, www.Revvellations.com
http://rawcast.rawkinradio.com

"Debbie is a vibrant raw goddess and is full of energy, most of it due to her raw vegan lifestyle and the other part is because she skates, jumps, bounces and runs all over the place, plenty of exercise. She has been a beacon of light carrying the torch on the front lines for raw and continues to glow in every way. I thank her for her ability to express herself with such force and commitment to raw veganism. I know her TV show will grow to maximum potential as she hits the

best seller list with her new book The Raw Truth to the Fountain of Youth *and I truly look forward to reading it. I love you, Debbie, keep it up!"*

—Brian Lucas
aka Chef BeLive (Gourmet Live Cuisine Master
Chef/Energy Healer) www.belivelight.com

"Debbie, as a health conscious individual, I greatly appreciate your contribution. You've shed light on areas most people aren't aware of and need to be."

—Bruce Fitzpatrick
Published Author and Screenwriter.

Debbie Merrill is a true shining star! She is always a joy to have at Whole Foods Market, Venice. She is so enthusiastic about her diet and lifestyle that it motivates everyone to want to live that way. She always talks so highly about the product she represents and does such a great job in representing them. We always invite Debbie to all of our different events because we know she'll be excited and have a huge smile on her face the whole time. Thanks Debbie for your hard work and commitment!

—Sylvia Gonzalez, Marketing Assistant
Whole Foods Market, Venice

"I have known Debbie Merrill for many years. She is and lives what she talks about and promotes. She is "IT" and her new book, The Raw Truth to the Fountain of Youth, *is a hit!"*

—Lucien Martin, D.C.
Doctor of Chiropractic

"When i first met Debbie I thought I was doing everything right. I was working out, not eating red meat and not drinking or smoking. Unfortunately my diet consisted of french fries, ice cream and huge amounts of coffee. My wake up call came when I was diagnosed

with prostate cancer. Soon after I was involved in a horrific car crash which landed me in the hospital for nine weeks. Thanks to Debbie's unlimited knowledge of raw foods and her super products, plus her loving, caring and positive outlook on life, after reading, The Raw Truth to the Fountain of Youth, I am re-inspired, motivated and excited about life again. I AM NOT ONLY CANCER FREE and having a rawesome recovery, but my goal of leading a productive life again and some day getting back on skates is a reality."

—Tary Jahn Duarte
Client/Student

"Creative, witty, charming, gregarious, talented, caring and did I mention ENERGY. Could it be her diet? Her energy is boundless. Glad this book is out so that I have a course to follow. You are the 'raw' deal. I mean real deal."

—Thomas DiGiacomo
Corporate Traveler of Champion-Nationwide

"Debbie Merrill is a dazzling example of health, vitality and spirit! In heels or on wheels, Debbie sparkles! Get ready for a success story that explodes like fireworks with her new book The Raw Truth to the Fountain of Youth!"

—Jeff Costa
fitness expert and creator of Cardio Striptease
www.cardiostriptease.com

"If you're looking for inspiration, look no further than Debbie Merrill. Her enthusiasm, perseverance and passion infuses all of her work in her new book, The Raw Truth to the Fountain of Youth. Her contribution to living healthfully is a gift to the community, worldwide."

— Teri Danz
Recording Artist/Vocal Coach, www.TeriDanz.com

"Debbie Merrill has come into her own knowing who she is and what she has to offer the world. Her journey and mission to take a stand for healing the planet through health of ourselves and respect for what God gave us, our life, is what her book is all about. It's a pleasure to read and it's about time someone is telling the truth. We are precious beings and the responsibility we have to life."

—Don Kidson
Hardware Humanitarian, Busy Bee Hardware
www healthyhardware.com

"Debbie's raw lifestyle is just like that of a gazelle. She dances, flows and glows glacially through life, healing and helping others transition to a healthier lifestyle. Her new book, The Raw Truth to the Fountain of Youth, *will definitely teach you how to uncook or be cooked. I highly recommend following her lead and picking up some speed."*

—Jessica Zaccaro
Internal Hygiene Specialist, www.transformyourhealth.NET

"Debbie has opened a whole new world in so many ways for me and helped change my life. Learning and being educated by her raw lifestyle and spiritual life has been so inspirational and eye opening. I love her new book, The Raw Truth to the Fountain of Youth, *it's the gift I've been waiting for, along with her delicious recipes and exotic products from around the world. Her beauty and brilliance is mesmerizing."*

—Louis Lewellen
Cameraman/age 72

"Debbie Merrill is the fountain of youth. She lives it, she gives it, and her book, The Raw Truth to the Fountain of Youth, *is all about it. I bought it, she sold it, I'm loving to live it. I like to think of her as Debbie Miracle!"*

—Pineapple Head
Raw food enthusiast. Myspace.com/pineappleheadlive

"If ever there was an energy magnet where normal life, health, speed, perception and health is colorful and irresistible, it is Debbie Merrill and her amazing focus on lifestyle. The Raw Truth to the Fountain of Youth *is an extension and recreation of herself in words, wisdom and guidance. Follow her brilliance! If she gets anywhere near you, you'll feel yourself changing, too, as I did!*

—Barry Helfanbein

Cruise Director

"I endorse Debbie's new book, The Raw Truth to the Fountain of Youth. *She has so much energy, vitality and love for her lifestyle of eating raw. All of the information and knowledge in this book comes from her hard work, her heart and spirit. She spends lots of time researching this and puts it in a truthful format of suggestions to help others. Debbie definitely walks her talk, she is a living example, leader and motivator in the raw vegan lifestyle and movement. We all need to support her vision, her journey and all she does and has done for the world for 25 years."*

—Janina Mikrut

Hollywood Set Designer

"Mother Earth has chosen Debbie as her ambassador. If we are wise we will listen to the wisdom of her message. The contribution that she makes way surpasses having it be about her and provides an incredible guide for all of us to live in coexistence with one another and the planet. The constraints that we have posed on ourselves in many areas are pushed to the limit, are broken through and a new ground is found with her guidance and light in her book, The Raw Truth to the Fountain of Youth."

—David Lalezar

Engineer/Businessman/Debbie's Student

"Debbie is quite a character! I say this in the most wonderful way as all animated souls that walk this wonderful path of health share with us a unique and amazing light. She has been entertaining us and sharing much of her light for along time. Now she touches us once again with new insights and more laughter in her book, The Raw Truth to the Fountain of Youth. *Thank you for your stamina, dedication and love."*

—John Schott
Sacred Symbiosis (John's Superfood Life Tortillas)

"Debbie has the magnificent quality of instant inspiration to make her listener listen to what she has to say. Her book, The Raw Truth to the Fountain of Youth, *is a reflection of her instant inspiration."*

—Robert Becker
Raw Food Enthusiast.

"Debbie's The Raw Truth to the Fountain of Youth *is an extra-ordinary piece of work, as is Debbie's extra-ordinary talent—a work of art."*

—Bob-e-true-love, Client

"Debbie is the most vibrant, energetic and charismatic person I know. She portrays all of this in her new book, The Raw Truth to the Fountain of Youth, *along with all her creative talents and knowledge of health and wellness. She makes reading this book fun and easy. I think it will help many people transition to a healthier lifestyle and benefit many to come. I can't wait for her next book!"*

— Kristen Noelle Heimo
Actress and Music Manager of Tracii Guns/L.A. Guns
www.LAGunsLive.com

Debbie's dedication to the raw food community and over all tenacious approach to health and fitness has allowed her to maintain her beauty and physical stamina which is unstoppable! Her energy radiates everywhere she goes. It is a real pleasure when she comes to Erewhon Natural Foods Market and shares her healthful knowledge experience and wisdom in her lectures and food demonstrations. The customers love her recipes, pristine quality product selection that she selects and our sales improve as well. Debbie is a great inspiration to all and so is her book, The Raw Truth to the Fountain of Youth *which we are happy to carry for our customers.*

—Vicky Osuna
Head Buyer, Erewhon Natural Foods Market

"We love Debbie's "raw" energy. We are glad to be providing her with sample cups and spoons made from sugar cane and corn. Thank you Debbie for being the host with the most compost…ables!"

— Allan and Herminia
Catergreen.com.

"I have been moved and inspired by Debbie's stand for creating a world of extraordinary health and quality of life. The Raw Truth to the Fountain of Youth *is an example of her consistent and sustained commitment, and is a must read by all. We need more Debbie's in the world!"*

—Mike/Michelle Dennis
Transgender Rights Advocate and Activist

"Debbie's boundless supply of energy and enthusiasm is infectious and a breath of fresh air. She never fails to entertain while she educates, motivates and rehabilitates you into a healthier, happier and more rewarding life. This book is an easy, flowing, simple read and I highly recommend it for all ages."

—Susan Jerrell
Entrepreneur

"*Debbie Merrill knows her stuff! Debbie is an expert at explaining and presenting the philosophy of raw foods. As a lifetime carnivore Debbie inspired me to try raw foods and surprised me with her absolutely delicious creations. She is an excellent speaker and engages our clients on a personal level. We had over 40 people attend the class and they didn't want to leave!*"

—Caroline Capizzano
Former Marketing Supervisor,
Whole Foods Markets, Santa Monica, CA

"*Debbie Merrill is our in-store demo diva! She has been representing my organic, raw food company, Lydia's Organics, in many natural food markets and Whole Food Markets stores in southern California over the last year. She is very knowledgeable about the raw food diet and making healthy lifestyle choices. Working with her is always a pleasure and a blessing!*"

—Lydia Kindheart
Lydia's Organics
lydiasorganics.com

"*The Raw Truth to the Fountain of Youth is a must-read for anyone interested in changing their life through raw living foods. Having been born with cerebral palsy, nutrition is a key factor in maintaining my own personal health and quality of life. Debbie's work has literally changed my life — physically, mentally and spiritually. Debbie Merrill's work is the "Bible" of raw food manuals, perfect for anyone, from beginner to expert who wishes to transform their lives through a raw food vegan diet.*"

—Rev. Dr. Jason Sheilds
Harbor of Light Ministries
jasonsheilds.org

Resources

Books, Websites, Markets, Restaurants, Videos, Vitamins, and other useful information for you to navigate your journey of extraordinary health, fitness, and well-being.

Markets

Erewhon Natural Foods Market, Hollywood, CA
www.erewhonmarket.com

One Life Natural Foods, Santa Monica, CA (310) 392-4501

Co-Opportunity, Santa Monica, CA, www.coopportunity.com

Whole Foods Market, wholefoods.com

Rainbow Acres. Los Angeles, CA, www. rainbowacres.com

Josh's Organic Garden, on Hollywood Beach, Hollywood, FL
954-456-3276

Glaser Organic Farms, Miami, FL, www.glaserorganicfarms.com

Raw Vegan Restaurants

Juliano's Raw Restaurant, Santa Monica, CA
www.planetraw.com

Leaf Cuisine Restaurant, Culver City, CA
www.leafcuisine.com

Rawvolution, Santa Monica, CA, www.rawvolution.com

Raw Makery, Las Vegas, NV, www.rawmakery.com

Cafe Gratitude, San Francisco, CA, www.cafegratitude.com

Books/DVDs

The Sunfood Diet Success System, by David Wolfe (Maul Bros Pub.) www.Sunfood.com

Conscious Eating and Spiritual Nation, by Gabriel Cousens, The Tree of Life Rejuvenation Center, www.treeoflife.nu

RAW (Regan Books), by Juliano, www.rawplanet.com

Rawvolution, by Matt Amsden (Regan Books) www.euphorialovesrawvolution.com

Raw Spirit: What The Raw Food Advocates Don't Preach and *Raw Success*, by Matt Monarch, www.rawspirit.org

Rawsome!, Beauty By Nature, and *The Desktop Guide to Herbal Medicine*, by Brigitte Mars, www.brigittemars.com

Eat To Live and Eat For Health, by Dr. Joel Fuhrman, www.DrFuhrman.com

Raw Food Diet Revolution and *Angel Foods, by* Cherie Soria, www.RawFoodChef.com

Hooked on Raw, by B. Rhio, www.rawfoodinfo.com

The Bragg Apple Cider Vinegar Miracle Health System, by Patricia Bragg, N.D., PhD., (Healthy Living), www.bragg.com

The RealFood Daily Cookbook: Real Fresh, Really Good, Really Vegetarian, by Ann Gentry (Ten Speed Press, Berkeley, CA) www.realfood.com

Living Foods for Optimum Health: Staying Healthy in an Unhealthy World by Brian Clement (Three Rivers Press) http://www.hippocratesinst.org/

Diet for a New America, by John Robbins

The Real Forbidden Fruit, by Jeff Popick, www.JeffPopick.com

Fast Food Nation, Eric Schlosser

Diet For All Reasons, (DVD), Michael Klaper, M.D.

Eating, (DVD), Michael Anderson

Super Size Me, (DVD), Morgan Spurlock

Raw For Thirty Days, (DVD), Mark Perlmutter,
www.rawfor30days.com

Book Stores

Barnes and Noble, Marina Del Rey, CA. For great writing and
research. www.bn.com

Novel Café, Santa Monica, CA. A great place to write.
www.novelcafe.com

Fitness

Crunch Fitness, Hollywood, CA. Where I sway my hips, gloss my
lips, jump my flips and do my strips. www.crunch.com Jeff
Costa, cardiostriptease.com

Debbie Merrill's Skate Great USA School of Skating, Santa
Monica, CA, 310-625-0059. Private and group classes, all
ages, all levels. www.skategreat.com

Santa Monica Y.M.C.A. Where I swim and stay trim.
www.ymcasm.org

Vitamins/Nutrients—Shop Online

Robert Williams, www.Ultimatesuperfoods.com

David Wolfe, www.Sunfood.com

www.NavitasNaturals.com

www.RejuvenativeFoods.com

www.LydiasOrganics.com

www.EssentialLivingFoods.com

E3live, Klamath Falls, OR, www.E3live.com

James Tejada, Ancient Sun Nutrition, www.ancientsuninc.com

Steve Meyerowitz, Sproutman, www.Sproutman.com

Holistic Enterprises LLC, Santa Ana, CA, Joanne Cuddigan and David Koren, www.MSMSupplements.com

Miscellaneous Services and Miracle Makers

Sergio Nicolas, 310-968-4014. Raw cleaning, and raw food catering and delivery.

Don Kidson, the Godfather of the raw living lifestyle, Living Light House, Santa Monica, CA, www.livinglighthouse.com and Busy Bee Hardware (for the best-cooked nuts and bolts) Santa Monica, CA www.healthyhardware.com

Raw Summit, www.RawSummit2.com

OHI, Optimum Health Institute, Lemon Grove, CA 800-993-4325, 619-589-4094

Hippocrates Institute, West Palm Beach, FL www.hippocratesinst.org

The Tree of Life Rejuvenation Center, Gabriel Cousens M.D., author of *Conscious Eating* and *Spiritual Nutrition*, www.treeoflife.nu

Sandra Mohr, Mohr Productions. Animal Rights Videos. www.mohr-productions.com

Perry's Café, Santa Monica, CA. For all your beach needs: skates, bikes, boogie boards and more. www.perryscafe.com

Nutrex-Hawaii, for great organic Spirulina. 800-453-1187 www.Nutrex-Hawaii.com

Jessica Zaccaro, Transformational Health, Santa Monica, CA (310)399-1722. Detox and Colon Hydro Therapy. www.Transformyourhealth.net

Herbal Detox Program, www.ariseandshine.com

Vita-Mix® Corp., Cleveland, OH, www.vitamix.com

CaterGreen, Zero Waste Solutions, 323-663-7747. For great natural, environmentally-friendly spoons, cups and containers for our planet and its people. www.CaterGreen.com

The Humane Society of California, www.humanecalifornia.org

John Wood, 21-day detox, www.naturaldoctor.com

Cherie Soria, author of *Raw Food Diet Revolution and Angel Foods*, and Director of Living Light Culinary Arts Institute, 707-964-2420, www.RawFoodChef.com

Chef Melissa, melissamango@gmail.com

Rawsheed, raw chef and alchemist of raw foods, rawsheedandjusticeteam@gmail.com

Brian Lucas, aka Chef BeLive, www. belivelight.com

Lucien Martin, D.C., Doctor of Chiropractic

P. Revati, www.revvell.com and www.rawcast.rawkinradio.com

Paul Nison, www.paulnison.com

Sign-Tist, Venice, CA, www.signtist.com

Yahoo Living Food Groups

Serenity Spaces, http://health.groups.yahoo.com/group/
serenityspaces

Traveling Raw Foodists, http://health.groups.yahoo.com/group/
travelingrawfoodist

Living Foods Groups

L.A.: http://health.groups.yahoo.com/group
LosAngelesLivingFoods

Orange County: http://health.groups.yahoo.com/group/Orange_
County_CA_ Living_Foods

San Diego: http://health.groups.yahoo.com/group/
SD-LivingFoods

And a special thank you to all the following who helped me, supported me, guided me, and whose faith in me never waivered...

Bethann Carbone

Time Warner Cable, Santa Monica, Hollywood, Westchester, Van
Nuys, Chatsworth, C.A. for hosting and airing *The Debbie
Merrill Show*. www.timewarnercable.com

Charter Cable, Malibu & Glendale, CA. www.charter.com

Gary Austin Los Angeles, CA. Rawsome, awesome acting coach.
www.garyaustin.net

Angela Hartman, A. Hartman, Inc.

Victoria Giraud, www.victoria4edit.com

Caryn Rae Robin, loving, supportive friend, youtube.com/carynrr

Alan Heinze, CEO, Imagelock West Communications. For great web design and hosting. www.usa-server.net

Uncle Frank from *Jimmy Kimmel Live!* www.ABC.com

Jane Velez-Mitchell, Celebrity Journalist and author of *Secrets Can Be Murder* (Touchstone).

Joe Olivas, Product Marketing Coordinator, Rollerblade USA. www.rollerblade.com. For great inline skates, and for sponsoring my *Learn to Inline Skate* DVD, available for purchase at www.SkateGreatUSA.com.

Teri Danz, Recording Artist/Vocal Coach, www.TeriDanz.com

Anina Mikrut, Creative Supporter/Set Designer

Kevin Janow, Photographer, www.kevinjanow.com

Denni Christopherson, Creative Artistry

Printing Palace, Santa Monica, CA. For all my cards and printing. 310-451-5151

Ann Gunder, writer and producer, www.anngunder.com

Creative Publishing Book Design, www.CreativePublishingDesign.com

Jason Mendez of Sir Speedy, Whittier, CA. jason@sswhittier.com

And to Kristen Noelle Heimo for being such a fabulous assistant, and music manager of Tracii Guns/L.A. Guns. www.LAGunsLive.com

About the Author

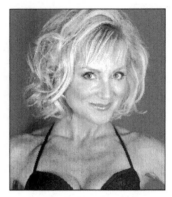

The unstoppable Debbie Merrill is proud to announce the publication of her new book, *The Raw Truth to the Fountain of Youth*. This book is the latest project for the award-winning dancer, international figure-skating star, actress, choreographer and lecturer. This dynamic, multi-talented woman is also an internationally renowned skating fitness expert and founder of Skate Great USA School of Skating in lovely Santa Monica Beach, California. Debbie's interest in fitness and good health led her to become a vegetarian over 28 years ago. As America's "Raw Veggie Vegan Diva," she has been promoting a healthy lifestyle ever since. With her public TV show, *Raw Foods on the Roll, Getting America Healthy*; and her fitness DVD, *Debbie Merrill's Learn to Inline Skate to Look and Feel Great*, Debbie has built a loyal fan base across the US and around the world. An extraordinary asset to her community, Debbie is passionate about her volunteer work with physically challenged children, sharing with them the liberating benefits of good health. You may meet, greet, and eat with her in a variety of health food stores throughout Southern California and across the country where she hosts fitness lectures, raw food demonstrations and un-cooking classes, featuring *The Raw Truth to the Fountain of Youth: Food-for-Life Plan* and her own unique recipes.

Made in the USA
Charleston, SC
17 November 2012